WORK, HEALTH, AND PRODUCTIVITY

WORK, HEALTH, AND PRODUCTIVITY

Edited by

Gareth M. Green
Frank Baker

New York   Oxford
OXFORD UNIVERSITY PRESS
1991

Oxford University Press

Oxford New York Toronto
Delhi Bombay Calcutta Madras Karachi
Petaling Jaya Singapore Hong Kong Tokyo
Nairobi Dar es Salaam Cape Town
Melbourne Auckland
and associated companies in
Berlin Ibadan

Library of Congress Cataloging-in-Publication Data
Work, health, and productivity /
edited by Gareth M. Green and Frank Baker.
p. cm.
Papers from the Johns Hopkins Conference on Work, Health, and
Productivity, held at Aspen on Wye, Oct. 21–23, 1987.
Includes bibliographical references and index.
ISBN 0-19-505778-3
1. Industrial hygiene—Congresses.   2. Work environment—Congresses.
3. Labor productivity—Congresses.   I. Green, Gareth M., 1931–   .
II. Baker, Frank, 1936–   .   III. Johns Hopkins Conference on Work, Health,
and Productivity (1987 : Aspen Institute, Wye Plantation)
HD7260.5.W66 1991
331.25—dc20   90-7607

9 8 7 6 5 4 3 2 1

Printed in the United States of America
on acid-free paper

Foreword

A great deal of my time has been spent with labor and management in the private sector and government resolving difficult workplace and labor market issues. I have also spent a lifetime in a university setting, and I understand something of the academic perspective. However, during all of those interactions I have felt woefully inadequate in knowing what the specialists in workplace medicine and hygienics have contributed to the understanding and resolution of work-health problems. I came to the 1987 Johns Hopkins Conference on Work, Health, and Productivity to look these specialists in the eye and to learn what they have to teach us.

It must be noted that it was a research conference; and it must also be noted that the questions of what problems or issues were particularly worthy and what methodologies were appropriate were matters about which I had some views. The following observations constitute a summary of my perspectives on these topics.

1. *There are a number of systems at work with regard to health care in the workplace; and there is a need to develop some way in which they can be examined and integrated.* There are several administrative arrangements for provision of health care for employees, including health insurance, Medicaid, and Medicare, as well as arrangements for ensuring occupational health in company policies, the Occupational Safety and Health Act (OSHA), state policies on disability and workers' compensation, and so on. My experience as an arbitrator has made me aware of how these various policies and administrative procedures are involved in a fair amount of counterplay and conflict and of the importance of finding some way to integrate these systems.

2. *Each workplace in the United States is in some respects different from others in terms of the ways in which their conditions impinge on health and safety.* There are literally millions of workplaces that differ in technology, age of plant and equipment, nature of raw materials and processes, state of repair and maintenance, training and supervision of workers, and formal programs in matters of health and safety and their vulnerability to accident, disease, and state of health. The relations and responsibilities of managers for workers range from that for employees, owner-operators, share-farmers, and subcontractors. The problems of setting and administering health and safety standards in small establishments are particularly difficult. Consider the issues that arise in various workplaces including processing plants, mines, construction sites, offices, laboratories, trucking operations, or farms. Although it is difficult to generalize about such a large and diffuse "universe," there are common parameters that can be used to treat these workplaces.

3. *The degree of health and safety of the workplace is fundamentally integrated into the main operations of the work process; the staff, however, are vital to its quality.* Safety and health at the workplace fundamentally derive from the technology of the plant and its capital equipment, the quality of materials, the quality and attention of supervision, and the training of the workforce. The degree of safety and health is derived from the managerial process and the relations between the supervisors and the workers.

4. *All regulation tends to change, or distort, the preexisting competitive relations among enterprises and workplaces.* This proposition applies to the regulation of health and safety conditions, whether by government or through collective bargaining. Leone (2) stated:

> Every act of government, no matter what its broader merits or demerits for society at large, creates winners and losers within the competitive economy. These gains and losses, which accrue to both individuals and corporations, become the objects of intense political attention at the same time they help shape the nation's international competitiveness, impart a direction to its research and development programs and generally shape the direction and pattern of growth of our economic institutions.

In itself, this iron law of public policy should not be construed as an argument against health and safety standards, only an indication of some consequences.

5. *Regulation of work standards at the workplace by government is seldom widely effective without acceptance of the standards by dedicated management in the absence of collective bargaining.* There are multitudinous workplaces, many of which are small. Government never allocates adequate resources for enforcement; and in any case there are genuine limits to what can be accomplished by an order on a piece of paper. Government workplace regulations are most effective when they are reinforced with a workplace labor organization (4).

6. *The regulatory process is more satisfactory if it is built on a common factual base and is accepted and agreed upon by the major concerned parties.* A factual basis is not mutually accepted if developed solely by scientific agencies and then imposed on management and labor representatives. To become a satisfactory base for effective policy decisions, factual data and their interpretation must command the respect of those required to live under a regulation. Procedures must be developed from the outset to induce such understanding and confidence.

7. *Increasing attention is being devoted to the development of health and safety standards by a consensus process and through negotiations among major interests.* The results are then likely to be more acceptable, achieve a higher degree of compliance, avoid litigation, and be more flexibly administered over time with changes in circumstances. Negotiated rule-making is an important tool to establish workplace health and safety standards. The methods of negotiation, however, are not likely to be successful or appropriate in all cases at present; they may also require new talents and skills among the administrators (1,3).

8. *Consideration should be given to developing a joint national forum of labor and management organizations in the United States with the purpose of considering major standard issues of policy regarding health.* Such a joint organization with experts selected by the parties for particular issues could materially advance under-

standing and agreement on contentious issues. Such a joint body should be funded by foundation support. Schools of public health might well have a role to play, with specialists drawn from various institutions depending on the problem.

9. *The development of wellness activities and other programs influencing life styles constitutes a major area for labor and management cooperation at the workplace.* These activities can be reinforced by joint participation with local community health care groups.

These issues are some of the ones I thought important to highlight at The Johns Hopkins Conference on Work, Health, and Productivity. I am pleased to see that Drs. Gareth Green and Frank Baker, who organized this forum and were co-chairs of the conference, have not been satisfied just to bring together experts from many disciplines to discuss the key issues in employee health and productivity but have continued their efforts in this volume.

In *Work, Health, and Productivity,* Green and Baker have brought together some of the key papers presented at The Johns Hopkins conference on this topic. The book summarizes the current state of the art, provides important examples of scientific research, and sets forth an agenda for further research in this critically challenging interdisciplinary field. The resulting volume is an important contribution to an area of vital concern to our nation at this time of technological change, industrial transition, discovery of workplace latent disease, and widespread concern about national competitiveness and productivity.

Lamont University Professor Emeritus   JOHN T. DUNLOP
Harvard University

REFERENCES

1. Administrative Conference of the United States. (1985). *Federal Register, 50*(249), December 27, 1985.
2. Leone, R. A. (1986). *Who profits, winners, losers, and government regulation* (p. 3). New York: Basic Books.
3. Perritt, H. H., Jr. (1987). Administrative alternative dispute resolution: the development of negotiated rulemaking and other processes. *Pepperdine Law Review, 14,* 865–928.
4. Weil, D. (1987). *Government and labor at the workplace: role of labor unions in the implementation of federal health and safety policy.* Ph.D. Thesis, Harvard University.

Preface

Beginning in the late 1960s and intensifying after 1973, a persistent decline in productivity growth in the U.S. economy as measured by the change in unit cost of goods and services has taken place. Many explanations have been offered, and some have suggested that it is the result of the interaction of peculiar technological, governmental, and labor/management factors that have occurred in the United States during this period. The concern for productivity has not been limited to the United States, however, or to this time period.

A concern for productivity is worldwide during this period of turbulent international competition. Whereas the United States has shown marked ambivalence in its earlier commitment to enhancing the work conditions and benefits of labor in the old-line industries in an effort to cut costs, Japan and Sweden have combined their concerns about productivity with a greater attention to the conditions of work and their effect on workers. In the United States the more innovative companies have shown an increased concern for maintaining and promoting worker health and fitness.

The uneasiness and concern about productivity at a time when goods and services have never been more plentiful for more people suggests that fundamental changes in cultural and national values and priorities are taking place in industrialized societies, perhaps in part because of the incredible material successes of industrialization. A quick review of the past 100 years reveals astonishing changes in the quality of health, longevity, and material well-being. At the same time there is growing concern over other quality of life measures, both material and nonmaterial; and societies have shown a willingness to forego some level of material well-being to protect their natural environments, elevate their underclasses, and better provide such social services as health, housing, child care, education, and recreation, with extensive development and renewal of urban communities, low-cost housing, privately and publicly financed entitlement programs, and so on. These developments suggest that the successes of industrialization have fostered an evolution of values toward a more humane, socially concerned, and environmentally conscious society with an expanded concept of productivity and a higher priority for health and the aesthetic qualities of life.

Viewed in these terms, some consider this society as becoming more, not less, productive; and they perceive the problem as the persistence of industrial definitions of productivity while we have moved into a postindustrial economy in which productivity is measured partly by human goals. The industrial society uses material resources, high energy, and assembly technologies to produce material goods for food, shelter, and security—which we measure as productivity. The postindustrial world uses uniquely human knowledge and information and communications technologies with low energy requirements to produce goods that are more useful for enlightenment, entertainment, cultural enrichment, and health. Perhaps it is time to review our measures of productivity and to incorporate values of health, environment, education, and cultural enrichment along with material goods in these measures.

This book focuses on the relation between health and productivity as necessary considerations in the design and development of the postindustrial workplace. It attempts to integrate the research in a paradigm based on the hypothesis that health, broadly defined, is a key variable that influences and is influenced by productivity, redefined.

The audience for this book includes researchers in the fields represented by the authors, including public health, occupational medicine, psychology, management science, industrial engineering, and economics. In addition to its relevance for researchers in the fields involved in studying aspects of workplace health and productivity, it may also be used for advanced courses in schools of public health, medicine, business, engineering, and arts and sciences. Given its relevance to widespread current concerns about productivity, leaders in business and industry will find this book of interest in the United States and abroad. Policy makers and governmental decision makers are included in the wider readership concerned with identifying a basis for fostering organizational excellence.

The book is divided into six major parts. The first section presents an overview of the literature, which reviews previous research dealing with work, health, and productivity, and a historical perspective based on two case studies. The second section reviews biological variables of susceptibility and physical and chemical hazards of the workplace as they affect worker health and workplace productivity. Major inputs to the workplace are examined, and chapters are included that deal with worker characteristics and the influence of life style issues and changes in technology on health and productivity.

In the third section of the book, the focus shifts to the workplace itself, and the chapters deal with the changing nature of the postindustrial work environment. The fourth section explores the growing significance of psychosocial aspects of the work setting in an emerging knowledge-oriented rather than labor-oriented economy. The fifth section deals with management techniques for improving health and productivity in the workplace and raises questions about their effectiveness and applicability in the health–productivity equation. The book concludes with the sixth section, which consists of a summary chapter by the editors and a final chapter that discusses the steps required to move research forward in the multidisciplinary area of work, health, and productivity.

Although broad in scope and integrative in its approach, a book of this length cannot comprehensively examine every issue; and so some gaps exist (employee assistance programs for example). The intent is to present sufficient depth in selected topics to validate the basic premise of the necessary interrelations of health and productivity in accomplishing the goals of our society.

Baltimore   G. M. G.
May 1991   F. B.

Acknowledgments

The idea and concepts for a book on work, health, and productivity grew out of a series of discussions among the faculty of The Johns Hopkins School of Hygiene and Public Health and members of the School's Health Advisory Council, representing private sector interests in manufacturing, industry, and health care organizations, and labor, management, legal, scientific, and business executives. These discussions culminated in a conference on research in work, health, and productivity held at The Aspen Institute at Wye Plantation, Queenstown, Maryland in October 1987. The participants at that conference were: Albert Ritardi, Allied-Signal, Inc.; Bertram Dinman, Aluminum Company of America; Michael P. O'Donnell, American Journal of Health Promotion; Diana Chapman Walsh, Boston University; George H. Cohen, Bredhoff & Kaiser; Marie Morell, University of California at Los Angeles; Lester Lave, Carnegie-Mellon University; Richard Evans, Children's Memorial Hospital; Gary S. Freedman, CIBA-GEIGY Corporation; Michael K. Allen, Dome Corporation; Duane Block, Ford Motor Company; Shlomo Breznitz, University of Haifa, Israel; John Dunlop, Harvard University; Carl Schramm, Health Insurance Association of America; Kiroya Kubota, Japan Productivity Center, Tokyo; Victor Dankis, Johnson & Johnson; Jonathan Fielding, Johnson & Johnson Health Management, Inc.; Manuel Dupkin II, Johnston Laboratories; Stuart W. Davidson, Kirschner, Walters, Willig; Paul Entmacher, Metropolitan Life Insurance Company; Donald Chaffin, The University of Michigan; Edward Emmett, National Institute for Occupational Health and Safety, Sydney, Australia; Larry Hirschhorn, University of Pennsylvania; Raymond Hunt, State University of New York at Buffalo; Eric Jannerfeldt, Embassy of Sweden; Gunnar Aronsson and Gunn Johansson, University of Stockholm, Sweden; Thomas Vischi, U.S. Department of Health and Human Services; Robert Worsfold; Susan Baker, Harvey Brenner, David Celentano, Jacqueline Corn, Morton Corn, Barbara Curbow, Ruth Faden, Alan Goldberg, Donald Henderson, Fusao Hirata, Jeffrey Johnson, Genevieve Matanoski, Alan Newman, Andrew Sorenson, Carol Sachs Weisman, Sylvia Eggleston, and John Kudless, The Johns Hopkins University.

Consequent to the conference, and because the participants agreed on the importance and general interest of the initiative, publication of this book was proposed and chapters solicited, with additional editorial material developed to provide thematic continuity.

The authors wish especially to acknowledge the stimulus, motivation, and unflagging support of Manuel Dupkin, one of the Health Advisory Council members and a member of the Board of Trustees of The Johns Hopkins University. A special debt of gratitude is owed to Jane Block, who managed the editorial process for the editors and prepared the manuscript for the publisher. In addition, acknowledgement is made to Gloria Schroeder for her help in typing correspondence and portions of the manuscript. Finally, the authors wish to thank Jeffrey House, vice president and executive editor of the medicine and science division at Oxford University Press, for his help and encouragement in seeing this book through the stages from idea to completed manuscript.

Contributors

Gunnar Aronsson, Ph.D.
Department of Psychology
National Institute of Occupational Health
S-171 84 Solna Sweden

Frank Baker, Ph.D.
Department of Environmental Health
Sciences
School of Hygiene and Public Health
The Johns Hopkins University
Baltimore, Maryland 21205

Susan B. Baker, M.P.H.
Department of Health Policy and
Management
School of Hygiene and Public Health
The Johns Hopkins University
Baltimore, Maryland 21205

M. Harvey Brenner, Ph.D.
Department of Health Policy and
Management
School of Hygiene and Public Health
The Johns Hopkins University
Baltimore, Maryland 21205

David D. Celentano, M.H.S., Sc.D.
Division of Behavioral Sciences and Health
Education
School of Hygiene and Public Health
The Johns Hopkins University
Baltimore, Maryland 21205

Don B. Chaffin, Ph.D.
Center for Ergonomics
The University of Michigan
Ann Arbor, Michigan 48109

Bernice H. Cohen, Ph.D., M.P.H.
Department of Epidemiology
School of Hygiene and Public Health
The Johns Hopkins University
Baltimore, Maryland 21205

Jacqueline K. Corn, Dr.A.
Department of Environmental Health
Sciences
School of Hygiene and Public Health
The Johns Hopkins University
Baltimore, Maryland 21205

Morton Corn, Ph.D.
Department of Environmental Health
Sciences
School of Hygiene and Public Health
The Johns Hopkins University
Baltimore, Maryland 21205

John T. Dunlop, Ph.D.
Lamont University Professor, Emeritus
Harvard University
Cambridge, Massachusetts 02138

Edward A. Emmett, M.B., B.S., M.S.
Worksafe Australia
National Occupational Health & Safety
Commission
Sydney, New South Wales 2000 Australia

Richard Evans III, M.D., M.P.H.
Division of Allergy and Immunology
Children's Memorial Hospital
Chicago, Illinois 60614

Jonathan Fielding, M.D., M.P.H.,
M.B.A.
Johnson & Johnson Health Management,
Inc.
Santa Monica, California 90404

Suzanne M. Fortney, Ph.D.
Research Physiologist
The Johnson Space Center
Houston, Texas 77058

Gareth M. Green, M.D.
Associate Dean for Professional Education
Harvard School of Public Health
Boston, Massachusetts 02115

Vicki S. Helgeson, Ph.D.
Department of Psychology
University of California, Los Angeles
Los Angeles, California 90024

Larry Hirschhorn, Ph.D.
Wharton Center for Applied Research
University of Pennsylvania
Philadelphia, Pennsylvania 19104

Raymond G. Hunt, Ph.D.
Department of Organization and Human
Resources
School of Management
State University of New York at Buffalo
Amherst, New York 14260

Gunn Johansson, Ph.D.
Department of Psychology
University of Stockholm
S-106 91 Stockholm Sweden

Hiroya Kubota
Institute for Mental Health
Japan Productivity Center
Tokyo Japan

Genevieve M. Matanoski, M.D., Dr.P.H.
Department of Epidemiology
School of Hygiene and Public Health
The Johns Hopkins University
Baltimore, Maryland 21205

†Harold A. Menkes, M.D.
Department of Environmental Health
Sciences
School of Hygiene and Public Health
The Johns Hopkins University
Baltimore, Maryland 21205

Marie A. Morell, Ph.D.
Beverley Hills Medical Center
Pain Care Center
Los Angeles, California 90035

Ann H. Myers, Sc.D.
Department of Health Policy and
Management
School of Hygiene and Public Health
The Johns Hopkins University
Baltimore, Maryland 21205

Carol A. Newill, Ph.D.
Department of Immunology and Infectious
Diseases
School of Hygiene and Public Health
The Johns Hopkins University
Baltimore, Maryland 21205

Gordon S. Smith, M.B., Ch.B., M.P.H.
Department of Health Policy and
Management
School of Hygiene and Public Health
The Johns Hopkins University
Baltimore, Maryland 21205

Megan E. Sullaway, Ph.D.
Department of Psychology
University of California, Los Angeles
Los Angeles, California 90024

Diana Chapman Walsh, Ph.D.
Department of Health and Social Behavior
Harvard School of Public Health
Boston, Massachusetts 02115

Contents

I
INTRODUCTION

1
Work, Health, and Productivity: Overview

Frank Baker and Gareth M. Green

A major goal of most organizations is enhanced productivity; without it, profit-oriented organizations cannot survive. In today's economic environment nonprofit organizations have to be concerned with improvements in output without a proportional increase in input. Of course organizations have multiple goals, and productivity is not their only concern. As society's values have changed, most organizations have also become concerned about the health and well-being of their workers, and they have come to acknowledge their responsibilities for the organization's customers, neighbors, and community at large. Thus in addition to the traditional role of the workplace to offer economic incentives and reasonable conditions of employment, there is now the incentive of enhancing worker health to achieve social as well as economic goals. This book is about these changing responsibilities for worker health and productivity in the workplace and the ramifications of the changes for industrial and health policies.

WORK

There is growing recognition of the fundamental importance of working life and its effects on the health and well-being of people in modern industrial societies. Most Americans, men and women, spend much of their adult lives on the job. Work is the source of much that is beneficial, as it provides a relatively enduring human community, experiences of psychological growth and mastery of skills, and potentially rich opportunities for creative activity. As a social institution, the workplace is often a source of stability, functioning as a major psychosocial resource.

WORK AND HEALTH

The work organization has important significance with regard to the health of its members. It is the place where workers acquire the resources for physical well-being and sometimes the know-how for maintaining health. Experience at work is a major determinant of adult behavior and personality, and hence it plays an important role in the development of both good and bad health behaviors.

One may even consider the school as an early work environment for children, where they learn about health behavior as well as supervised productive activity. Behavior learned there may continue into the adult work situation. School is also where young adults are prepared in terms of obtaining the skills that will support their productivity in the workplace.

WORKPLACE RISKS TO HEALTH

Workers are exposed to potentially adverse environmental conditions in the workplace, conditions that may increase their risks of acute and chronic diseases. The worker's health and safety are threatened by physical, chemical, and biological hazards in the work environment. In addition, there are various psychosocial factors in the organization that may have considerable influence on the physical and mental well-being of the worker.

Work has always carried risks of physical injury and even death, but the growing sophistication and complexity of twentieth century productive technology has multiplied the subtlety and complexity of those risks. Concern with toxic chemical and physical agents in the workplace may be divided into two phases: (a) high-dose, short-term exposures leading to acute illness or death, which characterized concerns during the first half of the century; and (b) low-dose, long-term exposures leading to chronic illness or lethal disease after long periods of latency (e.g., cancer), which dominated concerns in the years since mid-century. During the 1930s after several disastrous occupational exposures to silica dust—most notably the digging of the Gauley Bridge tunnel (49)—standards setting permissible exposure limits (PELs) to silica, and later to asbestos and other pneumoconiotic dusts, were established, and several states set up surveillance units to evaluate the effectiveness of those standards in terms of disease prevention. Experience in many settings and with many agents and diseases has firmly established the value of control of emissions according to scientifically determined standards for exposure as the cornerstone of occupational and environmental health policy. Health surveillance evaluates the effectiveness of exposure controls but is of diminished value where there is long latency from exposure to disease and the disease process is irreversible by the time it is detected, as with cancer. Therefore reliance has increasingly shifted to environmental monitoring of levels of exposure as the tool for ensuring compliance with established standards.

During the decades after World War II, with the growing awareness of the linkage between long-term exposure to chemical and physical agents in the working environment and delayed lethal diseases such as cancer, a vastly more difficult challenge to disease prevention through environmental control of the agent presented. First was the difficulty of proving the causative association between exposure to the specific agent and disease (e.g., lung cancer) appearing 15 to 25 years later. In many instances, the relation was established only after years of extensive epidemiological study in occupational groups experiencing the exposure in comparison to comparable workers not exposed or exposed at different levels. A good example is the relation between lung cancer and exposure to asbestos fibers. In other cases, the occurrence of a cluster of cases of a rare disease in association with a particular agent led to control of the agent within a matter of months, as in the case of vinyl chloride exposure and cancer of the liver (see Chapter 4).

The growing recognition that even low exposure to highly toxic chemicals can induce potentially disabling disease and death decades after exposure has fostered the concept of a strategy for prevention (69) based on prediction of potential toxicity according to (a) analysis of the structure of the substance and its relation to known compounds with similar structure or (b) evidence of toxic effects in experimental animals or in animal or human tissues tested in the laboratory. Many of these tests require additional research before their validity is securely established; moreover, they are time-consuming, are expensive, and delay the application of new chemical or process technology. An additional problem is that they impede productivity growth, at least over the short term. Furthermore, the benefits to the health of the workforce may not be seen for 10 to 30 years, when the worker may have long since moved to another job or retired and is no longer either a benefit to or the responsibility of the employer who incurred the expense. In addition, unless the control requirements are applied uniformly to all similar operations, in the same society or abroad, the regulated industry is at a competitive disadvantage because of the cost and delay of the control requirements. The societal benefit may be greater with regard to the production of a healthier working (and retired) population but lesser with regard to economic well-being.

Healthy workplaces were not a particular concern at the beginning of the industrial revolution when workers were seen as interchangeable cogs in a large production machine. Early in this century, Frederick W. Taylor's "Scientific Management Movement," with its emphasis on time and motion studies and getting the most work out of employees, had as an implicit assumption the belief that workers were replaceable. During these initial stages of the industrial revolution, the tendency of emerging industrial organizations was to exploit their employees in favor of increased productivity. A laissez-faire attitude prevailed, and there was a large supply of cheap immigrant labor readily available. Long work hours and low pay in relatively hazardous work conditions were common.

With the emergence of labor unions, changes in general social values, and other changes in society, there was more concern about the health and safety of the worker. However, the trade-off of worker health for increases in productivity and profitability continues as a problem to this day.

OCCUPATIONAL HEALTH

Changes in American society's views about issues of worker health were reflected in the development of the field of occupational health, the emergence of which in the United States dates back to the beginning of the industrial revolution. Levenstein (51), in a review of the history of this field, pointed out as a key event the creation by Massachusetts in 1867 of the first department of factory inspection in the United States and in 1877 enactment of the first safety law, which required guards for textile machinery.

After 1900 there was greater activity and concern for occupational safety and health particularly related to the use of lead and other toxic materials in factories. Around 1900 workers began to sue negligent firms in the courts and to win their cases. Concern for occupational health accelerated during World War I. Dr. Alice Hamilton, who studied toxic exposures in working people in industry in Chicago, helped to develop the field of occupational medicine from these early activities (33).

State workers' compensation laws originated during 1909 to 1911, but the first one in New York was pronounced unconstitutional. Later state compensation laws were upheld, and by 1948 all states had these laws (66). Such legislation provided income security to injured workers, and employers were encouraged through economic incentives to maintain safe working conditions.

Although attention was given to occupational problems at the national level during the 1930s, little substantial new attention was given to occupational health issues during the 1940s and 1950s. It was generally considered that workers' compensation legislation had dealt with the main problems. However, there was at least one significant event in the eradication of industrial hazards in 1941, when research showing chronic mercury poisoning among hatters led to a joint agreement of the manufacturers, unions, state health officials, and U.S. Public Health Service (PHS) to eliminate mercury from the hatting industry (26). Following World War II the political and economic strength of labor decreased, and it was not until the beginning of the environmental movement during the 1960s that widespread concern about pollution in the work environment developed.

Between 1961 and 1970 industrial accident rates went up 29%, and the death of 78 miners in a 1968 coal mine explosion in Farmington, West Virginia led to new political activity concerning industrial health and safety. The Coal Mine Health and Safety Act was passed in 1969. In 1972 the Black Lung Benefits Act was passed after considerable research had been conducted in Appalachia funded by the government (51). The Occupational Safety and Health Act was signed into law in 1970. The act created the Occupational Safety and Health Administration (OSHA) within the Department of Labor and the National Institute for Occupational Safety and Health (NIOSH) within the Department of Health and Human Services. The Toxic Substances Control Act was enacted in 1976 to regulate the production and use of potentially harmful chemicals (4).

Starting at the end of the 1970s and continuing into the 1980s, the position of occupational health on the list of the nation's priorities slid downward. However, the threat of hazardous waste gained new attention with the Love Canal incident, and the public became aware of the thousands of toxic waste dumps around the United States (52). The Three Mile Island nuclear reactor accident in 1979 stimulated widespread concern about technological disasters (63,78). The Bhopal incident in which tens of thousands of people living near a pesticide plant in India were exposed to poisonous fumes resulted in considerable apprehension about industrial toxicants (35). Certainly, more people today are aware of dangers to health produced by industrial production than anytime in the past.

WORKPLACE

At the same time that concerns about the effects of industry on the larger environment are growing, the character of industry in the United States has begun to shift from a focus on manufacturing, metals, chemicals, textiles, and other "smokestack" industries. It is now generally accepted that we are moving into a "postindustrial" era and that the central focus of work is shifting from the production of goods to the production of knowledge and delivery of services (7,75). This postindustrial society focuses on knowledge rather than human energy as the key factor in productive work. In turn, profound changes have begun to take place in the work sector and the larger society. There is evidence that we are just beginning to see the effects of some of the changes of the postindustrial age. For example, computerization of the workplace has had profound effects on the character of work and is expected to produce even greater changes in the near future (76). Robotics are increasingly being incorporated into manufacturing processes, and other major technological innovations on the horizons will have effects that are difficult to predict at this point (9). The use of automatic work processing and video display terminal operations may not only be a source of problems at work but may offer the means of inducing variety and challenge in traditional ways of working that have suffered from excessive routine and repetition.

Changes have helped to reveal that healthy workplaces create advantages for both employers and employees. As the postindustrial society evolves, there appear to be advantages to keeping difficult-to-replace workers healthy and productive. The long years of learning required of workers with special skills and knowledge in an economy based on information industries has led to more concern about the health of at least some of the workforce. In recent years large corporations have established risk reduction programs to protect the health of managers and their scientific and technical personnel.

LIFESTYLE CHANGES AND HEALTH

As we have grown increasingly concerned about stress and difficulties of adjusting to the environment, widespread concern has developed about the "quality of life" (5,14). In the workplace this trend was represented by the development of extensive research and discussion about the "quality of work life" (24).

The concern about quality of life extends into other aspects of our lives. Books and articles regularly appear comparing different cities in the United States regarding their relative merits in terms of quality of life (34), and there has been much discussion about the search and desire for improved "life styles" (54).

American concern about healthy lifestyles was further stimulated by the publication of the Surgeon General's report, *Healthy People* (13), in which the federal government gave much publicized recognition to the role of individual health behavior in preventing chronic disease. Lifestyle was described in companion documents as accounting for up to 50% of mortality from the ten leading causes of death, environmental factors and heredity contributing about 20%, and inadequate health care counting about 10% (38).

HEALTH PROMOTION IN THE WORKPLACE

The work organization is as central to the preventive thrust of adult public health as schools are central for children. The public health goals for the nation focus on these settings when trying to change health behavior and prevent the major causes of mortality and morbidity. One of the ways of tackling these goals is through encouraging worksite health promotion efforts.

As American society at large has become entranced with the benefits of exercise and diet, this trend has been recognized and promoted by advertising and marketing forces. Greater attention to healthy lifestyles has encouraged business organizations to extend the wellness programs that they originally developed as "perks" for their executives and professional staff to other employees (32,48). At the beginning of the 1980s, one author estimated that more than 1,000 companies were already spending more than two billion dollars annually on health promotion (41).

While considerable effort is being expended in workplace health promotion programs, systematic evaluation of these programs has lagged behind. Early evaluation tended to be anecdotal and nonrigorous. The clearest evidence of the effectiveness of worksite health promotion efforts has been in areas such as high blood pressure control (2,25,67) and smoking cessation (23,28,77). Most of the evaluations to date have focused on such single component programs. Recently, articles have begun to appear in the peer-reviewed literature reporting evaluations of comprehensive workplace health promotion programs. One of the most thoroughly evaluated comprehensive programs has been Johnson & Johnson's Live for Life program (10; also see Chapter 17). Another large-scale evaluation has recently appeared focusing on the impact of a comprehensive workplace health promotion program on absences at 41 intervention sites and 19 control sites with 29,315 and 14,573 full-time, hourly employees (8). Results from this study suggest that comprehensive worksite health promotion programs can reduce disability days among blue collar employees and provide a favorable return on investment. However, much remains to be done in developing adequate evaluations of workplace health promotion programs.

HEALTH AND ECONOMIC INCENTIVES

The expansion of health promotion and wellness programs has been motivated by the promise of decreasing the firm's employee medical care costs. A number of writers have commented on how these cost-containment concerns have affected an emphasis on health promotion and wellness programs for greater numbers of personnel in the industrial organization (27,61). Advantages for the organization have been claimed in terms of long-term health care cost savings, such as lower insurance premiums and fewer claims. However, few of these industrial health promotion programs have been adequately evaluated, and most of the economic data on these programs are not derived from long-term, well-controlled studies; they are simply descriptive (28,39).

Management's recognition of the possible benefits of overall cost reduction by maintaining a healthy workforce and decreasing health care expenses has been met with somewhat skeptical acceptance by labor. Labor leaders and others have expressed concern that focusing attention on workers maintaining their own health is a "blaming-the-victim" strategy that can be used by management to evade its responsibilities regarding the health and safety of workers (3).

Another impetus for growing attention to worker health and well-being has been the outstanding performance of the Japanese and an accompanying growing recognition of the underutilization of the potential of the American worker. A concern about exercise, diet, and involvement of workers in the organization also has been stimulated by the Japanese models of management. Interest in getting the most from American workers has stimulated serious attention to new forms of work organization and greater concern about worker health.

DEMOGRAPHICS

Several significant changes in demographics are projected that will influence the future of work in the United States. Over the course of the next two decades, the population will grow significantly larger and older, and it will include proportionately more women and minorities (56,58,60). Such changes will profoundly alter the labor force in the United States.

The U.S. labor force is expected to expand from approximately 115 million workers in 1985 to perhaps 150 million workers by 2010; and modification of immigration policies and related changes in population fertility may further boost these figures (60). Increases in life expectancy and aging of the population will create pressures to keep older people in the workforce longer. However, as the proportion of retirees grows, the social security system will be strained and pressure will exist for higher taxes to pay for the extended retirement periods that accompany longer life. Issues concerning the coverage of increasingly expensive medical care for this older population will put a strain on government's ability to pay, and it is likely that employers will be pressured to take greater responsibility for insuring health care for their employees throughout their lengthened lives (9).

Changes in the workplace have also been projected (43). Along with demographic trends, changes in technology, values, and overall economic performance will shape future demand for labor. It is projected that growth in new jobs will be balanced among professional, technical, clerical, and service workers (60). These office workers are subject to a range of psychosocial stressors that produce their own particular problems, as we discuss further below.

These changes in the workforce and the workplace itself will undoubtedly produce new pressures for attention to the health needs of employees. For example, as women appear in increasing numbers in the workforce, there are greater reproductive risks to workplace exposures and greater demands for maternity leave and day care at the workplace. Part of the argument made to management for providing day care is that having the children provided for in a reliable and safe environment close at hand reduces stress on the employee mothers and helps improve their productivity.

PRODUCTIVITY

How will these changes in the workforce and the workplace affect productivity? First, some attention should be paid to what is meant by productivity. There are a number of difficulties with the definition and measurement of productivity.

Productivity is generally regarded as an organizational or system variable. Some have viewed national or industrial productivity as a sum of organizational productivities. Human performance is conceptualized as an individual output that when summed across many individuals working together within the organizational context relates to productivity. Productivity also seems to be defined as a relation, or ratio, between input and output.

Sometimes the primary concern is with end results or final output, whatever the cost, whereas in other cases one is preoccupied with output relative to costs. Usually *performance* is defined in terms of levels of output achieved, and *efficiency* is used to refer to cost per unit of output. Hage (37) has observed that the essence of the matter is the usefulness in year to year comparisons when considering outputs achieved relative to the costs of achieving them in attempting to improve productivity.

Sutermeister (71), author of one of the major textbooks on organizational productivity, has defined productivity as "output per employee-hour, quality considered" (71, p. 5). He noted that productivity is not determined solely by either how hard or how well people work or by technical factors but, rather, by some interaction of both.

When considering the various possible approaches to productivity, one of the major issues is what unit of analysis to use. Does one focus on the society, sector, region, organization, occupation, or individual as a unit of measurement? It is not clear whether such measurement can be aggregated or disaggregated without introducing major distortion (73).

PRODUCTIVITY AND LEVELS OF ANALYSIS

Measures of productivity vary with the level of analysis used. For example, when one compares productivity across nations, the gross national product (GNP) per capita is used as an index of productivity, whereas in the comparison of productivity across individuals a variety of measures of job performance are used. It is difficult to use the measures developed in one level of analysis for another level of analysis (73). For example, it makes little sense to try to create a measure of GNP per capita. Another example is found in the demonstration by several social scientists that the index of output per hour of labor, which is used at higher levels of analysis, may not be meaningful at the level of the firm (36,37).

The discipline or background of the researcher influences the level of analysis chosen for research on productivity, but it is obvious that the measurement of productivity requires a multilevel approach. For example, if one focuses on organizations as the central unit of analysis, lower and higher aggregation levels need to be considered and factored into research designs that attempt to explain interorganizational differences in productivity. Pennings (62) has suggested that a multilevel approach can identify various "levers" that can be pushed for the sake of increasing productivity.

If aspects of organizational designs result in more productive firms, the organizational level should be the focus of social change. However, productivity for the society should consider the quality of the available workforce, including its level of skills, education, and health. To accomplish these goals, one might focus on such macrosocial levers as educational loans and fellowship programs, greater governmental support of schools and universities, and the funding of research on health promotion and disease prevention.

RESEARCH ON PRODUCTIVITY

Several trends have been observed in the study of productivity over the course of this century. As we noted above, the Scientific Management Movement earlier focused on productivity at any human cost. During the postwar period of the 1950s the Human

Relations Movement that developed placed a great deal of emphasis on democratic values in the workplace and the involvement of workers and their concerns in efforts to improve the organization as an environment for its membership. In recent years this concern has been translated into the concern for quality of working life mentioned above.

For a number of years the major variable to be related to human performance was job satisfaction. A vast literature developed over the conditions in the work environment that would contribute to the satisfaction of the employee with his or her work situation. However, reviews of the relevant research literature failed to reveal more than a small relation between satisfaction and level of performance or productivity (11,53). Rather than thinking about job performance as a response to satisfaction of workers with their jobs, the current view is to consider satisfaction or dissatisfaction with the job as linked to productivity as mediated by rewards that reinforce high levels of performance (64). In recent years the concept of "stress" has replaced job satisfaction as a key word for describing the relation between the organizational work environment and the performance of organization members.

Schneider (68) has shown that although industrial and organizational psychologists have relatively successfully developed reliable and valid measures of the job performance of an individual, there is little known about how they relate to productivity measures at a more aggregate level. An implication of this problem is that, if the reward structure of an organization is misspecified in terms of the key dimensions of a job related to organizational productivity, one may reward workers for performing activities that are not related to productivity of the firm. An example is rewarding a professor for productivity in terms of the number of his or her publications, a practice that may be counterproductive to negotiations with the state legislature regarding performance based on quality and quantity of teaching students from the state.

With regard to the multiple agendas of policy makers, governmental officials, owners, managers, and workers in industrial organizations, there are several key questions that may be identified as of central concern to applied research in the area of productivity. One would want to know how changing a policy variable at one level of analysis would affect productivity at another level. Also, it would be important to understand the relations of measures of productivity used at different levels of analysis. Finally, research should identify how changing a policy variable at one level of analysis affects attempts to adjust productivity under static and dynamic conditions (73).

PRODUCTIVITY AND HEALTH

The competitive nature of an industrialized world places a premium on productivity for economic well-being. Industry functions to provide material benefits to the society, the means of acquiring those materials through the financial rewards of employment, and material gain through profits to the employer. Profitability is determined in part by the amount received for a product, which is established through pricing and the cost of production—in many industries determined largely by the cost of labor.

As competition places downward pressure on prices, and demands for material gain by labor places upward pressure on the cost of production, the need to control costs, increased productivity, or both drives business policy. A common response is to cut costs through a reduction in safety measures. The inevitable consequence is increased hazard to the worker and increased injury, illness, and death. Rising social values make such practices ethically unacceptable; and as noted above, minimum safe working conditions have become mandated by the law of the land.

Opinions divide sharply as to whether the competition from abroad and a greater concern for productivity in American industry will involve a continued concern about an organization's members. Some forecasts predict that increased productivity means that many workers will lose their jobs or will have to work harder under more stressful conditions. Others argue that restructuring the workplace offers the opportunity for "rebirth into new careers and opportunities" (74).

As the United States and other developed nations have been moving to the postindustrialized society, the Third World has become increasingly industrialized. Applying a false historicism, some have argued that because industrialization in the past was accompanied by alienation and a decline in the quality of working life, developing countries will have to face these same consequences as a price of their industrialization.

INVESTING IN HEALTH FOR PRODUCTIVITY

Why would a company invest resources in preventing disease or optimizing health in its employees? Outside of value issues and moral concerns, it implies that the workforce is not easily replaceable. In a purely economic sense, irrespective of value considerations, it may be more understandable that corporations invest in the promotion of health of their workers. If the workforce is operating below par because of marginal health, the trade-off of investing in health-promotion activities may be easy to rationalize. Workers who are fit do not have to rely on drugs, have a high degree of mental alertness, and are more likely to turn in an effective performance and contribute to organizational productivity. Particularly with regard to executives who may take a long time to groom and who tend to come to their positions later in life, preventive intervention regarding their health may be the most straightforward investment. The health-promotion program most frequently offered by American corporations involves stress reduction because of the ready acceptance of this type of program by managers and coworkers and the general belief that we live and work in an increasingly stressful environment.

STRESS AND PRODUCTIVITY

Although stress at work may affect basic health processes, work environments are changing; as more is learned about the way work affects health, these changes may be for the better. For example, there is currently great concern about the effect of introducing new technology, e.g., automated processes in the application of electronics. Psychological stress and related health problems have been studied as associated with the introduction of these new technologies, which are intended to increase productivity.

One of the earliest experimental efforts to study the dynamics of productive behavior in the workplace was the extensive program of research carried out at the Hawthorne Works of the Western Electric Company between 1927 and 1932 (65). Although this group of researchers began by focusing on the physical aspects of work, such as lighting, color of walls, and the like, they ended up finding that the work group's social climate was a major determinant of productivity. One of the main findings of this research was that work group norms restricted productivity. Although these extensive studies focused on identifying characteristics of the most productive physical work environments, the studies are primarily remembered as a demonstration of the power and complexity of the social environment in its effects on productivity.

Stress in the workplace seems most destructive of health when workers have little control of their work environment. Participation in decisions about the work environment not only affects health, but this kind of worker control also seems to influence productivity. For example, Miller and Monge (55) conducted a meta-analysis of 25 studies containing estimates of the relation between worker participation in decision making and productivity. They found that participation does have an effect on productivity that appears to be more strongly demonstrated by field studies than laboratory research.

STRESS AT WORK AND EFFECTS ON HEALTH

The term *stress* has been used loosely to refer to an environmental condition that can be objectively defined and measured as well as to a subjective perception or appraisal of such an objective environmental condition. Studies have promoted the operational definition of stress as a subjectively appraised condition. Reviews of workplace stress in the literature have called for studies using both objective and subjective measures, with the pairing of subjective measures with objectively established environmental conditions (44,47,59).

Among the major factors in the work situation identified to produce stress (72) are the following:

1. Work overload.
2. Work pressure.
3. Responsibility for people.
4. Role conflict and role ambiguity.
5. Lack of social support at work.
6. Perceived inadequate work advancement.
7. Lack of control over work.

Caplan and Jones (15) observed that workers who perceive themselves as overloaded at work because they have too many tasks at which they must work too long and too hard feel more stressed and are at more risk with regard to their health.

Perceived pressure to work is also associated with stress and work overload (30). Role conflict and role ambiguity have been found to be associated with chronically high blood pressure and elevated pulse rates (29). Poor social relationships at work have repeatedly been found to be associated with job stress (40). Workers who are insecure about their job futures and whether they have been promoted appropriately experience more stress (18).

Lack of control over when or at what pace work is performed has been shown to be associated with stress reactions (42). In particular, the hypothesis that stress effects on health are increased in work settings where there is high job demand and low decision latitude has been tested in several studies. The results have indicated that this work situation is related to increased risk for heart disease (46). Karasek has worked with a group of Swedish researchers who have been the primary promoters of the Job Demands-Control Model (45).

A study by Caplan et al. (16) conducted for NIOSH on job demands and worker health showed that boredom, dissatisfaction with workload, and job satisfaction tended to occur together and appeared to be associated with underutilization of worker skills and abilities, low participation, high uncertainty about the future (job insecurity), and poor social support at work. Clear differences were found in the person–environment fit across occupations, suggesting that job environment may be a significant source of the poor fit between workers and environment.

Job environment is linked to health outcomes for workers in a growing literature. Some work has focused on linking work environment stress and immunosuppression (6). There are many problems with the studies that link immunosuppression competence and stress, including the use of weak research designs, dependence on retrospective reports, and difficulties assessing immunocompetence given the sheer complexity of the immune system. Also, the stress concept is tricky; it is more than measurement of "objective" work environment including physical stressors such as noise, heat, and crowding. Using one of the most popular psychological theories, stress was viewed by Lazarus and Folkman (50) as dependent on appraisal by individuals—both "primary appraisal" as to whether environmental stimuli pose a threat and "secondary appraisal" as to whether the individual has the resources to deal with them.

BOUNDARY BETWEEN WORK AND COMMUNITY

The worker is also exposed to stresses and toxic substances outside the workplace. These off-the-job exposures may have as great or greater effects on worker health than those encountered in the job situation. Workers carry the effects of stress and toxic exposures outside the job with them into the workplace, and there are interaction effects to consider as well. Earlier approaches to occupational health tended to focus on the work environment without dealing with what was going on at home and in the community at large. It was almost as if there were an integumented boundary around the work organization. That boundary is certainly seen as much more porous today (79). Occupational physicians and nurses, industrial hygienists, and others concerned with occupational health are now much more willing to recognize and attempt to develop programs to deal with these external exposures (1,12,22).

In particular, a focus on prevention and occupational health promotion by force of circumstances requires the occupational health professional to focus on activities outside the workplace. Health education efforts to change diet, exercise, and other health behaviors in order to be effective should involve the family. Dealing with smoking, alcohol consumption, and drug use in employee assistance programs requires consideration of off-the-job stresses.

The boundary between the workplace and the community has also been breached by the widespread recognition of the community's jeopardy from the possibly disastrous handling of toxic substances by industry. The company must now participate in community emergency planning and must effectively communicate with the public in the face of widespread fear about hazardous waste disposal, industrial accidents, and the possibility of spills when transporting dangerous materials.

As concern about technological risks has risen, greater effort has been made to improve methods of risk analysis and risk management. Behavioral and social scientists have developed a body of knowledge relevant to those responsible for risk analysis and decision-making. Studies of risk perception show that the judgments that both lay people and experts use are subject to bias in the evaluation of hazardous activities and technologies (19,31,70).

NEED FOR EFFECTIVE COMMUNICATION

In the attempt to respond effectively to community concern, communication about hazards has become a fast growing field combining research and theory from social psychology, decision sciences, and the field of persuasive communications with industrial hygiene, engineering, and risk sciences (17,20,21). Scientists and engineers have not been particularly effective in the past in dealing with community groups, local governments, and the media regarding concerns about industrial accidents and problems such as toxic waste dumps (52). The need for more effective community communication and interaction by industry is now recognized, and the translation of available theory and research to practice has begun (57). Much of the available research and theory has been based on college student samples in artificial situations, however, and there is considerable need for field research with industrial and community samples.

TOWARD A NEW PERSPECTIVE

Returning to our concern for the relation among work, health, and productivity, this review of some of the relevant history and literature suggests a need to change thinking about the meaning of productivity. Perhaps the postindustrial age requires a new perspective.

Although declines of productivity have been most dramatic in the United States, even Japan, whose products capture an increasingly larger share of the American market, has found it difficult to sustain the same level of productivity growth it experienced during the 1950s and 1960s. This point suggests a fundamental change in the nature of productivity in postindustrial society (37).

During the industrial age productivity was achieved by high volume produced at low cost. During the postindustrial age, different strategies may be involved in the achievement of productivity. Quality has become a concern, and consumers may prefer products and services with special characteristics produced in small batches. Initial price is not the only concern, and consumers are increasingly concerned about long-term durability and operating costs. Products and services are evaluated on the basis of attributes that were not a part of earlier considerations, such as if a product was organically produced, is free of pollution, consumes less energy, and so forth. Thus we need new measures of productivity that take into account the dimensions by which products are evaluated today.

Attempts to improve the efficiency of work organizations have neglected the consideration of long-term costs and false economies. The social and technical characteristics of work organizations, communities, and other social systems must be considered in order to achieve a balance between the goals of industrialization and community development.

REFERENCES

1. Alderman, M. H., & Hanley, M. J. (1982). *Clinical medicine for the occupational physician.* New York: Marcel Dekker.
2. Alderman, M., Green, L. W., & Flynn, B. S. (1982). Hypertension control program in occupational settings. In R. S. Parkinson (ed.). *Managing health promotion in the workplace: guidelines for implementation and evaluation* (p. 162). Palo Alto, CA: Mayfield Publishing Company.
3. Allegrante, J. P., & Green, L. W. (1981). When health policy becomes victim-blaming. *New England Journal of Medicine, 305,* 1528–9.
4. Anderson, F. R. (1983). Human welfare and the administered society: federal regulation in the 1970s to protect health, safety and the environment. In W. N. Rom (ed.). *Environmental and occupational medicine* (pp. 835–64). Boston: Little, Brown.
5. Andrews, F. R., & Withey, S. B. (1976). *Social indications of well-being: Americans' perceptions of life quality.* New York: Plenum.
6. Baker, F., Agnew, J., Curbow, B., Hirata, F., & Margolick, J. (1987). *Pilot study of the immunosuppressive effects of psychological job stress: plan for field investigation* (CDC/NIOSH contract No. 200-81-2538). Baltimore: Johns Hopkins School of Hygiene and Public Health, Department of Environmental Health Sciences.
7. Bell, D. (1973). *The coming of post-industrial society.* New York: Basic Books.
8. Bertera, R. L. (1990). The effects of workplace health promotion on absenteeism and employment costs in a large industrial population. *American Journal of Public Health, 80,* 1101–05.
9. Bezold, C., Carlson, F. J., & Peck, J. C. (1986). *The future of work and health.* Dover, MA: Auburn House.
10. Bly, J. L., Jones, R. C., and Richardson, J. E. (1986). Impact of worksite health promotion on health care costs and utilization. Evaluation of Johnson & Johnson's Live for Life Program. *Journal of the American Medical Association, 256,* 3235–40.
11. Brayfield, A. H., & Crockett, W. H. (1955). Employee attitudes and employee performance. *Psychological Bulletin, 52,* 396–424.
12. Brown, M. L. (1981). *Occupational health nursing: principles and practices.* New York: Springer-Verlag.
13. Califano, J. A., Jr. (1979). *Healthy people: the Surgeon General's report on health promotion*

and disease prevention. Washington, DC: U.S. Government Printing Office.
14. Campbell, A., Converse, P. E., & Rodgers, W. L. (1976). *The quality of American life.* New York: Russell Sage.
15. Caplan, R. D., & Jones, K. W. (1975). Effects of work load, role ambiguity, and type A personality on anxiety, depression, and heart rate. *Journal of Applied Psychology, 60,* 713–19.
16. Caplan, R. D., Cobb, S., French, J. R. P., Jr., Van Harrison, R., & Pinneau, S. R. (1975). *Job demands and worker health* (DHEW, NIOSH publication 75–160). Washington, DC: U.S. Government Printing Office.
17. Cohen, A., Colligan, M. J., & Bergner, P. (1985). Psychology in health risk messages to workers. *Journal of Occupational Medicine, 27,* 543–51.
18. Cooper, C. L., & Marshall, J. (1976). Occupational sources of stress: a review of the literature relating to coronary heart disease and mental ill health. *Journal of Occupational Psychology, 49,* 11–28.
19. Covello, V. T. (1983). The perception of technological risks: a literature review. *Technological Forecasting and Social Change, 23,* 285–97.
20. Covello, V. T., von Winterfeldt, D., & Slovic, P. (1986). Risk communication: a review of the literature. *Risk Analysis, 3,* 171–82.
21. Covello, V. T., von Winterfeldt, D., & Slovic, P. (1987). Communicating scientific information about health and environmental risks: problems and opportunities from a social and behavioral perspective. In V. T. Covello, L. B. Lave, A. Moghissi, & V. R. R. Uppuluri (eds.). *Advances in risk analysis. Vol. 4. Uncertainty in risk assessment, risk management, and decision making* (pp. 221–39). New York: Plenum.
22. Cralley, L. J., & Cralley, L. V. (1985). Rationale. In L. J. Cralley & L. V. Cralley (eds.). *Patty's industrial hygiene and toxicology. Vol. III. Theory and rationale of industrial hygiene practice* (pp. 1–26). New York: Wiley.
23. Dannaher, B. G. (1982). Smoking cessation programs in occupational settings. In R. S. Parkinson (ed.). *Managing health promotion in the workplace: guidelines for interpretation and evaluation* (p. 217). Palo Alto, CA: Mayfield Publishing Company.
24. Davis, L. E., & Cherns, A. B. (1975). *The quality of working life. Vol. 1. Problems, prospects and state of the art.* New York: Free Press.

25. Erfurt, J. C., & Foote, A. (1984). Cost-effectiveness of worksite blood pressure control programs. *Journal of Occupational Medicine, 26*, 892–900.
26. Felton, J. P. (1982). Occupational medicine in the United States: an historical background. In M. H. Alderman & M. J. Hanley (eds.). *Clinical medicine for the occupational physician* (pp. 3–24). New York: Marcel Dekker.
27. Fielding, J. E. (1984). *Corporate health management*. Reading, MA: Addison-Wesley.
28. Fielding, J. E. (1986). Evaluations, results, and problems of worksite health promotion programs. In M. F. Cataldo & T. J. Coates (eds.). *Health and industry: a behavioral medicine perspective* (pp. 373–96). New York: Wiley.
29. French, J. R. P., Jr., & Caplan, R. D. (1973). Organizational stress and individual strain. In A. J. Murrow (ed.). *The failure of success* (pp. 30–66). New York: Amacon.
30. French, J. R. P., Jr., Tupper, C. J., & Mueller, E. I. (1965). *Workload of university professors*. Unpublished research report. Ann Arbor: University of Michigan.
31. Freudenburg, W. R. (1988). Perceived risk, real risk: social science and the art of probabilistic risk assessment. *Science, 242*, 44–49.
32. Gebhardt, D. L., & Crump, C. E. (1990). Employee fitness and wellness programs in the workplace. *American Psychologist, 45*, 262–72.
33. Goodell, H., Wolf, S., & Rodgers, F. B. (1986). In S. Wolf & A. J. Finestone (eds.). *Occupational stress: health and performance at work* (pp. 8–23). Little, MA: PSG Publishing.
34. Gould, J. M. (1986). *Quality of life in American neighborhoods: levels of affluence, toxic waste, and cancer mortality in residential zip codes*. Boulder, CO: Westview.
35. Green, G. M. (1985). Crisis in Bhopal, India. Presented at 1985 Disaster Management Conference, Orlando, Florida.
36. Guth, W. D. (1984). Productivity and corporate strategy. In A. P. Brief (ed.). *Productivity research in the behavioral and social sciences* (pp. 252–67). New York: Praeger.
37. Hage, J. (1984). Organizational theory and the concept of productivity. In A. P. Brief (ed.). *Productivity research in the behavioral and social sciences* (pp. 91–126). New York: Praeger.
38. Harris, P. R. (1981). *Health United States 1980: with prevention profile*. Washington, DC: U.S. Government Printing Office.
39. Hollander, R. B., Lengermann, J. J., & DeMuth, N. M. (1985). Cost effectiveness and cost-benefit analyses of occupational health promotion. In G. S. Everly & R. H. L. Feldman (eds.). *Occupational health promotion: health behavior in the workplace* (pp. 287–300). New York: Wiley.
40. House, J. A. (1981). *Work stress and social support*. Reading, MA: Addison-Wesley.
41. Howe, C. (1983). Establishing employee recreation programs. *Journal of Physical Education & Dance, 54*, 34–52.
42. Hurrell, J. J., & Colligan, M. J. (1987). Machine pacing and shiftwork: evidence for job stress. *Journal of Organizational Behavior Management, 8*, 159–75.
43. Jackson, S. E., & Schuler, R. S. (1990). Human resource planning: challenges for industrial/organizational psychologists. *American Psychologist, 45*, 223–39.
44. Jick, T. D., & Burke, R. J. (1982). Occupational stress: recent findings and new directions. *Journal of Occupational Behavior, 3*, 1–3.
45. Karasek, R., & Theorell, T. (1990). *Healthy work: stress, productivity and the reconstruction of working life*. New York: Basic Books.
46. Karasek, R. A., Baker, D., Marxer, F., Ahlbom, A., & Theorell, T. (1981). Job decision latitude, job demands, and cardiovascular disease: a prospective study of Swedish men. *American Journal of Public Health, 71*, 694–705.
47. Kasl, S. V. (1986). Stress and disease in the workplace: a methodological commentary on the accumulated evidence. In M. F. Cataldo & T. J. Coates (eds.). *Health and industry: a behavioral medicine perspective* (pp. 52–85). New York: Wiley.
48. Kiefhaber, A. K., & Goldbeck, W. B. (1984). Worksite wellness. In *Prospects for a healthier America: achieving the nation's health promotion objectives* (pp. 41–56). U.S. Department of Health and Human Services. Washington, DC: U.S. Government Printing Office.
49. LaDou, J. (ed.). (1986). *Introduction to occupational health & safety* (p. 46). Chicago: National Safety Council.
50. Lazarus, R. S., & Folkman, S. (1984). *Stress, appraisal, and coping*. New York: Springer-Verlag.
51. Levenstein, C. (1983). A brief history of occupational health in the United States. In B. S. Levy & D. H. Wegman (eds.). *Occupational health* (pp. 11–12). Boston: Little, Brown.
52. Levine, A. G. (1982). *Love Canal: science, politics and people*. Lexington, MA: Lexington Books.
53. Locke, E. A. (1976). Nature and causes of job satisfaction. In M. D. Dunnette (ed.). *Handbook of industrial and organizational psychology* (pp. 1297–1349). Chicago: Rand McNally.
54. Matarazzo, J. D. (1984). Behavioral health: a 1990 challenge for the health sciences professions. In J. D. Matarazzo, S. M. Weiss, J. A. Herd, N. E. Miller, & S. M. Weiss (eds.). *Behavioral health: a handbook of health enhancement and disease prevention* (pp. 3–40). New York: Wiley.
55. Miller, K. I., & Monge, P. R. (1986). Participation satisfaction, and productivity: a meta

analytic review. *Academy of Management Journal, 29*, 727–53.

56. Naisbitt, J., & Aburdene, P. (1990). *Megatrends 2000*. New York: William Morrow.
57. National Research Council. (1989). *Improving Risk Communication*. Washington, DC: National Academy Press.
58. Offermann, L. R., & Gowing, M. K. (1990). Organizations of the future: changes and challenges. *American Psychologist, 45*, 95–108.
59. Payne, R., Jick, T. D., & Burke, R. J. (1982). Whither stress research? An agenda for the 1980s. *Journal of Occupational Behavior, 3*, 131–45.
60. Peck, J. C., Goldbeck, W. B., & Meyers, M. L. (1987). *The future of work and health*. Alexandria, VA: Institute for Alternative Futures.
61. Pelletier, K. R. (1986). Healthy people in healthy places: health promotion programs in the workplace. In M. F. Cataldo & T. J. Coates (eds.). *Health and industry: a behavioral medicine perspective* (pp. 351–72). New York: Wiley.
62. Pennings, J. M. (1984). Productivity: some old and new issues. In A. P. Brief (ed.). *Productivity research in the behavioral and social sciences* (pp. 127–40). New York: Praeger.
63. Perrow, C. (1984). *Normal accidents: living with high-risk technologies*. New York: Basic Books.
64. Rambo, W. W. (1982). *Work and organizational behavior*. New York: Holt, Rinehart & Winston.
65. Roethlisberger, F. J., & Dickson, W. J. (1939). *Management and the worker*. Cambridge, MA: Harvard University Press.
66. Rom, W. N. (1983). The discipline of environmental and occupational medicine. In W. N. Rom (ed.). *Environmental and occupational medicine* (pp. 3–6). Boston: Little, Brown.
67. Ruchlin, H. S., Melcher, M. A., & Alderman,

M. H. (1984). A comparative economic analysis of work-related hypertension programs. *Journal of Occupational Medicine, 26*, 45–49.
68. Schneider, B. (1984). In A. P. Brief (ed.). *Productivity research in the behavioral and social sciences* (pp. 174–206). New York: Praeger.
69. Sexton, K., & Perlin, S. A. (1990). The federal environmental health workforce in the United States. *American Journal of Public Health, 80*, 913–20.
70. Slovic, P. (1987). Perception of risk. *Science, 236*, 280–5.
71. Sutermeister, R. A. (1976). *People and productivity*. New York: McGraw-Hill.
72. Taylor, S. E. (1986). *Health psychology*. New York: Random House.
73. Thomas, A., & Brief, A. P. (1984). Unexplored issues in productivity research. In A. P. Brief (ed.). *Productivity research in the behavioral and social sciences* (pp. 285–301). New York: Praeger.
74. Toffler, A. (1980). *The third wave*. New York: Bantam Books.
75. Toffler, A. (1985). *The adaptive corporation*. New York: McGraw-Hill.
76. U.S. Congress, Office of Technology Assessment (December 1985). *Automation of America's offices* (OTA-CIT-287). Washington, DC: U.S. Government Printing Office.
77. U.S. Surgeon General. (1979). *Smoking and health*. DHEW(PHS) Pub. No. 79-50066. Washington, DC: Government Printing Office.
78. Walsh, E. J. (1987). Challenging official risk assessments via protest mobilization: the TMI case. In B. B. Johnson & V. T. Covello (eds.). *The social and cultural construction of risk* (pp. 85–101). Dordrecht: D. Reidel.
79. Zedeck, S., & Mosier, K. L. (1990). Work in the family and employing organization. *American Psychologist, 45*, 240–51.

2
Historical Perspective on Work, Health, and Productivity

Jacqueline K. Corn

The need for constantly rising levels of productivity has become a common premise in contemporary American social thought. Douglas C. North articulated this pervasive idea about the importance of ever-increasing production during the mid-1960s. He wrote, "The reason for the economic historian's concern with the overall growth of society should be apparent. How well-off people can be within a society depends on how much that society produces in the way of goods and services" (13). In a footnote to this statement North elaborated further: "The importance of increasing productive capacity cannot be overemphasized. Redistributing income or eliminating depressions would result in less gain for the poor or the whole society than they would derive from an even relatively short period of sustained economic growth" (13).

Although increased productivity has never been a panacea, the "cult of productivity" has led to exploration of the relation of productivity to technological complexities, management prerogatives, welfare, the extent of worker control, and other variables by labor, economic, and social historians. The variable neglected by historians has been health. Indeed, the impact of health on productivity and the reverse side of the coin, the impact of productivity on health, are just beginning to emerge as areas of history to be explored. Perhaps this phenomenon is best explained by the fact that historians have only recently begun to focus on the health of workers as an issue central to understanding the relation between industrial and social organization in America.

The primary objective of this chapter is to present a historical perspective on health, work, and productivity to further our current understanding of the relationship between health and productivity in the workplace. The chapter consists of two case studies. The first illustrates the perception of the relationship between worker health and productivity reflected in federal policy toward worker health and safety that existed during World War II. The second case study focuses on the Occupational Safety and Health Administration (OSHA) standard for vinyl chloride promulgated in 1974 and its resulting impact on both health and productivity.

Each study illustrates a different aspect of the relation between the health of workers and productivity. They both raise interesting questions about response to workplace hazards, how we assessed risk in the past, the hidden costs or benefits of new technologies, the relation between knowledge and action, and how we set priorities for the health and safety of working women and men in the United States. History suggests some troubling lessons.

WORLD WAR II

There is no more startling affirmation of the relation between health and productivity than the experience during World War II when federal policy for worker health and safety was based on the need for increased productive capacity. Desire to increase production took precedence over public health arguments to create a safe and healthy workplace.

Prior to World War II the United States, ill-equipped to fight, no less to win a war, urgently needed to develop war industries and production in order to equip its own armed forces and to assist other allied nations. In 1940 Congress had voted large sums of money to build a two-ocean navy as well as thousands of planes and equipment for an immense army. Lend-lease allowed the United States to make its shipyards available for the repair and reconditioning of ships of any nation whose defense the President deemed vital to the defense of the United States. The war had created a huge demand for increased production. The shipbuilding and repair industry, for example, faced the task of building and repairing ships faster than they were being lost at sea.

The U.S. Navy and Maritime Commission comprised one of the largest industrial employers in America. For example, from 1939 to 1945 approximately 5,777 ships were built. Ship construction consumed 25 million tons of carbon steel and engaged the labor of 1,750,000 workers at the peak of employment in 1943 (8). Shipbuilding represented only one segment of the growing industrial capacity of the United States.

Along with the demand for increased production, unprecedented in American history, came problems of shortages of both materials and qualified workers. The labor force, both men and women, needed to be kept productive. It seemed to follow that in order to keep workers productive they must be kept as safe and healthy as possible. The major, overwhelming, and all-consuming priority was to win the war.

All emphasis and activities directed toward ensuring safety and health in the shipyards and defense industries arose from the need to increase production and to remove all possibilities of slowing down the flow of tanks, ships, guns, planes, and ammunition. The wartime slogans "keep 'em flying," "keep 'em sailing," "keep 'em rolling" tell the story succinctly.

Thus industrial safety became a major wartime issue. Startling figures attest to this fact. Industrial casualties from Pearl Harbor to January 1, 1944 (two years) included 37,600 workers killed—7,500 more than the military dead. There were 210,000 permanently disabled and 4,500,000 temporarily disabled, 60 times more than the military wounded and missing. According to the Office of Labor Production, War Production Board, accidents caused approximately ten times as many lost man-hours as strikes; deaths and injuries occurred on the job at a rate of 270 million lost man-days a year. Estimates of losses sustained by labor, management, and the war effort because of diseases and illness placed figures at 400 million man-days lost, with an associated financial loss of $2 billion (12).

Because hazards to the health and safety of workers were considered to be among the chief causes of low labor productivity, the Office of Labor Production suggested improvement of unsanitary and unsafe conditions. The War Production Board established the Industrial Health and Safety Section in the Office of Labor Production to take appropriate action on behalf of the War Production Board. It is difficult to find evidence of a positive impact made by this organization on the health and safety of working men and women. They did collect safety statistics. The rhetoric was clear; it stated the health and safety policy and the reasoning behind the policy.

> The interest of the War Production Board in industrial hygiene is very real and vital. The War Production Board must have production. Industrial hygiene and preventive medicine are making a significant contribution in facilitating production by maintaining the health of workers. Each and every worker is increasing in value to our nation every day the war continues. Military success will come only if we win the battle of production. The War Production Board and the industrial hygienist are naturally drawn together by their mutual interest in a speedy victory and the welfare of the worker in industry [12, p. 34].

The priorities were also clear. In 1942 Surgeon General Thomas Parran addressed the National Conference of Governmental Industrial Hygienists (now the American Conference) at their annual meeting. He stated the prevailing rationale for a health and safety program.

> We must look ahead to the prodigious task which still lies in front of us. . . . You know much better than I the impact upon industrial health of the tremendously accelerated pace of production, the introduction of untrained workers, the longer hours, and in the future perhaps the rationing of foods. These factors make it important that every effort be made to conserve the health of the working population in this country [11, p. 3].

At the same meeting the chairman of the National Committee for the Conservation of Manpower in War Industries stated the following.

> Two years ago the Secretary of Labor, recalling vividly the industrial accident toll during the last world war, formulated this committee to develop a nationwide drive to stop manpower wastage through work accidents and injuries. May I point out here that the national safety program was from the beginning, and still is, directed solely to the objective of increasing production—not to the saving of compensation costs or even to the much more important prevention of human suffering and social distress. In other words, in advancing this program we do not ask management and labor to look upon the work injuries in terms of pain or money cost, but rather in terms of production loss and delayed delivery of urgently needed war supplies. If this seems a brutal approach, we have only to remember that individual suffering and money loss are of minor consideration in total warfare [11, p. 24].

The U.S. Navy and the Maritime Commission also set priorities and defined policy regarding health and safety in shipyards. Shipbuilding was one of the most important items in the war economy. In 1942 and 1943 German submarines took a heavy toll of allied shipping. During a 15-month period losses to submarines, air attacks, and marine casualties were close to 10 million tons. Ship production did not begin to replace the losses until the end of 1942. The task of building ships faster than the enemy could sink them continued throughout the war.

Faced with shortages of labor, the Navy and the Maritime Commission had to define and carry out a plan to keep workers safe, healthy, and productive. The immense increase in the number of ships being built and repaired and the expansion of the workforce served to make existing health and safety problems worse. The Navy and Maritime Commission were well aware of these issues. Their problem was one of how to initiate a workable and realistic safety and health program during a period of crisis and then what priority to give to developing and implementing that program.

The workforce continued to grow, and the accident situation in shipyards attracted much attention. (Accidents are more easily understood than health hazards.) Pressed by the need to maintain full operating forces to achieve maximum production, the Navy in cooperation with the Maritime Commission sponsored a joint project to survey the shipbuilding industry from the standpoint of accident prevention and control of industrial diseases. The Maritime Commission hired two consultants: Philip Drinker, a professor of industrial hygiene at Harvard University, was to make health surveys of the shipyards, and John Roche, an industrial safety engineer from the National Safety Council, was to survey accidents. Drinker and Roche completed their respective reports and made a series of recommendations based on their surveys.

Both men had found numerous safety and health hazards and an appalling lack of knowledge in shipyards about how to protect workers from accidents and illnesses associated with shipbuilding. The surveys revealed that accident and health problems were worse than originally thought (5). Both men recommended the writing of minimum standards for safety and health in the shipyards and proposed a two-day conference at the joint invitation of Secretary of the Navy Knox and head of the Maritime Commission Admiral Land. The purpose of the conference would be to discuss and then adopt the proposed standards. After the conference adopted them, the standards would be promulgated by the Navy and the Maritime Commission and a joint organization set up for advice and assistance and to ensure compliance with the standards, which would operate under the administrative direction of the Maritime Commission. The scheduled conference became the vehicle to establish the policy of the U.S. Navy and the Maritime Commission on occupational health and safety in the shipyards. The plan of action set in motion during late 1942 was based on a clear set of priorities. The minutes of the December 7–8 conference reveal that the number one priority was efficient building and repairing of ships (21).

Control of health and safety problems was a means to increase production. Daniel Ring, U.S. Maritime Commission, Director of Shipyard Labor Relations, made this statement when he presided over the first session on December 7. He said that the purpose of the meeting was to promote ". . . standardized programs to develop at least minimum requirements for the two, safety and health, for the million people who will be in the shipyards after the first of the year. We are building the ships to take the ammunition and supplies to the manpower of the nation, and it has been restricted and reduced in such a way that we must make sure that the farthest possible use must be made of every one of us who are able to work on the homefront." He said that the conference was dedicated to "promoting the greatest individual efficiency in shipyards throughout the country. Our objective is based upon production because everything is subsidiary to that" (21, p. 7).

At the conclusion of the conference the delegates recommended adoption of a set of minimum requirements for safety and industrial health in contract shipyards. The Navy and the Maritime Commission promulgated the agreed-on requirements immediately after the meeting (10). It was not clear what mechanisms would be utilized to enforce the requirements or if enforcement was ever intended. Indeed before, during, and after the conference the two terms "standards" and "requirements" were used as synonyms. "Standards" implies enforcement; "requirements" does not.

The document entitled "Minimum Requirements for Safety and Industrial Health in Contract Shipyards," signed by both Knox and Land, stated policy and priorities in the following manner.

> The necessity for conserving manpower and promoting physical welfare, health and safety of what shortly will amount to one million workers in shipyards requires that careful observance of standards for the prevention of accidents and protection of health be accorded. Aside from the weight which must be given humanitarian considerations, it is simply good common sense that as much care and attention be given to protecting the human factors in the war production program as is given machines [10, p. 1].

The requirements remained in effect from early 1943 to October 1945. According to Drinker, they served only as a guide and completely lacked enforcement provisions (6). It is difficult to know the extent of impact, if any, of the unenforceable, short-lived requirements on health and safety and productivity between 1943 and 1945.

The problems of scarce resources, including the workforce, at a time when it was imperative to increase production, had a tremendous impact on health and safety decisions during World War II. The problem was that action was not always taken, even though decisions were made. Nevertheless, a profusion of problems arose from the need to increase production and the concurrent growth of a labor force composed of large numbers of workers, many of them inexperienced and laboring in hazardous industries. Response to workplace health and safety hazards during World War II was based almost entirely on a need to produce. The health and safety "requirements" never became institutionalized. Furthermore, during the war there was lack of enforcement, little concordance between those charged with production and those charged with health, and an appalling lack of communication between the two. It made health and safety policy during World War II a paper sham.

VINYL CHLORIDE

The second case study focuses on the OSHA workplace standard for vinyl chloride promulgated in 1974 and its effect on the production of vinyl chloride as well as on the health of vinyl chloride workers. Vinyl chloride, an important component of a significant industry, represents one of many chemicals once considered safe but now known to cause cancer and other chronic illnesses.

After World War II vinyl chloride production levels rose rapidly, increasing from 45 million kilograms in 1943 to 2.4 billion kilograms in 1973. At that time 17 plants employing approximately 940 workers produced vinyl chloride. Forty plants produced polyvinyl chloride and employed approximately 5,600 workers (7). The greatest potential for harmful exposures occurs when vinyl chloride is polymerized to form polyvinyl chloride resins. The principal use of vinyl chloride is for the production of polyvinyl chloride, which in turn is utilized to manufacture a wide variety of plastic materials.

Human cancer was not associated with vinyl chloride before the 1970s, but other hazardous characteristics of the chemical were known. Its explosive and highly flammable nature could cause explosion or fire. During the 1940s vinyl chloride gas was utilized for medical anesthesia, but its use was quickly abandoned because it caused cardiac arrhythmias. From 1960 through 1963 scientific reports documented anesthetic effects in animals and humans as well as liver injuries in animals from chronic exposure. In 1962 Patty discussed the toxicity of vinyl chloride and summarized its accepted and then known adverse effects.

> Vinyl chloride appears to be a material of extremely low toxicity. The principal response seems to be one of central nervous system depression, which may result in symptoms of dizziness and disorientation that are somewhat similar to the response from ethyl chloride exposure. There is a possibility of some lung irritation occurring from chronic exposure as some edema is observed in acute vapor exposure. Most investigators do not observe kidney or liver damage. One group of authors indicated some hyperemia of the liver and kidneys from acute exposure. It is concluded that the material has essentially a narcotic effect, with some lung irritation and a possibility of organ injury. There has been quite extensive use of this material in the chemical industry but no clinical reports of injury [18].

During the 1960s a new clinical entity associated with vinyl chloride exposure appeared among workers engaged in the process of its polymerization to polyvinyl chloride. The disease, acroosteolysis, included symptoms of tenderness of the fingertips sometimes accompanied by gradual destruction of the bony integrity of the fingers. Workers with this condition exhibited a form of vascular disease known as Renaud's phenomenon. During the 1970s evidence of liver disease appeared among vinyl chloride workers. Effects of exposure to this substance were lumped together and labeled "vinyl chloride disease." Viola and colleagues first associated neoplasia with vinyl chloride in 1971 and reported malignant changes, including angiosarcoma, in animals (22). The American Conference of Governmental Industrial Hygienists had earlier adopted a threshold limit value (TLV) of 500 parts per million for vinyl chloride based on its acute liver toxicity (1). This TLV was adopted by OSHA in 1971 as a start-up standard.

In 1974 the B. F. Goodrich Company, a manufacturer of polyvinyl chloride, notified its employees, the National Institute for Occupational Safety and Health (NIOSH), and the Kentucky Department of Labor that three workers had died of angiosarcoma of the liver, a rare and incurable cancer. Because all three workers had been employed in the manufacture of polyvinyl chloride resins the suspicion arose that vinyl chloride caused angiosarcoma and that the disease was occupationally related. Angiosarcoma of the liver is one of the rarest human malignant neoplasms, with previous known incidence in the United States of only approximately 21 cases a year (9). The tumors appeared in Louisville workers 14 to 27 years from the onset of their exposure. This long latent period meant that past uncontrolled exposures would be reflected in tumors in decades to follow. After B. F. Goodrich disclosed its cases of angiosarcoma other companies also reported deaths from angiosarcoma among vinyl chloride and polyvinyl chloride workers. The growing number of known cases led to fear that it was only the tip of the iceberg. NIOSH began to develop a recommended occupational health standard, and on February 15, 1974 OSHA held an Informal Fact Finding Hearing on Possible Hazards of Vinyl Chloride Manufacture and Use to determine if the situation warranted an emergency standard.

On April 5, 1974, OSHA promulgated an Emergency Temporary Standard that reduced the permissible exposure level from 500 ppm to 50 ppm (17). The agency also established other temporary requirements such as workplace monitoring, use of air-supplied respirators if the new ceiling is exceeded, and impervious suits in some instances. OSHA based ceiling reductions on the findings of Maltoni, whose studies showed induction of angiosarcoma of the liver and other organs and the production of other cancers in rats exposed to vinyl chloride. His research confirmed vinyl chloride as a carcinogen and further confirmed its role in inducing the cancers observed in B. F. Goodrich workers (15).

In response to the vinyl chloride crisis a workshop entitled "Toxicity of Vinyl Chloride-Polyvinyl Chloride," sponsored by the New York Academy of Sciences, the American Cancer Society, the National Institute of Environmental Health Sciences, the National Institute for Occupational Safety and Health, and the Society of Occupational and Environmental Health, convened a large international working group of scientists to disseminate information on the toxicity and carcinogenicity of vinyl chloride. They presented information linking vinyl chloride to angiosarcoma and a variety of other diseases and tumors in sites other than the liver (19).

NIOSH began a major epidemiological study of vinyl chloride workers. The Manufacturing Chemists Association also sponsored a study. Meanwhile, the number of confirmed deaths due to angiosarcoma among vinyl chloride workers grew.

On the basis of evidence presented at the February 1974 hearings, the demonstrated evidence of the carcinogenicity of vinyl chloride in animal studies, and epidemiological studies, OSHA proposed a permanent standard of "no detectable level" on May 18, 1974. OSHA set the hearing dates for June and July, allowing a period of 30 days for public comment.

Records of the 8 days of hearings include pre- and posthearing comments, testimony at the fact-finding and rule-making hearings, records of OSHA inspections, an environmental impact statement, and economic and technical impact studies. OSHA received more than 600 written comments and more than 200 oral and written submissions. The record exceeds 4,000 pages. Employers, employees, labor unions, public affairs groups, physicians, and scientists submitted information and testified at the long and acrimonious hearings. The clearly adversarial relationship between labor and industry led each side to take opposing positions on the following key issues: Was the standard supported by medical evidence? Was the proposed standard technologically and economically feasible? In other words, the issues were clearly related to both health and productivity.

No one questioned the carcinogenicity of vinyl chloride; but representatives of industry believed that evidence did not support the "no detectable" level or 1 ppm exposure ceiling proposed by OSHA. The Society of the Plastics Industry (SPI) maintained that data did not exist to prove that the exposure provided under the Emergency Temporary Standard (50 ppm) was unsafe. Spokesmen from industry also pointed out that conclusions about human sensitivity to vinyl chloride could not be drawn from animal tests. They suggested the existence of a threshold for human carcinogenesis (16).

In contrast, cancer specialists from universities, the National Cancer Institute, and NIOSH and persons appearing for unions and public interest groups said that safe doses of carcinogens could not be scientifically determined. Experts testified that quantification of a safe concentration was not possible with the present state of scientific knowledge.

Representatives from industry testified that the permanent standard was not technologically feasible and would shut down the plastics industry if adopted (3). SPI estimated that a shutdown would result in the loss of 1.7 million to 2.2 million jobs and loss of production valued at $65 million to $90 million annually (14). SPI recommended less stringent standards.

Labor unions and the Health Research Group suggested that levels below 1 ppm were attainable and that means existed, or could be found, to maintain exposure below 1 ppm. Labor accused industry of attempting to blackmail OSHA into setting a lenient standard by exaggerating the difficulty and the cost of compliance and by predicting economic disaster and dislocation (2).

On October 4, 1974 OSHA promulgated the Permanent Standard for Vinyl Chloride. It accepted the principle of 1 ppm as the maximum possible exposure.

Representatives of the plastics and chemical industries had argued that if OSHA issued a permanent standard for vinyl chloride of 1 ppm the entire polyvinyl chloride industry would shut down. Instead, some of the control technology developed to reduce worker exposures to within allowable limits also cut costs and increased productivity by reducing worker exposures, improving product quality, reducing the time for cleaning the reactor vessels, and combining previously separate processes. The new production techniques were also sold to other companies. For example, B. F. Goodrich licensed its processes to other chemical manufacturers (20). By the time the standard became effective, major companies admitted that they could operate without curtailing production. Threatened shutdowns did not occur; and as mentioned above, major vinyl chloride producers licensed a variety of emission control devices. Industry's forecast of curtailment of production and economic ruin did not occur.

By 1979 vinyl chloride production capacity increased by 41% and polyvinyl chloride capacity by 85% over 1974 levels. Expansion of the vinyl chloride and polyvinyl chloride industry since 1974 has created an estimated 2,000 jobs, offsetting the job losses estimated by spokesmen for the chemical and plastics industries. During the years immediately after issuance of the standard, the growth rate for the vinyl chloride industry was above average for U.S. industry, and profits increased (20, p. 231).

It is not possible to judge the long-term health effects of the vinyl chloride standard using any measures of impact because of the long latent period of carcinogenic action, but a discussion of effects can be based on surrogate measures of effectiveness. When reviewing the accomplishments of OSHA, Corn and Corn used compliance efforts and reduction of exposure levels of employers exposed to carcinogens on the job as surrogate measures (4). In the case of vinyl chloride in 1973, exposure varied from 50 to 500 ppm. After OSHA promulgated its permanent standard for a Permissible Exposure Limit of 1 ppm in 1974, employees in the vinyl chloride industry could be considered to have experienced a subsequent exposure reduction of 98%. This reduction in exposure can be considered a measure of cancer reduction because the dose/response curves for carcinogens are assumed to be linear and to extend to zero in the absence of a threshold for the effect.

Thus the facts proved to be contrary to private sector manufacturing projections. It proved possible to have health and safety standards that protect working people and at the same time increase productivity.

CONCLUSIONS

These two case studies, although focusing on different aspects and outcomes of the relation between work, health, and productivity, were intended to illustrate the historical role of productivity in decision making to control occupational hazards. In the past, the two basic premises underlying control of occupational hazards were that (a) risks to health and safety could be alleviated by protective measures and (b) productivity and health were somehow linked. The first premise is a public health assumption that justifies intervention for control of health risks on the job. It has received much attention and more often than not has been the rationale for control. The second premise, the linkage between productivity and health, has received much less attention. Although it exists, it has been underestimated and neglected as an important factor in decisions to control occupational hazards.

The role of productivity in decision making to control occupational hazards reflects, in both cases, the social dimension of occupational safety and health policy. Action taken toward alleviating workplace hazards depended in part on technological and scientific factors. It was also directly related to how society perceived its problems and its social values.

There is no more dramatic illustration of the perception of the impact of health on productivity than the activity that occurred during World War II. The belief that keeping workers safe and healthy would lead to higher production levels, coupled with the necessity to increase production in order to win the war, led to activities, albeit limited and often unsuccessful, designed to bring about a safer, healthier workplace. The rationale that in order to maintain a productive workforce the worker must be kept as safe and healthy as possible was a reaction to the crisis of war. The policy did not continue after the war. It was shallow and based on expediency.

Given the historical context, i.e., the desire to win the war, the response to workplace health and safety hazards during World War II is easily understood. However, a policy based on crisis, cursory risk assessment, and limited social commitment could not and did not last after the war. We know now that a lasting policy leading to worker health and safety was not the outcome of the hectic, ad hoc, wartime health and safety activities. If there is a lesson here, it is that public health policy based mainly on expediency is short-lived.

In the second case productivity played a different role in the decision making process. Ideas about productivity presented at the hearings for a vinyl chloride standard reflected social values and perceptions of those involved, on each side, during the standard setting procedure. Decision making for regulating chemicals in the workplace has been evolving since the 1970s. There were two key questions associated with the vinyl chloride workplace standard: Could the proposed standard be supported by scientific evidence? Was the proposed standard technologically and economically feasible? The answers to these questions are still evolving.

Nevertheless, vinyl chloride is a success story. Compliance with the standard for health protection in a major United States industry led to preservation of health by eliminating hazards while increasing productivity. Other instances also can be cited where compliance with a health standard led to modernization of an industry and increased productivity. The cotton industry, where new technology and new production equipment increased productivity and reduced harmful exposures, is one (20, p. 99).

The case of vinyl chloride provides serious erosion to the pessimistic position that health and safety standards are a deterrent to productivity or have a negative impact on productivity. In the case of vinyl chloride, the private sector did not do its homework and miscalculated the effects of a significantly lowered standard on the industry. A repercussion of this miscalculation is that economic feasibility became one of the most difficult issues to resolve in future OSHA standards proceedings.

If history is prologue, the common denominator in both cases—the effect of health on productivity—should not be overlooked. One way or another, productivity was a factor in the decision to protect men and women at work. What is interesting about the two cited cases is that productivity was used as a rationale in one case to attempt to keep health and safety standards less effective; and in the other, increased productivity was the rationale to set requirements for health and safety in defense plants. During the standard-setting hearings for vinyl chloride, it was stated that lowering the standard for vinyl chloride might reduce cases of angiosarcoma but it would also close down the industry. That prediction was not fulfilled. The industry continued to grow despite the lower standard. On the other hand, during World War II productivity assumed a positive role, but actions taken were not lasting or institutionalized.

The most that can be said, although it cannot be stressed too much, is that health and safety decisions depend as much on the social setting as on technological and scientific factors. Another lesson, perhaps the most important one, has been learned: Health and safety standards need not adversely affect productivity. In fact, they can and often do have a positive impact on productivity.

REFERENCES

1. American Conference of Governmental Industrial Hygienists. (1962). *Documentation of threshold limit values*, Cincinnati.
2. *Business Week, 30* (2336) June 22, 1974.
3. *Chemical and Engineering News, 53*, 26. July 1, 1974.
4. Corn, J. K., & Corn, M. (1984). The history and accomplishments of the occupational safety and health administration in reducing cancer risks. In P. F. Deisler (ed.). *Reducing the carcinogenic risks in industry* (pp. 175–95). New York: Marcel Dekker.
5. Drinker, P. (1942). Talk before The Maritime Commission. October 20, 1942. Health and Safety, Shipyard Labor Relations, Record Group 178. Washington, DC: National Archives.
6. Drinker, P. (1943). The health and safety program of the United States Maritime Commission. *Journal of the American Medical Association, 121*, 822–3.
7. Environmental Protection Agency. Office of Research and Development. (1975). *Scientific and technical assessment report on vinyl chloride and polyvinyl chloride* (600/6-75-004, p. 3). Washington, DC: U.S. Government Printing Office.
8. Lane, F. (1951). *Ships for victory* (p. 6). Baltimore: Johns Hopkins Press.
9. Makk, L., Creech, J., Whalen, J., & Johnson, M. (1974). Liver damage and angiosarcoma in vinyl chloride workers: a systematic detection program. *Journal of the American Medical Association, 230*, 64–8.
10. *Minimum requirements for safety and health in contract shipyards*. (1943). Washington, DC: National Archives, U.S. Government Printing Office.
11. National Conference of Governmental Industrial Hygienists. (1942). *Transactions of the fifth annual meeting*, Washington, DC.
12. National Conference of Governmental Industrial Hygienists. (1944). *Transactions of the seventh annual meeting*, St. Louis.
13. North, D. C. (1966). *Growth and welfare in the American past* (p. 3). Englewood Cliffs, NJ: Prentice Hall.
14. Occupational Safety and Health Administration. (1974). Hearings on proposed standard for vinyl chloride. Exhibit 2Z (F). Statement of V. P. Ficcaglia, Manager of Economic Analysis and Forecasting. Cambridge, MA: Arthur D. Little.
15. Occupational Safety and Health Administration. (1974). Hearings on proposed standard for vinyl chloride. Exhibit 7 (hh). Preprint of ICS Series 322. Maltoni: Occupational carcinogensis.

16. Occupational Safety and Health Administration. (1974). Hearings on proposed standard for vinyl chloride. Exhibit 20D. Statement of A. Vittone, President, B. F. Goodrich Company.
17. Occupational Safety and Health Administration. (1974). New standard for vinyl chloride. In *Job safety and health*. U.S. Department of Labor.
18. Patty, F. A. (1962). *Industrial hygiene and toxicology* (2nd ed., Vol. II, pp. 1303–4). New York: Wiley.
19. Selikoff, I., & Cuyler, H. E. (eds.). (1975). Toxicity of vinyl chloride polyvinyl chloride. *Annals of the New York Academy of Sciences 246*.

20. United States Congress, Office of Technology Assessment. (1986). *Preventing injury and illness in the workplace* (OTA-H-256, p. 81). Washington, DC: U.S. Government Printing Office.
21. United States Maritime Commission. (1942). Stenographer's minutes before meeting in regard to *Minimum Requirements for Industrial Health and Safety*. December 7–8, 1942. Chicago: U.S. Department of Transportation, Maritime Administration.
22. Viola, P. L., Bigotti, A., & Caputo, A. (1971). Oncogenic response of rat skin lungs and bones to vinyl chloride. *Cancer Research, 31*, 516–19.

II

INDUSTRIAL ENVIRONMENT REGARDING HEALTH AND PRODUCTIVITY

A productive industrial society generates such a quantity and diversity of chemical and physical agents and hazardous conditions that it is intrinsically hazardous to health unless extraordinary efforts are made to control the exposures. During the course of this century, the industrialized societies have evolved systems to mitigate these hazards through the regulation of levels of emission according to exposure standards ideally derived from sound scientific data on dose-response relations. The risk to health of exposure to a hazardous substance or condition depends on the toxic properties of the agent, the duration (time) of exposure, and the level (concentration) of the agent or condition. These exposure factors, when corrected for the amount of the agent that fails to penetrate the target tissue because of barriers to penetration (e.g., skin), detoxification (or intoxification) by metabolism, and excretion before reaching the target tissue, constitute the dose of the agent available to produce an untoward effect.

People vary greatly in terms of the biological properties that determine dose and their vulnerability to a biologically toxic effect. Standards derived from data on observed dose-response relations in humans or in animals must allow for this wide range in biological variability and protect the more sensitive, or susceptible, members of the working population. Standards are ideally derived to reduce health effects below a socially acceptable proportion of the exposed population, e.g., one in a thousand, one in ten thousand, or one in a million chances of the untoward effect (e.g., mortality, cancer) over the lifetime of the workers.

Regulations protective of human safety and health to prevent illness require costly measures that may decrease the profitability of the business. An argument that has been advanced is that decreased injury and illness enhances the productivity of the employee and recoups at least some, all, or more than all of the employer's expenses incurred for establishing safety procedures by increasing the productivity of the worker and decreasing medical care and compensation costs. Although these measures may reduce absenteeism due to illness, which is costly to employers, it is not at all clear that they increase productivity in terms of the amount of work turned out by each working employee.

These issues are addressed in Part II. Emmett describes the physical/chemical agents released at the workplace and the workplace factors that lead to injury. The social value framework underlying the regulatory standards for physical/chemical agents is addressed by Morton Corn, as these values drive the relative stringency of environmental standards in different industries and societies. The extent to which societies differ in these values can influence their competitive status in the world economy as well as among companies in the same industry. A further advantage or disadvantage may accrue to the worker, employer, or industry based on factors of susceptibility to a given set of working conditions. What some of these susceptibility factors are and how they can be measured are addressed in the chapters by Evans et al. and Matanoski, who are primarily concerned with host factors of susceptibility that lower the range of acceptable exposure conditions and the means of measuring these factors. That injury can be prevented in the workplace is addressed by Baker and colleagues. Finally, Chaffin presents a systematic approach to the evaluation and prospective reduction of physical hazard to minimize the cost of injury and disability induced by overexertion and impact trauma in industry.

The many issues presented in these chapters are held together by three major themes. The first theme is the distinction between health as the absence of illness and health as a condition of maximal psychological, behavioral, and physical well-being. Not only are these concepts of health different conceptually and philosophically, but they may bear a different relation to productivity. The distinction is important as we explore the relation between health and productivity, the impact of different sets of working conditions on one aspect or the other of health, and the different emphasis that may be placed on these aspects as the nature of the workplace changes in the postindustrial economy. For example, the excess health-related costs in the workplace may be attributed to the direct or indirect costs of worker absenteeism, which in turn may be attributed more to job satisfaction than to worker illness. Because this definition of health is the absence of illness, this view attributes a lesser role of health for productivity. However, with the definition of health as a positive mental and physical state of well-being, even this model points to a potentially important relation between maximal health, including mental state, and productivity.

Emmett goes further in stating that productivity reflects good or impaired health of the workforce, a position supported by J. Corn in her two historical examples in the Introduction. To the extent that productivity reflects good or impaired health, it might itself be analyzed to assess health, especially if other contributors to impaired productivity can be simultaneously quantified. Emmett is emphatic regarding the distinction between optimal health and simply the absence of disease; mere absence of disease plays a relatively small role in productivity. Emmett gives several illustrations of how reduction in health without the presence of disease may impair the productivity of the workforce. His evidence suggests that optimal health may contribute to productivity, whereas the absence of disease may simply be a reduction in expense because it does not add the measure of health that contributes to productivity. It seems likely that most industry measures medical cost that reflects the absence of disease rather than its cost for health, which may reduce disease and contribute to productivity. Chapter 17, by Fielding, is a notable exception, but even he does not link health promotion to productive capacity.

The importance of these issues in economic terms and in industrial practice is illustrated by M. Corn in his explication of the Hatch diagram, which graphically illustrates the dependence of standards on social values and the importance of proving the linkage between health and productivity in gaining societal support for standards that enhance health, not merely prevent disease. If it should turn out that there is a positive relation between optimal health and productivity—and not between absence of disease and productivity—business values and societal values might come closer to agreement on the standards of exposure that serve the interests not only of improving health but also of maximizing productivity. Perhaps secondary standards of "minimal desirable concentration" in addition to the current threshold limit values could project the goal of optimal health while a maximum allowable concentration projects the goal of disease prevention.

A second major theme in this section on industrial environment and health and productivity relates to the relative obligations of the individual worker versus the employer versus society in managing the issues stemming from variations in susceptibility to workplace hazards and conditions. In Chapter 5 Evans examines a range of genetic, behavioral, and environmental factors that might influence the responsiveness of individual workers to a set of agents or conditions but that might elicit no response from most. Matanoski explores the epidemiological and toxicological tools of health surveillance that can be used to identify both the susceptibility and the early exposure and response of the worker.

Finally, a third major theme adds the variable of workplace heterogeneity to the equation and presages the transition to Part III of this volume (Changes in the Workplace: Results of the Postindustrial Revolution). In the Foreword, Dunlop stressed the importance of workplace heterogeneity in social as well as physical terms. Emmett, Baker et al., and Chaffin each emphasize the importance of the workplace in the relation between health and productivity and emphasize the heterogeneity of the workplace in terms of the differences in hazardous conditions that pertain as well as the differences in resources available to mitigate those hazards. Emmett points out that the occupational safety and health resources available in industry are determined by the size of the industry rather than by the relative hazard, with the large workplaces being relatively less hazardous and better equipped and the small workplaces more hazardous and less well equipped. Baker and colleagues emphasize the excess risk of small industries as a major remaining problem for health, as there are fewer financial resources for engineering interventions in small industries, raising the question of whether a different strategy is required for effective control in the small industries. These authors clearly emphasize the strategy of prevention and control through environmental engineering, which is appropriate for the large industries that have those resources in place but leaves small industries inadequately protected.

Workplaces are heterogeneous as to size, extent of industrial technology, age, intrinsic hazards, and differences in capital versus labor intensivity among other conditions. When assessing workplace hazards and their relation to health and productivity, there is a question of the appropriateness of using the same yardstick for vastly different employment conditions. Is it not far more likely that no single strategy will suffice and that distinct generic differences must be characterized and quantified with the strategies for control and for maximizing health and productivity tailored to the specifics of that particular workplace? Finally, as addressed in Part III, what are the implications for these considerations in a workplace environment that is vastly changed as a result of the postindustrial revolution where psychosocial hazards may far outweigh chemical and physical hazards in terms of their impact on health and on the productive capacity of the workforce?

3
Physical and Chemical Agents at the Workplace

Edward A. Emmett

Physical and chemical agents comprise two of the several categories of workplace factors that may influence health and productivity (Table 3–1). Although there is some overlap among these factors this chapter concentrates on chemical and physical exposures. Physical exposure may be of several types. This chapter deals with exposure to physical stressors, e.g., ionizing and nonionizing radiation, sound, vibration, temperature, and pressure; overt physical trauma resulting in accidental injury and death is covered elsewhere (see Chapter 8). Repetitive trauma and occupational overuse syndromes are generally regarded as ergonomic factors, as they involve job design.

The classification of workplace factors into these major categories helps define the professional roles of the toxicologist, health physicist, environmental physiologist, safety professional, biohazard specialist, ergonomist, and psychologist, allowing each professional to bring his or her unique skills to bear on optimizing workplace conditions. However, this categorization need not obscure the larger truth in occupational health and safety: that the whole is more than the sum of the parts. This platitude has a twofold impact: First, it is clear that although factors may act alone there are interactions between factors in different categories. For example, individuals exposed to a variety of organic solvents may have impaired psychomotor central nervous system function with a lowered reaction time and presumably are therefore more likely to become accident victims as a result of decreased vigilance and speed of response (2,3). Individuals exposed to chemicals that adversely affect the immune system may be more prone to develop pathological infections from biohazardous agents they contact at work, and so on. Second, we rarely have the power in clinical and epidemiological studies or in studies using statistical databases to distinguish clearly between various work factors as causes of disease. Thus we may determine that a particular group of workers has a higher incidence or prevalence of a particular disease, but generally we are not able to distinguish between the various factors and interactions that may have contributed to the outcome. Despite this limitation, investigators often attribute an outcome to a single workplace factor.

The narrower relations between chemical and physical agents and health and productivity may be viewed within the scaffolding of Table 3–2: workplace exposures to chemical and physical agents; the dosage of these agents received by the biological

Table 3–1. Major Workplace Factors that May Influence Health

Chemical exposures
Physical exposures
    Electromagnetic radiation, sound, vibration, temperature, pressure
    Overt trauma
Biological agents
Ergonomic factors
Psychosocial factors

target; biochemical, physiological, and pathological effects of this interaction; resultant disease, injury, or disordered health; and, finally, impaired productivity. Of course, productivity might be impaired in other ways, e.g., by cumbersome controls to prevent chemical and physical exposure or from justified or unjustified fears of effects that alter employee attitudes to the work. Productivity indicators appear to be novel and potentially useful measures for the purpose of monitoring workplace factors.

WORKPLACE EXPOSURES: U.S. NATIONAL OCCUPATIONAL HAZARD SURVEY

In the United States it is often stated that some 65,000 chemicals are in use in commerce and that some 700 new chemicals are introduced each year (12). Because some chemicals are presumably potentially toxic, given the right circumstances the potential for adverse impacts on working populations must be significant.

There is a relative paucity of information, however, on the extent of worker exposure to physical and chemical agents. Perhaps the most important source of information is the first National Occupational Hazard Survey (NOHS) conducted by the National Institute for Occupational Safety and Health (NIOSH) from 1972 to 1974 (15). A second survey was conducted from 1981 to 1983, but the full results from this survey are not yet available. The NOHS is a national data-gathering effort designed to provide baseline descriptive information. The sample of businesses used in the survey consisted of approximately 5,000 urban establishments in 67 metropolitan areas throughout the United States; mining, government activities, and agricultural operations were excluded. The survey of each facility consisted of two major segments. The first segment was information obtained during a questionnaire interview of management, profiling the Standard Industrial Classification (SIC) code and size of the facility

Table 3–2. Suggested Sequence for Considering the Relation of Physical and Chemical Agents at the Workplace to Health and Productivity

Workplace exposures
Biological dosage
Biochemical, physiological, and pathological effects
Disease, injury, and impaired health
Impaired productivity

along with any of its medical, safety, and industrial hygiene programs. The second segment, the bulk of the NOHS data, contained the recorded observations of the surveyor's management-escorted "walk-through" of all facility work areas. The surveyors were trained industrial hygienists. The surveyor listed, by job title, the number of employees who were potentially exposed to the same chemical and physical agents. The surveyor recorded all materials and physical agents encountered by each employee group regardless of toxicity, hazardous nature, conditions of use, and potential exposure. The surveyor also recorded the duration (full or part time), the intensity (detectable or undetectable to the five senses), the form (e.g., liquid, gas), the control utilized (e.g., no control, local ventilation, hand gloves), and if the control functioned. The existing conditions were recorded with no evaluation of the wisdom or safety of the situation. An attempt was made to indicate occupational exposures to specific subgroups of employees by the survey visitors.

Three types of exposure were defined as a basis for recording an observation: *Potential exposures* were described as any substances for which there was an intended control other than natural or dilution ventilation. *Actual exposures* were those observed to have existed. *Inferred exposures* were based on an observable accumulation (dusts or mists), which indirectly indicated that the substances were present in the air. These three types were recorded, but not necessarily distinguished, provided they met the general duration guidelines. It is important to note that exposures were not established by actual measurement. Therefore there are no doubt inaccuracies in the survey results, although a broad picture emerged.

The survey produced many interesting results. More than 8,000 hazards, mostly chemical agents, were identified by direct observation or by implication as a component of a generic or a proprietary product (about 70% of the chemical hazards were identified by trade name rather than chemical name). Exposure to multiple hazardous agents was the rule. The total number of employees represented by the survey was estimated from 1972 and 1973 payroll data to be 38,262,000, as shown in Table 3–3.

Table 3–4 indicates the number of these employees exposed to six of the most common hazards and the number who were estimated to be working without control measures. For these purposes, control measures could be respiratory protection, personal protection other than respiratory, local ventilation, other ventilation, or other controls. The proportion of workers for which no controls were available was high. Of course from a survey of this type we cannot determine if the controls (when used) were adequate, or if they would be required by current guidelines in cases where they were not in use. We may deduce from these results, however, that both the number of

Table 3–3. Employees Represented by the First NOHS Survey as Estimated from 1972 and 1973 Payroll Data

Type of employer	Total no. of employees
Small (8–249 employees)	15,394,000
Medium (250–500 employees)	10,883,000
Large (> 500 employees)	11,985,000
Total	38,262,000

Table 3–4. Employees Represented by the Survey (N = 38,262,000) Exposed to Most Common Hazards and those Exposed Without Control Measures

Hazard	Employees exposed	% Exposed with no control measures
Ethanol	8,144,000	92
Mineral oil	6,109,000	93
Isopropanol	6,016,000	93
Toluene	4,811,000	88
Continuous noise	4,203,000	82
Trichloroethylene	3,651,000	93

individuals potentially exposed to hazardous agents and the number of hazardous agents in use were high.

Results of the survey also showed that the major determinant of the use of preventive services to assess and control hazards was plant size and not, as might be hoped, the degree of hazard. Table 3–5 shows, for the 1972–1974 survey, the percent of plants and employees in plants for whom industrial hygiene services were available. It can be seen that the proportion of plants with industrial hygiene services was low in small plants but was over 40% in larger plants. As a result, more than one-half the employees in large plants but less than 3% of those in small plants were covered by industrial hygiene services.

Table 3–6 shows those plants and employees to whom coverage from a formally established health unit, either with or without a physician in-charge, was available. Almost 80% of employees in large plants had access to a formally constituted occupational health unit but only 3% of employees in small plants. The NOHS data clearly showed that the number of workers and plants without industrial hygienic and occupational health resources—full-time, part-time, or in the form of a consultant—was disappointingly high and was the rule in small and medium-sized establishments. Although not yet fully analyzed, the data from the second NOHS during the 1980s shows that the same pattern exists and that the provision of preventive services remains related to plant size and not to the degree of hazard (13).

Table 3–5. Plants and Employees in Plants who Receive Industrial Hygiene Services (1972–1974 NOHS survey)

Parameter	%
Plants	
Small	1.5
Medium	15.3
Large	42.3
Employees in plants	
Small	2.9
Medium	18.6
Large	56.6

Table 3–6. Plants and Employees in Plants that have an
Established Health Unit with a Physician in Charge

Parameter	With physician (%)	Without physician (%)
Plants		
Small	0.8	2.3
Medium	1.3	13.6
Large	26.5	70.0
Employees in plants		
Small	1.1	3.3
Medium	1.7	18.4
Large	45.0	79.6

HEALTH AND OCCUPATION

To this point we have been considering the effects of physical and chemical agents in relation to health. It is appropriate here to consider how we define "health" in this context.

"Health" has never been perceived in the same way by all societies or at any given time in history. In a primitive society, such as that of the early Australian Aborigines, an individual was considered healthy if his relationship with members of his family and with the land were good. The ancient Greeks, according to Pericles, defined health as that state of moral, mental, and physical well-being that enables man to face any crisis in life with the utmost facility and growth. Both these definitions of health could relate to the potential of a healthy individual to be productive. Toward the end of the last century and early this century, we developed a better understanding of disease processes and were thus able to define disease entities more precisely. "Health" became more synonymous with the absence of disease, and diseases themselves were carefully classified.

Much of our present approach to occupational health is still rooted in the pathological tradition. Our aims, insofar as regulation and control of the workplace environment are concerned, are still often interpreted as the prevention of definable occupational illness and disease. This point is well illustrated by the debate engendered by the regulation of formaldehyde by the U.S. Occupational Safety and Health Administration (OSHA). The OSHA Act of 1970 provided for "safe and healthful working conditions." Formaldehyde is a substance that produces pronounced eye and nose irritation in virtually all individuals at air levels well below 1 ppm. It also is a skin allergen, produces irritant dermatitis, and may produce alterations in behavioral and psychomotor functions at levels well below 1 ppm in the air. Yet OSHA proposed that two air concentrations be considered a permissible exposure level (PEL): a PEL of 1 ppm if formaldehyde was regulated on the basis that it was a human carcinogen or a PEL of 1.5 ppm if the compound was regulated as if it were not a human carcinogen (16). Such an approach, in which endpoints other than cancer are given little emphasis and where "safe and healthful work conditions" are those that could affect both comfort and productivity, is clearly rooted in "a serious-disease prevention" approach rather than a "health and productivity" orientation.

More recently, definitions of health have taken pains to differentiate health from the mere absence of disease. Thus the World Health Organization has defined health as a state of complete physical, mental, and social well-being and not merely the absence of disease. The Organization for Economic Cooperation and Development (OECD) went further and stated that "health appears as a physical, psychological, mental and social state of tolerance and compensation outside the limits of which any situation is perceived by the individual . . . as the manifestation of a morbid state . . . as far as the individual is concerned; his opinion is the only one that counts." These definitions are global; and although they do not mention productivity directly, they certainly define a state of health that, at least in theory, permits maximum productivity.

Rigorous scientific studies in occupational health have attempted to relate specific occupational diseases to causal agents. There has been relatively little study using health as an endpoint, presumably because it is much more difficult to define and quantify. Yet productivity may well relate more to health than to the absence of disease.

EFFECTS OF EXPOSURE

Chemical and physical agents must reach an appropriate biological target to cause injury. Generally the target is an intracellular component of the body such as an enzyme, DNA, or some other biochemical target or receptor. Radiation or vibration damages directly to the extent that it penetrates the target. In the case of physical agents, the dose at the target tissue can generally be calculated from the amount of radiation reaching the surface of the body and the attenuation by overlying tissues. The situation is more complicated with chemical agents. There are three main routes of absorption in the workplace: through respired air, through skin, and oral absorption resulting from contamination of food, cigarettes, or the surfaces of the mouth and lips. We now realize that percutaneous and oral absorption are more important than previously believed. For example, we had previously considered that polychlorinated biphenyls (PCBs) had been largely absorbed through inhalation, but studies have now indicated that the major part of industrial exposure is contact with skin rather than inhalation (9), and that skin absorption is rapid (4). Furthermore, some PCB congeners are volatile, whereas others are much less so and tend therefore to accumulate on surfaces and contact skin; the latter congeners are those that predominate in human tissues (7).

The relations between the dose at the target organ and the development of disease may be complex. Chemical and physical agents may affect the structure or function of organs, resulting in changes that may be reversible or irreversible. Some damage may be repaired, and biochemical or physiological compensatory mechanisms may allow an organ to function normally despite some damage. For a number of fundamental reasons individual susceptibility may vary widely, a subject dealt with in other chapters. The specific factors that modulate the toxicity of chemicals are complex and outside the scope of this chapter; they are discussed in standard textbooks of toxicology (8).

In addition, interactions may occur between toxic chemicals that may enhance or reduce damage. The number of possible interactions is great. With more than 8,000 hazardous workplace chemicals in use, and considering interactions where only two chemicals are involved, more than 65 million combinations could theoretically be considered. Such calculations emphasize the difficulty and indeed the practical impossibility of considering all chemical interactions individually.

OCCUPATION-RELATED DISEASE

Occupational disease is a term customarily reserved for the classic illnesses of occupation, e.g., lung cancer from asbestos, pneumoconioses, and contact dermatitis. They are defined, well recognized conditions that usually have (or are considered to have) a single, identifiable predominant cause and that in turn are recognized for workers' compensation purposes in most jurisdictions. The International Labor Organization (ILO) has constructed a list of accepted occupational diseases.

Table 3–7 lists representative occupational diseases caused in whole or in part by physical or chemical agents at the workplace. Unfortunately, it is apparent that there is a poor accounting of the number of occupational diseases that occur. A study in Oregon and Washington utilized environmental surveys, a medical questionnaire, and medical examination to determine if surveyed individuals had occupational diseases. Of 1,116

Table 3–7. Representative Occupational Diseases Caused in Whole or in Part by Physical or Chemical Agents at the Workplace

Cancer of many organs
Respiratory disease
    Asthma
    Chronic obstructive pulmonary disease
    Pneumoconioses
    Interstitial lung disease
Nervous system disease
    Psychogenic brain syndromes
    Peripheral neuritis
Noise-induced hearing loss
Skin disease
    Dermatitis
    Acne
Musculoskeletal diseases
    Repetitive strain disorders
    Acute injuries
Cardiovascular disease
    Coronary heart disease
    Arrhythmias
Reproductive disorders
    Birth defects, miscarriage
    Infertility
Systemic chemical poisonings
Occupational infections
Occupational eye diseases
    Conjunctivitis and corneal injury
    Cataracts

cases of occupational disease diagnosed in this way, only 2% were recorded by the Bureau of Labor Statistics (11). It is clear that official published figures, such as those from the Bureau of Labor Statistics, are virtually useless for indicating the extent of the burden of occupational disease from chemical and physical agents; this absence of data creates a difficult position in that we cannot estimate with any reliability the incidence and prevalence of these diseases when we wish to consider their relation to productivity.

Work-related disease, a more recently introduced term, refers to the large number of illnesses or diseases that appear to be related to work because their distribution is unequal among occupational groups. To the extent that there is an excess of illness in any particular occupational group(s), the excess may be considered work-related. To illustrate this point: the differences in mortality for those with different occupations are still marked, even in developed countries. For example, McMichael (10) studied the mortality of Australian males aged 15 to 64 years during the 1970s. Unskilled or manual workers had age-standardized mortality ratios almost twice those of professionals or executives. The premature death rates for unskilled or manual workers were 1.5 times higher for cancer, 1.5 times higher for cardiovascular disease, 4.9 times higher for mental disorders, 4.9 times higher for diseases of the nervous system and sensory organs, 3.1 times higher for diseases of the respiratory system, 1.6 times higher for diseases of the genitourinary system, and 2.9 times higher for accidents. Of course, many factors may play a part in the genesis of work-related illness, only some of which may be related to occupation. In addition, the role of workplace, if any, may be direct (e.g., through exposure to hazardous chemical and physical agents) or indirect (e.g., through factors such as nutrition, which in turn is influenced by income, differences in habits such as smoking among different trades, and the like). Nevertheless, for all work-related illness we must consider both the potential for resolution by attention to workplace phenomena and the potential effect on productivity. We have few data on the precise magnitude of work-related illness, although it is clearly substantial.

CHEMICAL AND PHYSICAL EXPOSURES AND PRODUCTIVITY

To what extent do workplace physical and chemical agents affect productivity through occupational diseases, work-related diseases, or impaired health? There has been little direct study of this question, but personal anecdotal experience suggests that in some circumstances substantial productivity disruptions occur, even apart from disease-induced absences from work.

Two examples follow, both investigated by the author, of situations where chemical exposures were likely to have resulted in productivity losses. The first involved employees of a chemical plant (14) where dimethyltin chloride was manufactured. As a result of apparent equipment failures, 12 of the 22 male employees who worked in the area had been heavily exposed to dimethyltin dichloride and a highly neurotoxic contaminant trimethyltin chloride. [As a matter of background, experiments in rats had shown that trimethyltin chloride causes tremors, hyperexcitability, convulsions, and particularly aggressive behavior (1).] The workers who were heavily exposed to trimethyltin dichloride developed a variety of symptoms including forgetfulness, fatigue and weakness, loss of motivation, headaches, sleep disturbance, and alternating rage and deep depression. These mood changes lasted a few hours to a few days. Neuropsychological testing confirmed defects in memory, hand-eye coordination, visuomotor integration, and learning and emotional disturbance. Consequently, workers often quarreled with each other while at work and with family members at home. As a result of difficulty with short-term memory, they forgot valve settings and other important details of the industrial operation. As a result of rage and frustration, they described setting gauges and controls wrongly. Although we could not directly substantiate the phenomena, we were led to believe that these actions caused the chemical reactions to proceed in unwanted directions, resulting not only in upset chemical reaction products and poor product yields but overproduction of the neurotoxic trimethyltin chloride at the expense of the intended dimethyltin dichloride product.

The second example comes from studies of commercial roofers, who were working with coal tar pitch, which sensitizes the worker to sunlight. Such exposure caused them to develop photosensitive keratoconjunctivitis, with eye pain, visual impairment, and painful dermatitis (5,6). Because roofing is outdoor work where further sun exposure cannot easily be avoided the condition became debilitating. The subsequent impaired vision was likely a factor in the high accident rate observed among these roofers, and it was not uncommon during the summer for several members of the crew to be away from work until their eye symptoms had abated. While at work they experienced pain in the eyes, which occurred within seconds of direct exposure to sunlight, resulting in substantially altered work practices in order to avoid the sun.

In neither of these two examples did we measure or adequately address productivity changes as a result of the investigated chemical hazards. Yet in both cases the potential for diminished productivity appeared real. For future investigation of this type of hazard, adequate methods to quantify productivity changes could be used, so that the full impact of workplace chemical and physical exposures can be described in a social and economic as well as in a health context. Such information should provide an additional incentive, where one is needed, to control harmful exposures.

CONCLUSION

Unfortunately, there is little information on the effects of chemical and physical agents that is pertinent to the relations between work, health, and productivity. Nevertheless, the following general conclusions are possible.

1. Workplace exposure to hazardous chemical and physical agents is widespread. Services that might control and ameliorate these exposures are unfortunately distributed on the basis of factors other than the posed hazard.

2. There is generally little information available on the extent of human "dosage" related to this exposure.

3. Chemical and physical agents cause a variety of identified "classic" occupational diseases; but partly because of weaknesses in workers' compensation statistics, we have no reliable information regarding the extent to which these diseases occur in the United States today.

4. A broader and probably more important category of disease is work-related disease. This category includes diseases that may be related to physical and chemical exposures in the workplace, other hazards of the workplace, or factors beyond work-

place hazards (alone or in concert). We have no good estimates of the total burden of work-related disease in the United States.

5. Health differs from the absence of disease. In the past most studies of the effects of workplace physical and chemical exposures have examined their relation to work-related or occupational disease. Studies that address "health" rather than disease may be more meaningful in terms of understanding variations in productivity.

6. Investigators should develop and incorporate measures of productivity into studies of the effects of workplace chemical and physical agents.

REFERENCES

1. Brown, A. W., Aldridge, W. H., Street, B. W., et al. (1979). The behavioral and neuropathologic sequelae of intoxication by trimethyltin compounds in the rats. *American Journal of Pathology, 97,* 59–76.

2. Cherry, N., Hutchins, H., Pace, T., & Waldron, H. A. (1985). Neurobehavioral effects of repeated occupational exposure to toluene and paint solvent. *British Journal of Industrial Medicine, 42,* 291–300.

3. Elofsson, S., Gamerale, F., Hindmarsh, T., et al. (1980). Exposure to organic solvents: a cross-sectional epidemiologic investigation on occupationally exposed car and industrial spray painters with special reference to the nervous system. *Scandinavian Journal of Work Environment and Health, 6,* 239–73.

4. Emmett, E. A. (1984). The skin and occupational diseases. *Archives of Environmental Health, 39,* 144–9.

5. Emmett, E. A. (1987). Cutaneous and ocular hazards of roofers. *Occupational Medicine, 1,* 307–22.

6. Emmett, E. A., Stetzer, W., & Taphorn, B. (1977). Phototoxic keratoconjunctivitis from coal tar pitch volatiles. *Science, 198,* 841–2.

7. Fait, A., Grossman, E., Self, S., Jefferys, J., Pellizzari, E. D., & Emmett, E. A. (1989). Polychlorinated biphenyl congeners in adipose tissue lipid and serum of past and present transformer repair workers and a control group. *Fundamental and Applied Toxicology, 12(1),* 42–55.

8. Klaassen, C. D., Amdur, M. O., & Doull, J. (1986). *Casarett and Doull's Toxicology* (3rd ed.). New York: Macmillan.

9. Lees, P. S. J., Corn, M., & Breysse, P. N. (1987). Evidence for dermal absorption as the major route of body entry during exposure of transformer maintenance and repairmen to PCBs. *American Industrial Hygiene Association Journal, 48,* 257–64.

10. McMichael, A. J. (1985). Social class (as estimated by occupational prestige) and mortality in Australian males in the 1970s. *Community Health Studies, 9,* 220–30.

11. National Institute for Occupational Safety and Health. (1975). *Pilot study for development of an occupational disease surveillance method.* University of Washington, Department of Environmental Health. DHEW publication (NIOSH) 75-162. Washington, DC: U.S. Government Printing Office.

12. National Toxicology Program. (1984). Toxicology testing: strategies to determine needs and priorities. Washington, DC: National Academy Press.

13. Radcliffe, J. M., Halperin, W. E., Frazier, T. M., Sundin, D. S., Delaney, L., & Hornung, R. W. (1986). The prevalence of screening in industry: report from the National Institute for Occupational Safety and Health, National Occupational Hazard Survey. *Journal of Occupational Medicine, 28,* 906–12.

14. Ross, W. D., Emmett, E. A., Steiner, J., & Tureen, R. (1981). Neurotoxic effects of occupational exposure to organotins. *American Journal of Psychiatry, 138,* 1092–5.

15. U.S. Department of Health Education and Welfare. (1977). *National occupational hazard survey.* Washington, DC: U.S. Government Printing Office.

16. U.S. Department of Labor, Occupational Safety and Health Administration. (1985). Occupational exposure to formaldehyde: proposed rules and notice of hearing 29 CFR Part 1910. *Federal Register, 50,* 50412–99.

4

Meeting Regulatory Standards for Physical and Chemical Agents

Morton Corn

Current technical and managerial options available for meeting U.S. regulatory standards for physical and chemical agents are influenced by underlying concepts of the interaction between the agents and the human receptor. Because these underlying concepts are different in different nations, the regulatory agendas may also differ. A prominent illustration of the results of these conceptual differences is the differences in standards for airborne toxic chemicals in the United States and the USSR (19) (Table 4–1). The data in Table 4–1 illustrate the fact that Russian standards of occupational exposure to airborne toxic agents can be 2 to 70 times lower than U.S. standards on the basis of the time-weighted average (TWA) exposure for an 8-hour period (TWA = 8 hours) in the United States and ceiling values in the USSR.[1] Such differences in standards are confusing to developing nations and cause innumerable difficulties when these countries are developing their own regulatory programs. The World Health Organization has attempted to explain the basis for these differences, but the selection of standards on one list or the other by developing nations appears to be related more to political alignment with either the USSR or the United States than to scientific considerations.

Perhaps the best way to describe the philosophical and conceptual differences in establishing a permissible exposure concentration for airborne toxic chemicals and for physical agents is to review the concepts proposed by Hatch (8). Figure 4–1 shows the relation between impairment and disability proposed by Hatch.

> In Figure [4–1] a distinction is made between impairment and disability, the two scales represented by the abscissa and ordinate, respectively. Impairment is the underlying disturbance of the physiological system; the consequence of such disturbance in terms of identifiable disease. Starting with normal health, the individual progresses, for one reason or another, along the scale of impairment and that of disability, ultimately to death. Early departures from health (impairment) are accompanied by little disability. At the low ends of the scales, normal homeostatic processes insure adequate adjustment to offset stress. For a distance beyond this early zone of change, compensatory processes maintain the overall function of the system without serious disability. Further increments in impairment beyond the limits of compensatory processes, however, are accompanied by rapidly increasing increments in disability; the individual moves into the region of sickness and

45

Table 4–1. Selected Work Environment Hygiene Standards for Airborne Contaminants in the USA and USSR

Contaminant	USA–OSHA 1974 (mg/m³)[a]	USSR 1972 (mg/m³)[b]
Acetaldehyde	360	5
Ammonia	35	20
Carbon monoxide	55	20
Carbon tetrachloride	65	20
Chloroprene	90	2
DDT	1	0.1
p-Dichlorobenzene	450	20
Epichlorohydrin	19	1
Ethylenediamine	25	2
Formaldehyde	2	0.5
Phenol	19	5
Propylaldiol	500	10
Thallium	1	0.1

Source: U.S. Department of Labor (17).

[a]Eight-hour time-weighted average.
[b]Ceiling value.

disability, terminating in death. A healthy individual, functioning at point A on the curve and subjected to a given type and degree of stress may respond with relatively minor and temporary disturbance, returning to his/her starting position when the stress is removed. An individual at point B, on the other hand, may find the same kind and degree of stress intolerable and, in consequence, move rapidly up the curve to a position of serious disability and even death. In our past, concern with occupational disease, relationships were established between conditions of exposure and degrees of disability and objectives were to bring the stresses of the job within limits which would prevent such disability. For the future, concern must be with impairment, rather than disability, and relationships have to be demonstrated between the stresses of the job and the subtle physiological disturbances. The degree of impairment must be kept within limits well below the level of disease (8).

Figure 4–1 and the concept of impairment versus that of disability represent a well articulated rationale for establishing permissible exposure concentrations in human populations. Paull (14) traced the origin of the threshold limit value to Rudolph Kobert, who published data concerning harmful concentrations of air contaminants in 1912. The limits were based primarily on acute toxicity and were derived from animal experiments. The concept of a dose, or integrated amount of chemical in the body, was not part of the reasoning by Kobert in establishing the permissible concentration. The U.S. Bureau of Mines, in a technical paper (6) derived mostly from Kobert's work, addressed 33 compounds, most of them acting acutely. The idea of a permissible exposure concentration continued throughout the 1920s with maximum exposures to lead based on animal experiments, to benzene, and to dust-containing free silica in the granite industry. The permissible exposure concentrations for benzene and airborne free silica dust were based on observations in human populations; the exposure concentrations that existed for these agents were unchanged for several decades. Thus once again the concept of an integrated dose was not addressed (5).

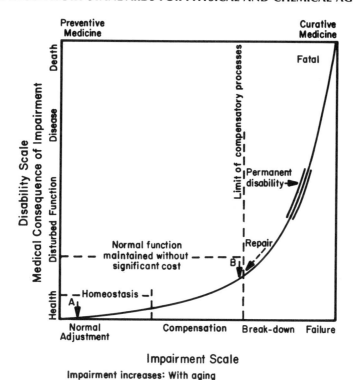

Figure 4–1. Suggested relation between impairment and disability. There is considerable movement along the scale of impairment accompanied by relatively little disability. Basic man–environment relations are between environmental stress and impairment, the precursor of disease. From Hatch (8).

The practical problem of defining what was "harmful" began to be formalized during the 1940s. In 1943 Sterner (15) commented that "gradually a considerable body of data has been accumulated for a variety of compounds giving levels of exposures which have not been associated with injurious effects. The values more generally used are those which apply to a continuous exposure. By the term "maximum allowable concentrations" (MAC) is meant the upper limit of concentration of an atmospheric contaminant which will not cause injury to an individual exposed continuously during his working day and for indefinite periods of time." Sterner presented a list of 56 MACs.

The codification of all available data on MAC's and presentation in one publication is attributable to Cook (2). The table of maximum allowable concentrations was made a continuing activity by the American Conference of Governmental Industrial Hygienists, and the concept of the threshold limit values (TLVs) was born (4). The TLVs have been incorporated into federal regulations in the United States, first in the Walsh Healy Public Contracts Act of 1956 and then in the Occupational Safety and Health Act of 1970. The TLVs are not consensus standards; that is, they are not subject to public input and discussion prior to resolution. They are the work of an expert committee that considers all of the available evidence and then makes its judgments. For this reason the Occupational Safety and Health Administration (OSHA) must engage in public rule-making to change any of the TLVs in the 1968 list that was adopted under the 2-year permit given to OSHA to adopt as permanent standards all standards preexisting in federal legislation; it was this 2-year "window" that permitted OSHA to adopt the 1968 TLVs because they existed in the Walsh Healy Public Contracts Act. Any changes in the current TLVs require Administrative Procedures Act rule-making procedures.

The TLVs have a disclaimer to the effect that "nearly all workers" are protected if values are adhered to. The TLVs have always embraced the concept that there is a small percentage of those exposed who are indeed affected by exposure. There is no mention of employee productivity in the TLVs. It is an article of faith that if health is not affected productivity is most certainly maintained or increased.

DECISION TO CONTROL

It is not feasible here to review the history of voluntary effort by employers to provide satisfactory conditions in U.S. workplaces. The reader is referred to the biography of Alice Hamilton, *Exploring the Dangerous Trades* (7), the U.S. Department of Labor document *Protecting People at Work* (16), and Mintz's *OSHA: History, Law and Policy* (11), which briefly reviews U.S. legal recourse during the early part of this century. A host of publications by J. K. Corn should also be consulted (3). It can be concluded from these references and others that, at east in the United States, voluntary compliance has not been highly successful—in contrast to another cultural norm, that of Sweden, where the situation was reviewed by Kelman (9), who concluded that because of the different historical tradition of the Swedes voluntary compliance through a collective bargaining process between management and labor can indeed work. Several incentives for voluntary compliance in the United States can be cited, including improved corporate image, reduced workers compensation and insurance costs, avoidance of tort liability, and increased productivity. Documentation of increased productivity through improved working conditions has not been an investigatory focus in the past, and evidence is sparse.

In this discussion it is assumed that some guideline, TLV, or regulatory standard has been established as a target for the concentration of the potentially toxic agent in the working environment. This target has been derived with some philosophical reference to the Hatch curve and the availability of epidemiological and animal data. It is often mistaken in the United States that when there is a permissible exposure limit under OSHA regulation the risk is zero. This assumption is not accurate. The current reduced asbestos standard of 0.2 per cubic centimeter (f/cc) is associated with 6.85 lung cancer and mesothelioma deaths per 1,000 workers following a 35-year exposure (17). The current $2 \ mg/cm^3$ respirable mine dust standard enforced by the Mine Health Safety Administration is associated with one first stage simple pneumoconiosis case per 100 workers for every 40 years' exposure. Each of our standards is a compromise among technical feasibility, cost, and health impact. As Lowrance has stated (10), that which society deems acceptable risk is called "safe". All of our guidelines and standards are associated with a measurable level of risk, judged to be safe by the regulatory agency, deliberations of experts, or consensus groups, or by negotiation (18).

In the United States, under the Occupational Safety and Health Act of 1970, standards for toxic agents are promulgated, if it is possible, to technically achieve the permissible exposure limit. Economic feasibility is not a determining factor in the consideration of acceptable risk at the workplace. This interpretation of the OSHA Act of 1970 statutory language was made by the U.S. Supreme Court (1). In its decision the Supreme Court held that the Act does not require cost-benefit analysis, which is in direct contrast to other federal statutes, such as the Clean Air Act and the Toxic Substances Control Act, where Congress directs the Environmental Protection Agency to perform cost-benefit analyses. Thus insofar as national policy is concerned, the approach to acceptable risk differs depending on the specific statute invoked as the basis for regulation.

MANAGEMENT/CONTROL OPTIONS

After an acceptable level of risk has been targeted (TLV or PEL) and the decision to control reached, options for control are evaluated for the most cost-effective approach to control. The control alternatives have been codified (5). Table 4–2 indicates the available options. Options 1 through 7 are considered engineering controls. The "hierarchy of controls" refers to the supremacy of engineering controls over the other options listed in Table 4–2 (13). Engineering controls are preferred because they do not involve the hour to hour, day to day, year to year constant attention of the employee; in contrast, work practices, personal protective equipment, dust suppression, and so on do require such attention. Engineering controls require periodic maintenance and, if so maintained, generally function with little attention. This argument also assumes that the engineering controls are appropriately designed for the task at hand.

The achievement of a guideline or target concentration usually necessitates the invocation of several of the options listed in Table 4–2. One gains a small amount of ground with each approach. It is seldom that any one or even two approaches can achieve the desired result. For example, control of lead in the environment of primary and secondary battery facilities mainly utilizes engineering controls, including process design and local exhaust ventilation. Control of lead also requires concentrated attention to housekeeping, periodic maintenance, work practices, personal protective devices, and environmental and medical surveillance to achieve the required result.

COMMENT

The above discourse is a terse statement of our ability to get the job done when a standard or guideline exists. We have never focused on the "payoffs" of getting the job done because most of the incentives to utilize the controls listed in Table 4–2 were driven by regulations. With few exceptions in the history of U.S. occupational safety and health, voluntary compliance did not lead to major utilization of the techniques listed in Table 4–2 or to significant impact on hazards in the work environment. The progress with improving workplace conditions in the United States since 1970 when the OSHA Act was passed, albeit slow, has been a major improvement over pre-OSHA primarily voluntary compliance. Prior to 1970 only six states boasted respectable regulatory programs. There is good reason to believe that there has been a substantial impact on worker health and safety since 1970 despite incomplete statistics (12).

Table 4–2. Methods for Control of Toxic Chemical, Physical, or Biological Hazards in Human Environments

---

Engineering controls

1. Elimination: of the toxic substance, hazardous condition, biological agent, or the source, e.g., use of alternate fuels to eliminate sulfur
2. Substitution: of a less toxic substance, e.g., toluene for benzene, glass fiber for asbestos fiber on thermal insulation
3. Isolation: use of distance or shielding, e.g., as in hot cell controls for radioactive materials or barriers and restricted access to carcinogenic or biohazardous operations
4. Enclosure: totally, as in a glove box, or partially, as in a booth or hood
5. Ventilation: general dilution or local exhaust
   a. Hood, enclosure, or extraction connection at the source
   b. Ductwork
   c. Industrial air and gas cleaning device
   d. Air-moving device
   e. Stack or ducted outlet
   May also include ancillary systems or functions for operation, control, recirculation of exhaust, and waste disposal
6. Process change: use of change in manufacturing method or machine, or process or operation to reduce or eliminate hazard; soft energy technologies; closed system versus open kettle operation
7. Product change: process research to reduce benzene yield in petroleum refining; reduced free vinyl chloride content of polyvinylchloride

Other controls

8. Housekeeping: keeping all surfaces clean of contaminants, as in biological, radiological, or chemical carcinogen hazard control to prevent their redispersion or to eliminate personal contacts
9. Dust suppression: wetting down dusty sources; wet drilling; use of soil, stock, or waste pile stabilizers, windbreaks, and the like
10. Maintenance: continued maintenance of effective control system performance, as well as of process, operational, or manufacturing equipment to reduce or eliminate inadvertent release of hazardous materials
11. Sanitation: use of hygienic principles to reduce or eliminate hazardous materials from the person, as with clothing changes, shower-in or shower-out, sterilization, chlorination, and pasteurization
12. Work practices: specification of proper work procedures to reduce or control release, dissemination, or inadvertent exposure to hazardous substances or conditions
13. Education: of worker, management, and the public to the nature of a hazard and how properly to minimize risk; most importantly, education of engineers to discover, develop, and design products, processes, and systems with minimum hazard to workers or users
14. Labeling and warning systems: for use in conjunction with other methods, e.g., education
15. Personal protective devices: for use where other control methods are not technically or economically feasible, e.g., use of respiratory protective devices during firefighting procedures or when painting the inside of a tank, ship, hull, or rail car
    a. Head protection
    b. Ear protection
    c. Eye protection
    d. Respiratory protective devices
    e. Hand and arm protection
    f. Trunk, body, or apron-type protection
    g. Lower torso, thigh, leg protection
    h. Foot protective devices
16. Environmental monitoring: use of intermittent or continuous atmospheric sampling and analysis methods for the hazard by area sampling, personal sampling, or process or duct sampling; each type used to determine characteristics of the emission, level of human exposure, or operational condition

---

(continued)

Table 4–2. (*Continued*)

17. Waste disposal practices: to reduce or eliminate redistribution of discharged contaminant or process waste streams to other receptors, including solid waste disposal in effective incinerators or landfills, liquid waste disposal to appropriate treatment and dilution, and atmospheric dilution and dispersion of gases or vapors after effective removal of contaminants, e.g., as in disposal of asbestos wastes, sulfur oxide scrubber sludges, or stack gas discharges

18. Administrative control: reduction of time of exposure of receptor to the contaminant, as in supplemental control strategies by the use of fuel switching to reduce sulfur oxide emissions or use of annual accumulated radiation dose of 5 REM/year for worker and removal from exposure when exceeded; may include plant location or setting and plant layout

19. Medical control: to reduce or eliminate effects of human exposure to hazardous substances, conditions, or agents through medical surveillance
    a. Preplacement screening to restrict high-risk persons
    b. Biological monitoring (e.g., for lead in blood)
    c. Medical removal
    d. Medical exclusion
    e. General reviews and treatment

20. Management program: formal organization with authority and responsibility to provide control program activities; plan, organize, implement, control

Source: Corn (4).

The introduction of productivity data to provide incentives for bettering working conditions may well speed the pace of improvement, and such dialogue is welcomed by most health professionals. However, vigorous enforcement of standards appears to be the heretofore successful approach to better working conditions in the United States. Relaxation of enforcement would be an error until evidence of voluntary compliance is persuasive.

NOTE

1. Concentrations of toxic contaminants in air and water tend to fluctuate. A TWA of 8 hours is the average concentration for that period of time and is a meaningful measure of exposure for those contaminants that physiologically act slowly to produce or aggravate disease. Rapidly acting agents cause asphyxiation or irritation of the respiratory tract, and exposure is best described by shorter-term average concentrations. A ceiling value refers to the peak concentration permitted for the briefest feasible measurement period, usually expressed in minutes. Thus it is important to state the time base for any measures of concentration utilized in a standard.

REFERENCES

1. American Textile Manufacturers' Institute v. Donavan. (1981). U.S. Supreme Court. 452 U.S. 490.

2. Cook, W. A. (1945). Maximum allowable concentrations of industrial atmospheric contaminants. *Journal of Industrial Medicine, 14,* 936–46.

3. Corn, J. K. (1981). Byssinosis: an historical perspective. *American Journal of Industrial Medicine, 2,* 331–52.

4. Corn, J. K. (1990). Protecting the health of workers: the American conference of Governmental Industrial Hygienists, 1938–1988. Cincinnati: ACGIH.

5. Corn, M. (1983). Assessment and control of environmental exposure. *Journal of Allergy and Clinical Immunology, 72,* 233–41.

6. Fieldner, F. L., Katz, S. H., & Kinney, S. P. (1921). Gas mask for gases met in fighting fires. Paper 248. Pittsburgh, PA: Bureau of Mines Technology.

7. Hamilton, A. (1943). *Exploring the dangerous trades.* Boston: Little, Brown.

8. Hatch, T. F. (1962). Changing objectives in occupational health. *American Industrial Hygiene Association Journal, 23,* 1–7.

9. Kelman, S. (1981). *Regulating Sweden, regulating America.* Cambridge, MA: MIT Press.

10. Lowrance, W. W. (1974). *Of acceptable risk* (p. 75). Los Altos, CA: W. Kaufmann.
11. Mintz, B. W. (1984). *OSHA: history, law and policy.* Washington, DC: Bureau of National Affairs.
12. National Academy of Sciences. (1983). *Risk assessment in the federal government: managing the process* (pp. 29–40). Washington, DC: NAS.
13. Office of Technology Assessment. (1985). *Preventing illness and injury in the workplace* (OTA-H-256, 175-188). Washington, DC: U.S. Government Printing Office.
14. Paull, J. M. (1984). The origin and basis of threshold limit values. *American Journal of Industrial Medicine, 5,* 227–38.
15. Sterner, J. H. (1943). Determining margin of safety—criteria for defining a "harmful" substance. *Journal of Industrial Medicine, 12,* 514–18.
16. U.S. Department of Labor. (1980). *Protecting people at work.* Washington, DC: U.S. Government Printing Office.
17. U.S. Department of Labor. (1986). Occupational Safety and Health Administration. 29CFR Parts 1910 and 1926: Occupational exposure to asbestos, tremolite, anathophyllite and actinolite; final rules. 51 *Federal Register* No. 119, 20 June, 1986, pp. 22611–22790.
18. Wilson, R., & Crouch, E. A. G. (1987). Risk assessment and comparison: an introduction. *Science, 236,* 176–270.
19. Winnell, M. (1984). An international comparison of hygienic standards for chemicals in the work environment. In M. E. LaNier (ed.). *Threshold limit values: discussion and thirty-five year index with recommendations* (pp. 253–256). Cincinnati: American Conference of Governmental Industrial Hygienists, Annals Series.

5
Biological Indicators of Susceptibility

Richard Evans III, Suzanne M. Fortney, †Harold A. Menkes,
Carol A. Newill, and Bernice H. Cohen

Occupational factors such as work facilities and environmental agents affect the health and productivity of workers but do so to a variable degree. Whether acute or chronic health effects develop because of conditions in the workplace depends on the workplace factors and the biological characteristics of the worker. Whether a worker maintains a state of health, which supports his or her potential as a productive individual, or converts to a state of disease, which interferes with productivity, is influenced by his or her innate and acquired susceptibility to the conditions at the workplace (Fig. 5–1).

In this chapter we focus on two questions: First, why are some individuals at increased risk or more susceptible to occupational factors than other individuals? Second, how can that risk be better estimated to prevent the adverse health effects and loss of productivity that may result from the interplay of occupational factors and worker susceptibility? We draw on results from large, population-based studies and from small, clinically based studies to illustrate principles of susceptibility.

Worker characteristics that reflect increased susceptibility to workplace agents and conditions may be genetically determined and therefore fixed from the time of birth, or they may be acquired as environmental agents act on the genetically susceptible host (Fig. 5–2). Most of the biological indicators of susceptibility to be discussed represent the effects of environmental factors in the susceptible host. Examples of these factors are presented in Figure 5–3.

Health responses to workplace factors occur at multiple biological levels and involve specific genes, enzymes, cells, or organ systems. Examples of attempts to isolate, assay, or sample biological links to susceptibility at different biological levels are (a) the search for the specific gene associated with α_1-antitrypsin deficiency or cystic fibrosis, (b) the target cell associated with bronchogenic or cervical carcinoma, and (c) the organ system abnormality associated with congestive heart failure or renal insufficiency. This chapter describes studies that focus on organ systems at an integrated level. We attempt to relate results to events that occur at the cellular, biochemical, or genetic level. For example, the underlying reason for male-female differences in sweating rates must lie in genetically-determined, sex-linked factors. Similarly, the crucial missing link determining α_1-antiprotease levels in serum may lie in an abnormal liver enzyme, and the underlying lesion of airways reactivity in asthma

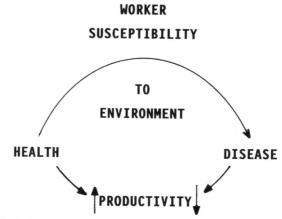

Figure 5–1. Biological indicators of susceptibility. Whether an individual worker passes from a state of health to a state of disease depends on his or her biological susceptibility. The state of workers' health or disease then affects their productivity.

may be found in the epithelial cell of the airways. Although this discussion of biological indicators is limited to studies dealing with physiological measurements of organ system function in human subjects, these studies provide important clues and insights into molecular and cellular origins of susceptibility.

When evaluating biological susceptibility, it is informative to utilize clinical studies that include assessment of small numbers of individuals in a controlled laboratory or clinical setting. It is also informative to utilize population studies that include

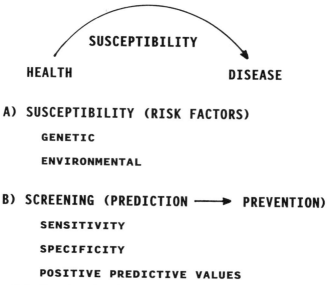

Figure 5–2. Genetic and environmental factors affect biological susceptibility.

GENETIC FACTORS

SEX

ABO BLOOD TYPE

PI TYPE

ENVIRONMENTAL FACTORS

SMOKING

FITNESS

SOCIOECONOMIC STATUS

Figure 5–3. Genetic and environmental factors that contribute to biological susceptibility.

assessments of large numbers of subjects derived from epidemiological or occupational settings.

Three studies are discussed. The first focuses on stress physiology in human subjects. Physical stress or exercise in the workplace taxes multiple systems in the body. The cardiovascular, pulmonary, and thermal regulatory systems play major roles in determining how an individual responds. Whether these systems respond appropriately or adequately depends on the sex, age, and fitness level of the individual at risk. Although differences attributable to sex are frequently cited when explaining individual responses to exercise, biological susceptibility due to fluctuations of sex hormones are probably overestimated and receive an inappropriate amount of attention. In contrast, the effects of age and fitness on responses to exercise are profound and deserve special attention for two reasons: (a) our working population is growing older; and (b) fitness level can be assessed and modified.

The second and third studies described in this chapter deal with a specific organ system, the lung. Because lung disease is often associated with exposures in the workplace, these studies are used to illustrate how risk factors are assessed, to address some of the complexities of genetic–environmental interactions, and to discuss risk assessment for screening and preventing disease.

PHYSIOLOGICAL STRESS DURING EXERCISE: EFFECTS OF SEX, AGE, AND FITNESS

Individuals in the workplace exert themselves physically and may be exposed to extremes of temperature and humidity; their responses, however, vary. A commonly held but poorly supported belief is that women sweat less than men (5) because of a direct inhibiting action of the female sex steroid, estrogen, on the output of sweat glands (16). However, in a study that characterized sweat production in women with and without supplemental estrogen during cycle ergometer exercise in a warm environment (30°C, 50% relative humidity), there was no difference in the sweating threshold (the core temperature at which sweating started) or the sweating sensitivity (the slope of the sweating/core temperature relation) when estrogen supplements were given. In addition, there was no significant difference in the exercise-induced rise in deep body temperature associated with estrogen treatment.

An important risk factor for heat stress is level of fitness (23). Reports in the literature (2) indicate that heat tolerance in women is not significantly different from that in men when subjects are matched for relative levels of fitness. If these studies included women with lower maximum aerobic capacities owing to their smaller body size and generally more sedentary life style than their male counterparts, at a given absolute exercise intensity, the workload would have been relatively greater for the women than for the men and would account for the higher heart rates and body temperatures observed in the women. Thus fitness level may be a more important determinant of thermal responses to physical stress than estrogens and should be taken into consideration when assessing the placement of women (or men) who are exposed to physical stress in the workplace.

Endurance exercise training is associated with increased sensitivity of skin blood flow and sweating responses (22). Part of the improvement in thermal responses after training may be due to increased plasma volume (12). To determine if the impairment in thermal tolerance seen after deconditioning can be prevented by the maintenance of plasma volume, the exercise responses of women after 11- or 12-day programs of bed rest were studied. In a study that included 12 subjects, plasma volume decreased an average of 19% during the 11-day bed rest protocol, and peak oxygen consumption decreased an average of 11% at 24 hours after bed rest. Submaximal exercise responses were significantly reduced by bed rest (Fig. 5–4).

In another group of seven women, supplemental estrogen was given. Although their loss of plasma volume during bed rest was attenuated, the exercise responses of this group were similar to those seen in the control (non-estrogen-treated) group, and the rise in esophageal temperature and the heart rate response was similar in the two groups. Thus it appears that the loss of plasma volume that occurred during bed rest was not responsible for the impairment in exercise responses that developed during bed rest. These results suggest that a normal state of hydration alone is inadequate to compensate for the heat and exercise intolerance that occurs in the deconditioned state. If in addition to loss of fluid during bed rest the cardiovascular system becomes deconditioned (e.g., if the vessels lose their ability to regulate tone), simply replacing fluid may not reverse abnormalities of cardiovascular function. These studies pointed out that multiple factors contribute to the compromise in thermal regulation that occurs in the deconditioned state.

Do similar factors play important roles in responses of older subjects whose cardiovascular function is limited by the aging process as well as by the fitness level of the subjects? Early epidemiological studies (13) indicated that during heat waves most fatalities associated with high temperatures occur in individuals over 50 years of age. A study by Phillips et al. (21) indicated that older individuals may be less able to sense a body water deficit and to maintain body hydration. The resultant dehydration could reduce skin blood flow and sweating during thermal stress and contribute to an older individual's increased susceptibility to heat stress.

To determine if thermal regulation is impaired in otherwise healthy older individuals, five young and five older men with equal age-adjusted fitness levels exercised in a warm room (30°C, 50% relative humidity) while measurements were obtained of

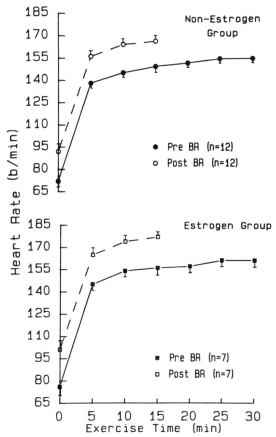

Figure 5–4. Heart rate plotted as a function of exercise time for 12 women who did not receive estrogen (Premarin) supplement (top panel) and 7 women who received estrogen supplement (bottom panel). The mean ± standard error is shown for exercise tests performed before bed rest (Pre BR) and immediately after bed rest (Post BR).

their skin blood flow response, deep body temperature, and chest sweating. The young men exercised at an average absolute exercise intensity that was 30% greater than the older group, which produced a similar relative exercise stress. Although the older subjects worked at a considerably lower absolute exercise intensity, they had a rise in body temperature similar to that of the younger group. Because the older individuals produced less heat yet had similar body temperatures, it is reasonable to conclude that the older men were less able to lose body heat during exercise, a conclusion supported by Figure 5–5, which shows a decrease in the slopes of both the sweating and the skin blood flow responses in older men. The heat loss responses of older individuals may become less efficient with increased age, thus placing the older individuals at greater risk when exposed to high thermal loads at work.

These examples illustrate that even though gender is not an important risk factor, age and fitness are. As the working force becomes older and more sedentary, these factors should receive greater consideration. If an aging individual retains an active life

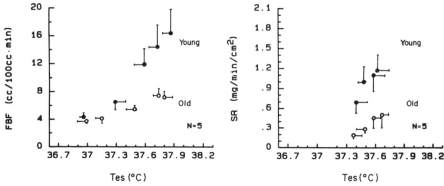

Figure 5–5. Forearm blood flow (FBF; left panel) and sweating responses (SR; right panel) plotted as a function of the esophageal temperature (TES) for the young and old subjects. Each point represents the mean of the values obtained at rest and at 5-minute intervals during 20 minutes of cycle ergometer exercise.

style, it is possible that the rate of decline in fitness can be slowed, as assessed by maximum oxygen consumption (7). Does it mean that the individual can reduce his or her susceptibility to heat as well as other physical stresses?

RISK FACTORS AND AIRWAYS OBSTRUCTION

Chronic obstructive pulmonary disease (COPD) is commonly attributed to workplace exposures. In 1971 a multidisciplinary study of COPD was initiated to assess environmental and genetic factors that contribute to the development of airways obstruction and to develop better methods of characterizing individuals at increased risk of developing airways obstruction. The study had a modified case-control design. A group of patients with airways obstruction (defined as COPD) were selected. Their family members, as well as a number of comparison groups, were then assembled for study. The study population has been described previously (9,10). The analyses discussed here are based on a sample of 2,539 adults from which all "patients" were excluded.

Study participants underwent pulmonary function tests, blood and saliva studies, and a detailed interview regarding demographic, medical, family, and other epidemiological information. More than 14 variables were examined as potential risk factors or confounding factors for COPD, including (a) age, gender, and race; (b) cigarette smoking, socioeconomic status, and coffee, tea, and alcohol consumption (environmental factors); (c) the genetic factors of protease inhibition, or Pi (α_1-antitrypsin) type, ABO blood group, ABH secretor status (ability to secrete in water-soluble form into the body fluids "A," "B," and "H" antigens), phenylthiocarbamide taste ability, and amylase type; and (d) being a first degree relative of a COPD index case. In results to be presented, the effect of each factor is given as an adjusted value that simultaneously considers all other factors in the model.

Cross-Sectional Observations

As with many of the chronic disorders, older age and smoking were associated with a higher frequency of impaired pulmonary function (8) (Fig. 5–6). Being of low socioeconomic status (SES), being a first degree relative of a patient with COPD, and being male were also associated with significant differences; racial differences were questionable. The familial component is seen by comparing first degree relatives of COPD patients with first degree relatives of nonpulmonary patients and other nonpatient subjects including neighbors, teachers, and various family members of subjects other than first degree relatives of pulmonary patients. Genetic factors, e.g., carrying at least one Z allele in the Pi system, having an A blood group antigen, or being an

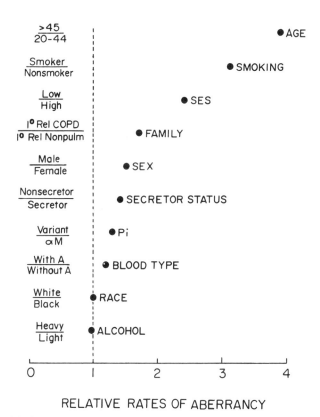

RELATIVE RATES OF ABERRANCY

Figure 5–6. Risk factors and aberrancy of forced expiration (FEV$_1$/FVC <68%). Ratios of adjusted rates of aberrant forced expiration are shown for comparisons of old subjects (>45 years) to young subjects (<45 years), smokers of one or more packages of cigarettes daily to those who never smoked, low socioeconomic groups to high socioeconomic groups, first-degree relatives of patients with lung disease to first-degree relatives of nonpulmonary patients, males to females, nonsecretors of ABH antigens to secretors, variant protease inhibitor types to MM types, subjects with blood type A to subjects without A, Whites to Blacks, and heavy drinkers to light drinkers. From Cohen et al. (10).

ABH nonsecretor (especially in Whites), appeared to be associated with poor pulmonary function.

For the environmental factors, coffee intake (but not tea) appeared related to pulmonary impairment; increased alcohol consumption was not (Fig. 5–7). The effects of the familial component and coffee consumption were assessed separately in smokers and never-smokers. A familial component in airways obstruction is observed in non-smokers as well as smokers (11), particularly nonsmokers who are first degree relatives of COPD patients compared to nonsmokers who are neighborhood controls. A smoker–nonsmoker difference in response was found in the association of airways obstruction with coffee intake in smokers but not in nonsmokers. Perhaps the personality factors associated with heavy coffee intake are those that influence the inhalation patterns in smokers, causing greater exposure of the lungs to the smoke.

Longitudinal Observations

A 10-year follow-up assessment of 1912 of the 2,539 individuals in the initial cross-sectional sample of nonpatient subjects was performed. When assessing longitudinal changes, the decline in FEV_1 was examined directly and expressed in terms of an absolute fall in volume as a function of time (4).

Age, smoking, and the presence of type A red blood cell antigen had an effect on FEV_1 in women (Fig. 5–8, top panel). It is noteworthy that race, SES, family association, ABH secretor status, PTC taste ability, and coffee intake, some of which were

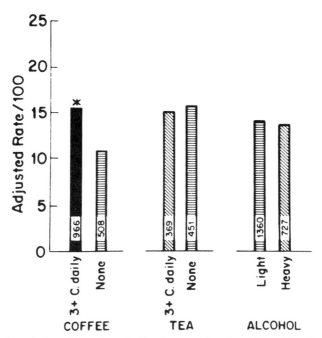

Figure 5–7. Association of impairment of pulmonary function with coffee, tea, and alcohol consumption. 3+ c. = three or more cups daily. From Cohen (8).

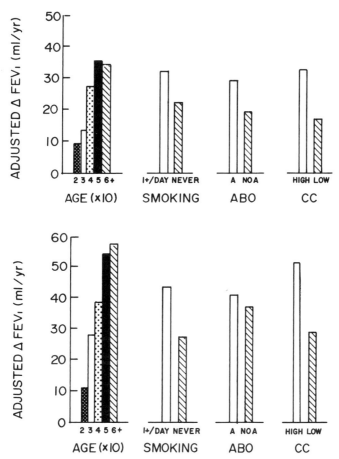

Figure 5–8. Adjusted change in FEV$_1$ values for women (top panel) and men (bottom panel) by age, smoking, ABO type, and closing capacity (CC). Data were obtained in only 669 of the 893 women and in only 805 of the 1,019 men included in the other categories. From Strydom (23).

significant in the cross-sectional evaluation, failed to provide a significant independent contribution to the longitudinal decline in function. An additional factor, the test of closing capacity, was also correlated with the longitudinal decline in function in women. The closing capacity reflects the lung volume at which small airways begin to close. The notion that abnormalities of small airways indicate early stages in the development of COPD is supported by these results. Men do not show a significant relation between ABO type and decline in function, although the direction of deviation is similar to that in women (Fig. 5–8, bottom panel). When all of the risk factors that proved to be significant were considered (including closing capacity), only 16.7% of the variation in fall in FEV$_1$ could be accounted for in women and 11.6% in men. Thus although this analysis provides insight into potential risk factors as well as the pathophysiology of disease, little can be said for an individual to predict his or her loss of function over a 5-year period.

Atopy and airways reactivity, two potentially important risk factors that were not included in this study but that are included in the Johns Hopkins animal worker study (see below), could play an important role. Airways reactivity was measured in a small subseries of selected subjects (6); and although this testing was performed at the end of the observation period, it was done without knowledge of the initial FEV_1 or the magnitude of the decline in FEV_1. Twenty subjects were identified who were adult male relatives of individuals with COPD, were under age 30 at the time of entry into the long-term study, and had pulmonary function data available from two visits. The subjects underwent a methacholine chloride inhalation challenge.

Surprisingly, 9 of 20 healthy, presumably normal sons of patients with COPD were reactive to methacholine; the other 11 were not. Over an average 4-year observation period, the reactors had lost pulmonary function at a mean rate of 150 ml/year, five times the rate of loss in the nonreactive group ($p < 0.001$). There were no differences in age, height, and forced vital capacity between the groups, although in retrospect it was noted that baseline FEV_1 had been significantly lower in the reactive group when they entered this longitudinal study. These results suggest the potential importance of a risk factor—airways reactivity—in the development of COPD. As is shown below, this risk factor may also be critical in the development of "asthma" in animal workers. However, caution is needed when interpreting these findings, as the challenge was done at the end of the observation period, not at the beginning.

Lung Disease and Mortality

Epidemiological studies in Tecumseh (15), Framingham (1), Sweden (24), and San Francisco (14) have demonstrated a relation between decreased forced expiratory volumes and mortality. This relation is not limited to mortality from respiratory disease but includes deaths from nonpulmonary processes as well. Of the 2,539 nonpatient adults studied between 1971 and 1976, 108 (4.3%) had died as of 1981 (3). A multiple binary regression model was examined to estimate the impact of potential risk factors on mortality. These risk factors included age, sex, smoking, ABO blood type, alcohol, socioeconomic status, Pi type, coffee consumption, ABH secretor status, and family relationship. Of these factors, age, sex, race, and smoking habits influenced mortality. At a minimum, these factors must be considered when assessing the impact of pulmonary function on mortality. Adding pulmonary function impairment to this predictive model gave an adjusted frequency of deaths among impaired individuals that was almost twice as great as the adjusted rate among nonimpaired individuals (69.3/1,000 versus 38.3/1,000).

To estimate the impact of each factor on the probability of dying, multiple logistic regression models were then examined. This analysis provided predicted risk curves for death during the follow-up period. Figure 5–9 shows the results of this analysis for white men and white women. (Blacks produced similar results.) It can be seen that although the mortality curves in women were shifted by almost a decade compared with those of the men, impaired individuals (men and women) had higher mortality rates than did unimpaired individuals. Because these curves incorporate adjustments for age, smoking, and time of follow-up, these findings confirmed the strong association between pulmonary function status and risk of dying.

In this sample, only 3 of the 108 deaths were attributed to COPD. Of the others,

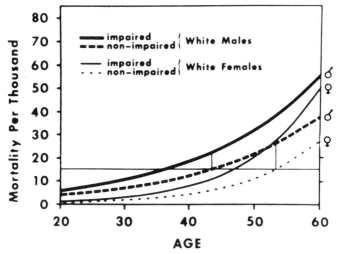

Figure 5–9. Predicted risk curves for mortality in impaired and nonimpaired white men and women based on multiple logistic regression models. From Beaty et al. (3).

69% had cardiovascular-renal disease or neoplasms listed as the underlying cause on the death certificates. When comparing cause of death between impaired and nonimpaired subjects, no significant differences were found. Thus although impaired subjects were dying more frequently than unimpaired subjects, the causes of death in the two groups were similar. In a later analysis of pulmonary function and mortality (18), we found that the slope of phase III of the single-breath nitrogen test of lung function was strongly associated with mortality, even more so than tests of forced expiration. Because the single-breath nitrogen test is performed at a slow rate (unlike forced expiration) and reflects peripheral lung function and not expiratory effort, these results provide further evidence indicating that lung function may be a strong predictor of mortality.

Two possible explanations for the striking relation between abnormalities of lung function and subsequent overall mortality that is largely from nonpulmonary disease have been proposed. First, it is possible that the lungs may serve to protect other systems of the body. Therefore poor pulmonary function may contribute to a number of disease processes leading to death. Second, it is possible that lung function may merely reflect existing disorders in other systems of the body, and the observed association between mortality and pulmonary function is a reflection of nonpulmonary diseases. In either case, tests of lung function could prove useful for screening not only for lung disease but for potential disorders of other systems in the body.

AIRWAYS REACTIVITY, ATOPY, AND OCCUPATIONAL EXPOSURE

Asthma and allergy to laboratory animals among persons who work with animals have become recognized as a significant occupational disease. Cross-sectional surveys of workers exposed to animals in their occupation indicate prevalence rates of allergic symptoms ranging from 19% to 30% (17). Among those with allergic symptoms, asthma is frequent, occurring in as many as 30 to 40%. Of additional concern is the observation that nearly one-half of those persons who develop allergic symptoms to the animals are forced to leave their job.

In 1983 a study began at The Johns Hopkins Medical institutions to evaluate factors contributing to the risk of asthma in persons exposed to animals in the laboratory. Five hundred persons who work with laboratory animals were followed, some for as long as 2.5 years. Of the first 305 subjects challenged with methacholine at entry to the study, 78 (26%) had airways hyperreactivity (a 20% decline in FEV_1). Of the 305 subjects, 208 reported having past or present symptoms of allergic rhinitis, 45 had a self-reported lifetime history of asthma symptoms, and 122 had positive skin tests (Table 5-1). Allergic rhinitis and positive skin tests showed odds ratios of 3.7 and 2.9, respectively, for the association with hyperreactive airways. The odds ratio for those reporting a history of asthma symptoms was 3.5. This finding is surprising, as the characteristic feature of asthma (some consider it pathognomonic) is airways hyperreactivity. Thus one would expect an even higher relative odds of a history of asthma in persons with a positive methacholine challenge test. Although the explanation for these surprising results is not clear, one possible explanation is based on worker selection into the study. Any individual who previously experienced symptoms of asthma when exposed to laboratory animals was excluded from participation in the study. This admission criterion could have selectively excluded participants with airways hyperreactivity and a history of asthma.

During the first 2.5 years of this study, four persons developed occupational asthma (10% decline in FEV_1) to laboratory animals. Characteristics of these subjects with occupational asthma to laboratory animals were (a) a history of allergic rhinitis; (b) a history of asthma not associated with animals; (c) at least one positive allergen skin test; and (d) a positive reaction to methacholine challenge. These observations were made at the initial visit of three of the subjects; the other subject had negative skin tests to all allergens tested at that time. The duration of exposure prior to the first symptom of occupational asthma and the animal species involved varied: Two subjects developed asthma in response to the rat, with 56 and 373 weeks of exposure to the animals, respectively; one subject developed asthma to the mouse, with 26 weeks of exposure; and one developed asthma to the guinea pig, with 27 weeks of exposure. Three subjects had positive skin tests to the research animals; and the fourth, who reacted to mouse exposure, showed an equivocal or weak reaction to mouse antigens.

The finding of bronchial airway hyperreactivity and atopy in all four of the subjects who developed occupational asthma due to laboratory animals is striking. It is

Table 5–1. Cross-Sectional Analysis of Risk Factors at Initial Visit Associated with Hyperreactive Airways

Risk factors	Total	With HRA[a]	Without HRA	Odds ratio	(95% C.I.)
Total	305	78	227		
History of allergic rhinitis[b]	208	67	141	3.7	(1.9, 7.4)
History of asthma[b]	45	22	23	3.5	(1.8, 6.7)
Positive skin test	122	46	76	2.9	(1.7, 4.9)

[a]HRA = hyperreactive airways; C.I. = confidence interval
[b]Self-reported lifetime history

Table 5–2. Prospective Analysis of HRA and Atopy at Initial Visit as Risk Factors for Development of Occupational Asthma

Condition	Asthma[a]	No asthma	Total
Atopy[b]			
HRA	3	43	46
No HRA	0	76	76
No atopy			
HRA	1	31	32
No HRA	0	151	151
Total	4	301	305

[a] Asthma induced by occupational exposure to animal(s).
[b] Atopy = a positive direct allergen skin test to any allergen (see text).

also noteworthy that all four had histories of allergic rhinitis and asthma symptoms. Table 5–2 depicts the association of hyperreactive airways and atopy at initial visit with the subsequent development of occupational asthma. Although four cases of occupational asthma is not a large number, three of the four cases of asthma were among the 46 who were both atopic and had hyperreactive airways at the time they were first evaluated and when they did not have occupational asthma. Not one case of occupational asthma developed in an individual with atopy alone and no airway hyperreactivity (76 subjects; see Table 5–2) or with neither hyperreactive airways nor atopy (151 subjects). This observation supports the hypothesis that both immunological and airway reactivity factors are necessary for allergen-induced asthma. It is noteworthy that most individuals with hyperreactive airways in this study were atopic as judged by positive skin tests (46/78 versus 76/227; $p < 0.01$). It is anticipated that further allergen exposure associated with increased length of time of exposure will result in more cases of asthma.

These observations suggest that a lifetime history of asthma and allergic rhinitis symptoms in the presence of nonspecific airway hyperreactivity to methacholine together with a positive allergen skin test may place an individual at increased risk of developing occupational asthma resulting from prolonged exposure to animals in the workplace. Implications of these observations when assessing screening strategies are discussed in the next section.

SCREENING

The data from the four individuals who developed occupational asthma when they were working with animals in the laboratory suggest that atopy and hyperreactive airways might be useful as screening criteria in the selection of persons for employment in that occupational environment. There are epidemiological methods that can be applied to the assessment of potential screening criteria (19,20). It will become evident that the primary intention (goal) of screening must be defined before deciding upon screening criteria. The definitions of parameters useful in screening are given in Figure 5–10. The positive predictive value helps to identify persons who are themselves at high risk; specificity helps to identify a large proportion of applicants at low risk; and sensitivity

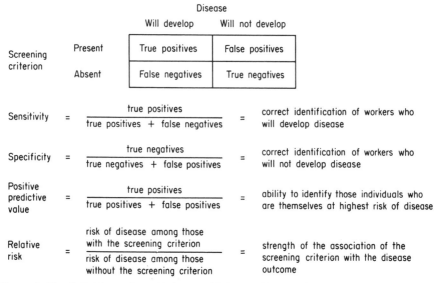

Figure 5–10. Definitions of sensitivity, specificity, positive predictive value, and relative risk applied to preemployment screening. From Tibblin et al. (24).

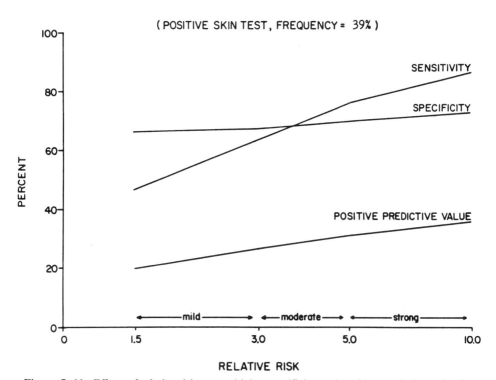

Figure 5–11. Effects of relative risk on sensitivity, specificity, and positive predictive value for screening criterion of a positive allergen skin test.

helps to identify a large proportion of applicants at high risk. These parameters cannot be maximized at the same time. They depend on the frequency of the criterion, the disease frequency, and the strength of the association of the screening criterion with the disease outcome (relative risk).

For purposes of this discussion, the following assumptions are made: (a) the cumulative incidence of asthma to laboratory animals is 15%; (b) the frequency of positive allergen skin tests among job applicants is 39% (from our data); and (c) the frequency of hyperreactive airways among job applicants is 26%. These frequency estimates (b and c) are derived from the 225 study subjects (of 305) who were in the first year of employment in their current job. This figure approximates the frequency in the job applicant pool. The strength of the association (relative risk) of these criteria with asthma to laboratory animals is not known. Therefore several calculations of relative risk from 1.5 (mild association) to 10.0 (strong association) can be made.

In the example of screening for a positive skin test with a criterion frequency of 39%, it can be seen from Figure 5–11 that specificity, the correct identification of workers who will not develop disease, is generally constant at 65 to 72% in association with relative risk. Sensitivity, the correct identification of workers who will develop

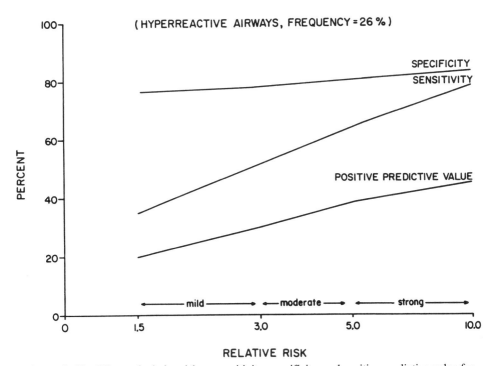

RELATIVE RISK AND SENSITIVITY, SPECIFICITY, AND POSITIVE PREDICTIVE VALUE

Figure 5–12. Effects of relative risk on sensitivity, specificity, and positive predictive value for screening criterion of hyperreactive airways.

disease, rises rapidly with relative risk. Sensitivity increases from 46% at a relative risk of 1.5 to 85% at a relative risk of 10.0. However, the positive predictive value, the ability to identify those individuals who are themselves at highest risk of disease, is low, reaching no more than 35% with a relative risk of 10.0.

The criterion, hyperreactive airways, with a frequency of 26% is more specific and less sensitive than the criterion of a positive allergen skin test (Fig. 5–12). The positive predictive value of airway hyperreactivity to methacholine is probably better than the allergen skin test, yet it remains below 50% at a relative risk of 10.0. If a combination of the two criteria is indeed strongly associated with occupational asthma, as Table 5–2 suggests, screening for this combination may have high potential for use in a screening program intended to identify those workers who are themselves at highest risk of disease, i.e., positive predictive value (Fig. 5–13).

All of these estimates of sensitivity, specificity, and positive predictive value depend on the relative risk, i.e., the association of the criterion with the disease. At this time, the relative risk estimates are based on insufficient evidence. For that reason it is concluded that preemployment screening for risk factors for the development of asthma

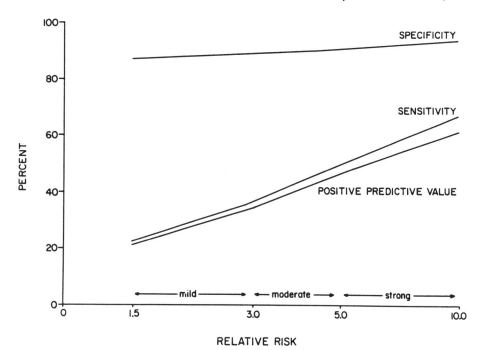

RELATIVE RISK AND SENSITIVITY, SPECIFICITY, AND POSITIVE PREDICTIVE VALUE

(HYPERREACTIVE AIRWAYS AND POSITIVE SKIN TEST, FREQUENCY = 16 %)

Figure 5–13. Effects of relative risk on sensitivity, specificity, and positive predictive value for screening by the criteria of positive allergen skin tests and hyperreactive airways combined.

to laboratory animals is not yet warranted and would not be recommended until firmer data regarding the evaluation of relative risks are available.

SUMMARY

Occupational health and productivity are affected by conditions of the work environment and by the biological susceptibility of the workers. Biological susceptibility is related to genetic and environmental factors. It is important to estimate biological susceptibility in order to define and thus predict the risk of individuals prior to their developing progressive or irreversible disease. To illustrate how it is done, we have referred to three studies designed to assess biological susceptibility.

The first study centered on physiological evaluations performed in small numbers of well defined groups exposed to variable but controlled environmental stress. From this study it was concluded that age and fitness level, but not gender, are major contributing factors in the responses to exercise or physical stress. Inasmuch as the working population includes older subjects, and because physical fitness can be modified, these factors deserve careful consideration when assessing biological susceptibility in occupations where physical stress is an important feature.

The second study centered on epidemiological evaluations of lung disease in large groups of individuals with varying genetic and environmental backgrounds. From this study it was concluded that genetically determined factors (e.g., gender, blood type, protease inhibitory capacity) and environmental factors (e.g., socioeconomic status, smoking) determine risk for the development of lung disease. Because working populations are frequently exposed to airborne toxic insults that affect the lungs, genetic and environmental risk factors should be considered in the evaluation of biological susceptibility to lung disease in an occupational setting.

The third study centered on a group of workers with environmental, job-related airborne exposures to animal dander. This study concluded that atopy and airways hyperresponsiveness are important risk factors for the development of occupational asthma. These factors are biological indicators of susceptibility that can be assessed when an individual enters the workforce. They provide attractive approaches for estimating the risk of developing lung disease in an individual who begins employment as an animal handler. Despite extensive knowledge concerning the risk of groups of individuals when placed in an occupational setting, the ability to screen for and to estimate individual risk is limited. Indeed, if serious mistakes based on clinical impressions are to be avoided, more detailed and rigorous estimates of specificity, sensitivity, and positive predictive values for biological indicators of susceptibility are needed.

REFERENCES

1. Ashley, F., Kannel, W. B., Sorlie, P. D., & Masson, R. (1975). Pulmonary function: relation to aging, cigarette habit, and mortality. *Annals of Internal Medicine, 82,* 739–45.
2. Avellini, B. A., Kamon, E., & Krajewski, J. T. (1980). Physiological responses of physically fit men and women to acclimation to humid heat. *Journal of Applied Physiology: Respiratory Environmental and Exercise Physiology, 49,* 254–61.
3. Beaty, T. H., Cohen, B., Newill, C., Menkes, H. A., Diamond, E. L., & Chen, C. J. (1982). Impaired pulmonary function as a risk factor for mortality. *American Journal of Epidemiology, 116,* 102–13.
4. Beaty, T. H., Menkes, H. A., Cohen, B. H., &

Newill, C. A. (1984). Risk factors associated with longitudinal change in pulmonary function. *American Review of Respiratory Disease, 129*, 660–67.

5. Bittle, J., & Henane, R. (1975). Comparison of thermal exchanges in men and women under neutral and hot conditions. *Journal of Physiology, 250*, 475–89.

6. Britt, E. J., Cohen, B., Menkes, H., Bleecker, E., Permutt, S., Rosenthal, R., & Norman, P. (1980). Airways reactivity and functional deterioration in relatives of COPD patients. *Chest, 77*, 260–1.

7. Buskirk, E. R., & Hodgson, J. L. (1987). Age and aerobic power: the rate of change in men and women. *Federation Proceedings, 46*, 1824–9.

8. Cohen, B. H. (1980). Chronic obstructive pulmonary disease: a challenge in genetic epidemiology. *American Journal of Epidemiology, 112*, 274–88.

9. Cohen, B. H., Ball, W. C., Jr., Bias, W. B., et al. (1975). A genetic-epidemiologic study of chronic obstructive pulmonary disease. I. Study design and preliminary observations. *Johns Hopkins Medical Journal, 137*, 95–104.

10. Cohen, B. H., Ball, W. C., Jr., Brashears, S., et al. (1977). Risk factors in chronic obstructive pulmonary disease (COPD). *American Journal of Epidemiology, 105*, 223–32.

11. Cohen, B. H., Diamond, E. L., Graves, C. G., et al. (1977). A common familial component in lung cancer and chronic obstructive pulmonary disease. *Lancet, 2*, 523–6.

12. Convertino, V. A. (1983). Heart rate and sweat rate responses associated with exercise-induced hypervolemia. *Medicine and Science in Sports and Exercise, 15*, 77–82.

13. Ellis, F. P., Nelson, F., & Pincus, L. (1975). Mortality during heat waves in New York City: July, 1972 and August-September, 1973. *Environmental Research, 10*, 1–13.

14. Friedman, G. D., Klatsky, A. L., & Siegelaub, A. B. (1976). Lung function and risk of myocardial infarction and sudden cardiac death. *New England Journal of Medicine, 294*, 1071–5.

15. Higgins, M. W., & Keller, J. B. (1970). Predictors of mortality in the adult population of Tecumseh. *Archives of Environmental Health, 21*, 418–24.

16. Kawahata, A. (1960). Sex differences in sweating. In H. Yoshimura, K. Ogata, and S. Itoh (eds.). *Essential problems in climatic physiology* (pp. 169–84). Kyoto: Nankodo Publishing Company.

17. Lutsky, I., Kalbfleisch, J. H., & Fink, J. N. (1983). Occupational allergy to laboratory animals: employer practices. *Journal of Occupational Medicine, 25*, 372–6.

18. Menkes, H. A., Beaty, T., Cohen, B., & Weinmann, G. (1985). Nitrogen washout and mortality. *American Review of Respiratory Disease, 132*, 115–19.

19. Newill, C. A., Evans III, R., & Khoury, M. J. (1986). Preemployment screening for allergy to laboratory animals: epidemiologic evaluation of its potential usefulness. *Journal of Occupational Medicine, 28*, 1158–64.

20. Newill, C. A., Khoury, M. J., & Chase, G. A. (1986). Epidemiological approach to the evaluation of genetic screening in the workplace. *Journal of Occupational Medicine, 28*, 1108–11.

21. Phillips, P. A., Rolls, B. J., Ledingham, J. G. G., Forsling, M. L., Morton, J. J., Crowe, M. J., & Wollner, L. (1984). Reduced thirst after water deprivation in healthy elderly men. *New England Journal of Medicine, 311*, 753–9.

22. Roberts, M. F., Wenger, C. B., Stolwijk, J. A. J., & Nadel, E. R. (1977). Skin blood flow and sweating changes following exercise training and heat acclimation. *Journal of Applied Physiology: Respiratory Environmental and Exercise Physiology, 43*, 133–7.

23. Strydom, N. B., Wyndham, C. H., Williams, C. G., Morrison, J. F., Bredell, G. A. G., Benade, A. J. S., & Von Rahden, M. (1966). Acclimatization to humid heat and the role of physical conditioning. *Journal of Applied Physiology, 21*, 636–42.

24. Tibblin, G., Wilhelmsen, L., & Werko, L. (1975). Risk factors for myocardial infarction and death due to ischemic heart disease and other causes. *American Journal of Cardiology, 35*, 514–22.

6
Screening and Monitoring for Susceptibility and Health: Techniques for Assessing Exposure and Response

Genevieve M. Matanoski

Occupational medicine specialists in industry once attended to illnesses among workers regardless of whether those illnesses were job-induced. As in any clinical practice, the physician provided individualized care to the patient who had identified himself or herself as ill. Times have changed, however, and industry today has allotted health care a surveillance role. In this situation, all workers are monitored for the potential or actual presence of disease. This approach to health involves the discipline of epidemiology. The total population of workers, most of whom are healthy, is the target of constant monitoring. Evaluation of rates of disease and of statistical differences between the working population and a comparison group or between subsets among the workers is the focus of the health program. The epidemiological issues related to screening of populations, such as ethics, cost-effectiveness of long-term programs, appropriate models for predicting the future prevention of disease in the population, become important considerations. Because the total population is the focus of study, variations in host characteristics and exposures are major points of emphasis.

At present, all testing of worker populations tends to be classified under the single term "screening." However, some tests actually measure the presence of an environmental agent, e.g., lead. Other tests determine potential host susceptibility to disease, e.g., sickle cell trait. Still other tests measure suspected early stage disease, e.g., cytological abnormalities. Others simply determine physiological changes that probably bear some relation to disease, e.g., cholesterol level and coronary heart disease. In some cases the relation between the test and the disease is less direct than that, for example, between cytological changes and cancer. Each of these types of testing requires different considerations regarding course of action, ethics, use in predicting disease, and evaluation of effectiveness. This chapter discusses some of the techniques for testing in occupational settings and the basic differences between the various methods of testing and the expected long-term results of using the programs. The

discussion emphasizes the principles of epidemiology that apply to these health surveillance programs.

MONITORING FOR EXPOSURE

Exposure measurements are the most straightforward types of testing. Commonly,
exposure testing in the past took the form of direct sampling of agents in work areas
where the materials might be present. Less frequently, personal sampling of individuals
throughout a working day was used to assess exposure. With the exception of radiation
monitoring, in which all individuals in the workplace are given badges, most environmental sampling has not focused on measuring the exposure of each worker. In fact, in
most cases, when assessing past exposures of individuals, epidemiologists have had to
rely on samples obtained in a haphazard manner, usually where it was convenient to
test or where potential problem exposures had been identified. The samples were
collected without regard to biostatistical issues such as variance. Thus little attention
was given to the number and location of collected samples, which would be necessary
to characterize the worker's environment within a narrow range of variation. The
industrial hygienists are increasingly aware of the need to provide sufficient samples at
appropriate locations to characterize the working population (4). However, personal
sampling, using an instrument to measure the external environment of each individual
worker, is still infrequently used. Although there may be variation in external exposures for individuals in the same work area, the differences are often predictable
based on the specific location of the worker at the site. The only problem is that
personal control devices and local area controls may alter individual worker exposures.
Therefore external measures based on area or even individual personal sampling have
been considered crude assessments of the true internal dose of each subject.

Biological monitoring involves the testing of tissues or body fluids from all
potentially exposed individuals for the presence of the hazardous substance or its
metabolic by-products. Blood or urine samples are the usual sources of test materials.
For most biological testing, each individual in the potentially exposed population
undergoes the test rather than sampling a few representative workers whose levels
characterize an entire exposure area. Biological monitoring may produce extensive
variation in results. The sources of variation include environmental changes in the
substance, multiple sources of the agent, and physiological differences in the host's
handling of the material. The importance of these sources of variation when planning
and interpreting biological monitoring is the focus of the following discussion.

ENVIRONMENTAL FACTORS
INFLUENCING BIOLOGICAL MONITORING

Before considering the host factors that introduce variability, it is important to consider
the environmental factors that can influence the results of biological monitoring. The
interaction of multiple substances in the environment may influence the composition of
materials presented to the subject and thus the type and level of material that may be
detected in biological tests. These interactions can be chemical, physical, or both. The
simplest example that frequently is overlooked is the oxidation of a substance in the

atmosphere. For example, reactive oxidative agents such as arsenic or chromium are reduced quickly to more stable substances (9). Each form of a substance may be handled differently by the human's metabolism and storage. Likewise, concerns have been raised regarding the toxicity of formaldehyde as it relates to the surrounding physical environment. Although this highly reactive agent is rapidly changed into formate or formic acid in tissues, questions arise whether binding of the gas to particles in the environment may prevent its rapid breakdown (2). Thus an exact characterization of the kinetics of the multiple agents in the environment and how they present to the worker are essential steps before biological monitoring is attempted.

The results of environmental monitoring are usually reported as a time-weighted average for an 8-hour day and possibly a peak value. Whereas a daily average is important in setting standards, the dose rate also may be an important consideration if we wish to explain differences in measured levels in individuals. Overloading the human system at any point in time could change biological pathways of chemical detoxification. Repair mechanisms and tolerance of biological systems could be overwhelmed. For example, massive loading of particles into the lungs could change clearance mechanisms in the respiratory tract (7). Thus the amount of substance that can be detected by biologically monitoring the individual may vary by dose rate independent of the environmental average daily dose.

OTHER FACTORS INFLUENCING RESULTS
OF BIOLOGICAL MONITORING

Even in situations in which we are aware of the agent's environmental form and dose rate, we must still consider the feasibility of testing for that agent. Biological monitoring has been useful in the past for metal exposures. In general, these materials occur naturally in humans at low levels. Thus detection of the agents at more than trace levels in an individual indicates an unusual exposure. The task of studying the toxicokinetics of these substances has been relatively straightforward; sites of storage are identifiable because the original metal can be measured. However, even in this situation, it is necessary to consider the human factors that may change the apparent level of the substance. For example, the deposition of lead in bones depends on the turnover rates of the bone structure. Age, sex, hemoglobin level, and physical activity of the subjects may play a role in bone deposition, which in turn would influence the level of lead detected at other sites of storage and in transport systems, such as in the blood and urine. Thus blood lead, although closely correlated with lead intake, may be influenced by individual host variability. The individual's total lead burden is represented not only by the current blood lead levels but by all the accumulated lead at storage sites. When interpreting the results of monitoring for such a substance, we must determine what test represents toxicity for the subject and how levels at other sites may act to change the test results, e.g., the factors that may activate lead stores and raise a nontoxic to a toxic blood lead level.

Organic chemical exposures present further difficulties. Such chemicals may be difficult to trace in human systems because they often are metabolized to compounds that are natural by-products. For example, detection of formaldehyde is difficult because humans form formaldehyde during normal metabolism; and once formed, all formaldehyde quickly converts to formic acid. Measuring a small excess of formaldehyde over a background level is not a simple task. The toxicokinetics of the substance in the human may be difficult to determine. The use of radioactively labeled compounds in animal models may provide limited information on human metabolism. However, methods of detoxification of chemicals in animal systems may not be the same as in humans. The classic example is the case of 2-naphthylamine, which causes bladder cancers in humans. This substance is not metabolized to the toxic orthoaminophenol in most animal species; humans and dogs handle the chemical in a similar way (14).

Individuals may vary from one another in regard to the enzyme systems available to metabolize chemicals. These differences might be referred to as genetic host variability or susceptibility. The best known examples of these problems come from the field of pharmacology. For example, patients given isoniazid (INH) for tuberculosis treatment accumulate different levels of the drug depending on their ability to inactivate the drug through acetylation. The U.S. population, both Blacks and Whites, have an equal distribution of rapid and slow isoniazid inactivators. Eskimos and Orientals, on the other hand, are all rapid inactivators. Because one-half the U.S. population accumulate high levels of the drug and thus are subject to toxic neuropathy and possibly other side effects, all patients should be treated as if they are slow inactivators (8). The relation between the genetic constitution of an individual and his or her handling of drugs is referred to as pharmacogenetics. Less is known about whether similar relations between chemical metabolism and genetic susceptibility can explain individual differences in toxicity from workplace exposures. It is likely that genetic differences in detoxification of chemicals may explain some of the variation in levels seen in exposed workers.

Host factors other than genetics can also influence chemical levels in biological monitoring of populations. Blood lead levels appear to be higher in children than adults. Some of this difference may be due to the rapid turnover of stored lead. Sex may play a role because of variation in physiological characteristics or other factors (10).

Individual differences in the level of an agent could arise if activation of an enzyme has occurred because of the presence of another exposure. Personal characteristics of individuals, such as smoking, alcohol consumption, and exposure to other agents, may activate the P-450 liver enzyme system, for example, which in turn could facilitate breakdown of chemicals found in the workplace. This situation too could lead to individual variability in the results of biological monitoring.

When individual biological measurements of agents showed variation in the past, the emphasis has been on trying to explain the differences on the basis of exposure. Attention must also focus on the host variation in handling the chemical.

Biological measurements should play a major role in monitoring worker populations for potential toxicity. Direct assessment of the exposure level within the individual is the relevant measure of the risk related to an agent regardless of the source of the agent (industry, home, hobbies) or its interaction with host characteristics. What must be considered is the implication of such monitoring in industrial populations. How much variation results from individual differences in the handling of an agent? When individuals are above the norm for the population, the steps now include investigation of specific workplace and nonindustrial exposures. If this action does not indicate another source of the agent, how far should industry carry investigations of host characteristics that may influence these levels? This research could be important in identifying individuals who are at high risk of excess exposure to toxic agents even with optimum environmental controls.

EXPOSURES LESS AMENABLE TO BIOLOGICAL MONITORING

As more is understood about the metabolism of chemicals, the development of biological markers of exposure will increase. However, although chemical exposures may be measured by either environmental sampling or biological monitoring, exposure to physical agents such as radiation, electromagnetic fields, and physical forces are still measured primarily via environmental sampling of exposures or assessment of outcomes. The measurement of ionizing radiation exposure has been carefully standardized. There are even methods of measuring the biological stores of internal emitters. Interest in potential risks of cancer from exposure to electromagnetic fields has led to the development of an instrument that records on a miniature computer the changes in fields over an 8-hour period (EMDEX Instrument, Electric Power Research Institute, 1987). These recorded variations in electromagnetic field strengths are then downloaded to a larger computer from which cumulative dose, dose rate, peak levels, and other measures are calculated. This instrument is being used in current studies of communication workers as well as in other studies of exposed workers in the electric power industry. Future adaptations of this instrument should reduce its size to that of a wristwatch, which would widen the potential for individual exposure assessment. Unlike the situation with ionizing radiation where chromosome breaks are considered to be an early measure of outcome, there are no established persistent biological effects related to low level exposure to electromagnetic fields. Therefore it is essential to have a reliable environmental measure of exposure.

In The Johns Hopkins University study of amateur boxers (13), the investigators were faced with the problem of developing an environmental measure for a physical force to link with the neurological assessment of function, which is an outcome measure. Final work is in progress on developing an accelerometer the size of a die that can fit into the boxer's mouthpiece. This device should solve the problem of measuring a physical force when no tool for biological monitoring of the force is possible. This development may prove useful for other acute impact situations in individuals. It may also be adaptable to other types of physical impact, such as a slow continuous force.

Despite the extensive pursuit of biological measures of exposure, we still need to use external environmental measures for several important exposures. However, these measures too are being developed to use on individual workers to characterize personal exposures. In such cases the variability of individual measurements will be larger than if environment area sampling were used, but it still will not be as widely variant as biological tests where host characteristics play a role. In any case, the physician, epidemiologist, and biostatistician are likely to be involved increasingly in the future to provide interpretation and analysis of data that involve extremes, outliers, and subgroup evaluation.

SCREENING POPULATIONS

Screening must be considered a separate activity with a purpose different from that of biological monitoring for exposure. Screening measures a physiological dysfunction in subjects. It may include such tests as cytology for the early detection of cancer or spirometry for impaired lung function. In the past, the term "screening" was limited to testing for conditions known to be predictors of eventual disease. The tests had to identify conditions that through early treatment or removal from exposure would prevent serious illness, long-term disability, or death from the disease. The role of screening in occupational health programs has expanded this concept to include testing for: (a) genetic traits that are permanent characteristics; (b) chromosome abnormalities and sister chromatid exchange that have an indefinite relation with specific cancer risks; and (c) existing disease, such as back problems that might alter the worker's vulnerability to injury.

Epidemiologists have established principles that relate to screening of healthy populations. Eddy enunciated the implications of rescreening for cancer in populations and discussed the ethical and financial problems related to this practice (5). These principles apply to programs for health surveillance in workers. Industrial populations are generally closed groups with a small proportion of the workforce terminating annually and being replenished with new, young workers. Most workers have repeated tests over many years. The information on changes in the individual's tests over time and the factors that predict eventual disease in a previously healthy population are important data for evaluation.

Screening for prevention is a relatively new area of medicine. There are several principles distinguishing it from clinical practice. The population is generally healthy, and thus "disease" or "abnormality" is defined on the basis of the results of a test. Screening identifies a condition in the host regardless of the cause of that condition. Therefore it does not tie exposure to the measured outcome in the individual. The purposes of various screening tests differ. Those that detect physiological changes or early disease in the subjects, e.g., lung function testing, versus those that measure hereditary characteristics, e.g., deficits in lung enzyme function, carry different implications for relating exposures and outcomes.

Screening for Host Susceptibility

Screening for host susceptibility may be appropriate in industries in which there is potential exposure to hazardous substances. The purpose of such testing would be the detection of individuals who, by hereditary predisposition or preexisting conditions, have an increased risk of disease when exposed to specific substances. This type of prescreening is already used by industry in employment examinations for appropriate job placement. This screening needs to be done only once to identify the susceptible individuals and eliminate their exposure to potential hazards. Often, however, it is not known if the test has actually identified a susceptible individual (12, pp. 98–99). Do individuals with the hereditary hemoglobin abnormality thalassemia have an increased risk of blood disease when exposed to benzene (6)? Does an individual with a history of joint pains have an increased risk of back injuries on the job?

The scientific community is moving toward the development of tools that can detect individual susceptibility, especially that which is genetically predetermined (15). Some examples were already presented in the discussion of pharmacogenetic susceptibility to toxicity. In that section, we addressed the problem of hereditary traits playing a role in the detoxification and accumulation of agents. There are also genetic traits, however, that increase the susceptibility to disease without altering the agent. One important example to consider is that of the genetically determined deficiency of α_1-antitrypsin, which plays a role in panlobular emphysema. Serum immunoelectrophoresis is used to classify the protease inhibition (Pi) system. Normal individuals are designated as PiM and have normal levels of antitrypsin. Homozygotes for the deficiency allele PiZ have low levels of antitrypsin and are known to have associated emphysema in adults and liver disease in children. Other individuals have inherited other Pi types with intermediate antitrypsin function. Heterozygotes who have deficient Pi systems may be at increased risk of emphysema because of their inability to protect the lung against endogenous enzyme activity. Whereas the homozygote with PiZ presents early with disease and thus is not a likely candidate for employment in dusty occupations, individuals with less severe forms of the disorder may not show overt signs during early life. It is unknown if these individuals with compromised pulmonary physiology are susceptible to workplace dusts or chemical agents.

Other examples of hereditary disorders that might deserve consideration in future employment screening include glucose-6-phosphate dehydrogenase (G-6-PD) deficiency, which is a disorder of erythrocytes common to persons of African and Mediterranean descent. Hemolytic anemia as well as other manifestations may occur in individuals with this disorder when exposed to primaquine, vitamin K, fava beans, and other substances. There is limited information about whether this abnormality, which occurs in about 10% of males and 1% of females with these ethnic backgrounds, triggers manifestations of disease following workplace chemical exposures. There is in vitro evidence that aromatic amino and nitro compounds such as naphthalene and TNT may cause a problem (12, pp. 90–91). Investigators have suggested that in selected populations, e.g., black men, in whom the prevalence of the deficiency is high, screening should be done before exposing them to welding fumes or hemolytic chemicals (3).

Most screening tests for genetic susceptibility are practical only when the prevalence of the trait is high. Thus genetic screening must be tailored to fit the ethnic characteristics of the available employee pool. In addition, for many of these genetic conditions the associations between an increased risk of occupationally induced disease and genetic susceptibility are limited. More information is needed from countries other than the United States: The pure characteristics of the genetic pool of another country may increase the prevalence of the genetic trait and the probability of identifying an existing association.

Many of the screening tests are complicated and time-consuming, and so their use has been limited. The Departments of Biochemistry and Epidemiology at Johns Hopkins have been jointly involved in research that has developed a relatively simple test for identifying deficits in the endonuclease needed to repair DNA (1). It is known that patients with xeroderma pigmentosa are at increased risk of skin cancer when exposed to ultraviolet (UV) light. All of their cells have the same genetic susceptibility, but because only skin cells are exposed to UV light cancers occur predominantly at that site. It has been possible to develop a test for DNA repair deficit using peripheral lymphocytes. The cells are transfected with a UV damaged plasmid containing a marker foreign to human cells. The ability of the cells to repair the plasmid DNA in the next generation is a measure of excision repair proficiency. The test is simple and can be performed rapidly. It is postulated that "normal" individuals may have variation in the level of repair capacity. If so, we may eventually be able to relate this repair deficit to the risk of cancer (12, pp. 96–97).

What is the future for these tests of host susceptibility in job placement? General tests used in the past have been practical only for preexisting disease. Hereditary screening could become important if the screening test is simple and can be done on readily available body materials, which has not been the case in many situations in the past. The second factor to consider is the frequency of the defect in the population. If the disease is rare and manifests only in homozygotes (not in heterozygotes), screening is impractical. If heterozygotes exhibit an intermediate form of the disease, use of a screening test to detect heterozygotes or minor stages of the defect in normals, as may be the case with endonuclease repair deficit, may be important. Furthermore, in industries that may employ a large number of workers with a high frequency of the hereditary trait, the cost efficiency of screening will be increased.

Screening for Nongenetic Conditions

The usual screening test does not detect a permanent condition such as a genetic trait but identifies a point in a progressively changing physiological or pathological state. For that reason, individuals must be repeatedly rescreened to determine changes in that state that eventually might constitute "disease." However, because the screenee is healthy, the provider must decide on the definition of "disease." Whatever severity of change is selected as "disease," individuals will be found who reach that level of severity on one occasion but subsequently revert to less serious states. Therefore we are dealing with a dynamic process.

In addition, many characteristics selected for screening, e.g., blood pressure, hearing, and respiratory function, are known to demonstrate progressive change with increasing age. In the past, we have defined an "action point," which is some predetermined level of function as measured by the test that triggers either treatment of the person or his or her removal from exposure. Methods of analyzing data by rate of change in function and subsequent use of these measures to predict disease require new techniques in the field of epidemiology and biostatistics; and they will become important for screening programs in industry. For example, a rapid decrement in pulmonary function may be a better and earlier predictor of future problems of chronic lung disease than is a fixed level of impaired pulmonary function defined by the age and sex of individuals.

These screening tests simply measure stages of disease without tying the results to a causative agent. This situation is in contrast to the tests described previously in which one detects the presence of a potentially hazardous material in human tissue, an agent-specific adduct of DNA, or a metabolic product. Multiple agents can cause the same screening results. If one is simply trying to prevent disease in a population, as may be the case in a health promotion program, it is not a problem. If, however, one is trying to determine which cases are industrially related in order to develop environmental controls, it is important. Cytological abnormalities of lung cells cannot be attributed directly to smoking, infections, or workplace asbestos exposures of individuals. Epidemiological analyses of data from persons with and without each of these exposures can determine the relative contribution of the occupational agent for the group but not for an individual. Unfortunately, workplace screening programs often do not include occupationally unexposed workers; so there is no information on a comparison group. All abnormalities then tend to be attributed to the industrial agent, as the contribution of the other exposures to the outcome cannot be identified.

Epidemiological Principles Applied to Screening

No screening test can predict with 100% certainty the individuals who do and do not have disease. Cytological screening for cancer is one of the better tests because cells are directly examined for precancerous and cancerous changes. Such lesions should represent an early stage of cancer and, depending on the specific point in the natural history of the cancer at which the abnormal cells can be detected, might represent a reversible lesion or one that could be treated to prevent overt disease. Even cytology is limited in regard to the types of cancer that can be detected by this means. Other screening tests, such as chromosome abnormalities and sister chromatid exchange, are often considered early tests for cancer. They fall into a class of abnormalities, however, that are not clearly predictive of a cancer outcome. These abnormalities may identify an exposure to certain carcinogens as radiation and chromosome damage. However, the frequency of chromosomal aberrations declines within a few cell generations. In most situations, it is not clear where these abnormalities fit in the natural history of disease.

Because no test is 100% effective in identifying individuals with and without disease, epidemiologists characterize screening tests by the terms sensitivity and specificity. *Sensitivity* is a measure of the proportion of the persons with disease who test positive, as shown in Figure 6–1. Thus of those with the disease, a portion test positive and others falsely negative. *Specificity* is a measure of the proportion of persons without the disease who test negative, as shown in Figure 6–2. Usually screening defines disease by selecting an arbitrary cut-off point along a continuum of test values, and this cut-off point is supposed to separate a population into diseased and non-diseased groups. It is possible to change the sensitivity and specificity by simply changing this point. Any alteration in the value that redivides the population as classified by the test is reflected by opposing effects in sensitivity and specificity. For example, if we decide to offer dietary behavioral modification to individuals at a lower screening level of cholesterol than a currently accepted cut-off point, we identify a higher proportion of those who may have incipient heart disease. However, we also include in the programs an increased number and proportion of individuals who will never develop the disease because we have lowered the specificity of the screening test. This fact may not be a serious problem when the disease carries no stigma and the intervention (e.g., dietary modification) causes no serious side effects. These problems are more severe if the test screens for a disease such as cancer and a positive test results in the need for extensive diagnostic testing.

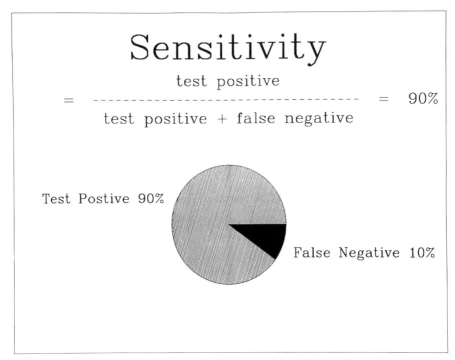

Figure 6–1. Sensitivity: the probability that a screening test will identify persons with disease.

As a general rule, the earlier the stage of detection in the natural history of disease, the less specific is a test in identifying individuals with future disease. It is especially true for tests that measure a changing physiological state such as pulmonary function. The capacity of the lung to exchange air can be measured by the forced expiratory volume within a fixed time period, e.g., 1 minute (FEV_1). Extensive testing of adults and children are used to determine not only if there are existing lung abnormalities, but also if individuals who fall on the extremes of the test distribution for the population are the ones who eventually have compromised lung function. For example, a child with a minor deficit in FEV_1 compared to the child with "normal" or average function for that age may not develop respiratory disease during adulthood. In fact, among the group of children who have a deficit at any point in time, some return to normal levels of function subsequently and others remain in the low percentiles of test results. How can we then use this test as a predictor of disease, as there would be many false positives? In fact, deficits during childhood may not foretell eventual disease. On the other hand, a screening test in adults, such as production of morning sputum for 3 months in a year, is considered a good predictor of individuals who will eventually have compromised respiratory function (11).

Recognizing this problem, the medical community has resorted to the use of multiple tests to reduce the problem of false positives. To classify a person as diseased, an individual must be positive on two or more screening tests. For example, multiple elevations of blood pressure are required before further diagnostic procedures are undertaken. Whereas this practice eliminates the false positives and increases the

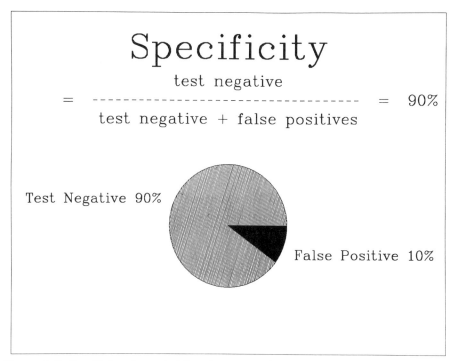

Figure 6–2. Specificity: the probability that a screening test will identify persons without disease.

specificity, it also reduces sensitivity, so some of the individuals with disease are missed.

What do these facts mean to those who may institute screening programs in a population? If the test does not specifically relate an outcome to the occupational exposure of interest, detected cases will include background cases as well as those related to the industrial agent. Instituting control of exposure eradicates some cases of disease but not all. Thus background cases continue to occur. It may be difficult to determine if they represent a "normal," or expected, number of cases of early disease in the general population, as comparable screening programs often are not available to establish the level of disease.

Predictive Value of Screening Tests in the Working Population

The capacity of the screening test to predict disease is another important facet to consider before undertaking a long-term program in a working population for the purpose of assessing health. The problems with such programs are similar to those found in the general population. If the prevalence of the disease is low, the predictive value of a positive test, i.e., the test's ability to distinguish persons with the disease from among all of those with positive tests, may be low. The predictive value of a test is defined by the number of individuals with incipient disease who test positive out of the total who test positive, i.e., the true positives and the false positives. Working populations differ somewhat from a general population in that they are relatively closed groups. Young, healthy workers enter the work force and are screened, and many terminate employment within a short time. Any working population that has a young average age necessarily has a low rate of chronic disease. The predictive value of a screening program is thus low.

Workers who are likely to have positive tests in a screening program are those who remain in the work force into advanced ages, often until retirement. At that point, screening stops. This aging, working population is continuously rescreened. Even in this group, with any program that screens for chronic disease in an active population the prevalence or frequency of the disease is low, as is the predictive value of the test.

Rescreening Workers

The issues of rescreening in closed, industrial populations must be carefully considered before undertaking these programs. Figures 6–3, 6–4, and 6–5 examine a hypothetical population of 10,000 workers that has no new entries into the workforce over the period of three screenings. For example, this screening program might be aimed at stable workers over age 40. When the program is first instituted, all stages of disease exist in the population, from incipient to advanced disease, and they are identified in the first wave of screening. In this example, the prevalence of disease initially is high, with 20% of the population having the disease, such as might occur with hypertension. If the test were 90% sensitive and 90% specific, 18% of the population would test positive and have the disease, and 8% would test positive and not have the disease.

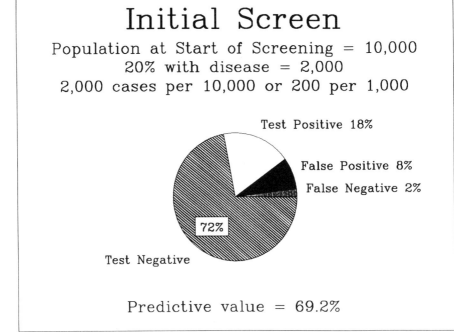

Figure 6–3. Classification of persons by test results after first screening.

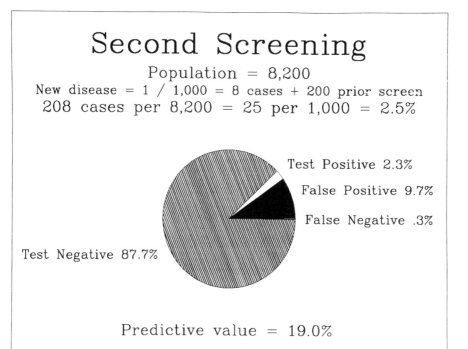

Figure 6–4. Classification of persons by test results after second screening.

(The latter figure occurs because the specificity is 90%; therefore 10% of the 80% nondiseased population is called positive incorrectly.) Two percent of the population test negative even though they have the disease. The overall predictive value of the test is thus 69.2% (i.e., 18% true positives divided by the 26% who test positive). This program would be considered highly effective: a large number of subjects prove to be positive (26%), and among these positives a high percent (69.2%) will be diagnosed as having disease when referred for further testing (predictive value).

In each successive screening (Figs. 6–4 and 6–5), the true cases previously diagnosed are removed, and we are left with new cases of the disease that become test-positive in the interval between tests plus the false negatives that remain from the previous screening cycle. Thus the prevalence of disease in the population decreases. In the example in Figure 6–4, with a high incidence of new cases (1/1,000) in the interval between screenings and the residual 200 false-negative cases from the initial screen, the prevalence has dropped to 2.5%. The proportion of the population that tests positive drops from 26% to 12%, as might be expected; but among those who are positive and are sent for further tests, only 19% are identified to have the disease. The example of a third screening suggests that about the same proportion of the population continue to test positive at subsequent screenings, but the proportion of positives detected with true disease, as indicated by the predictive value, is almost zero. Thus in any closed population with continuous rescreening for disease, the number of positive tests decreases slightly but the proportion of true cases among those who test positive decreases markedly. Eventually most individuals who test positive by screening will

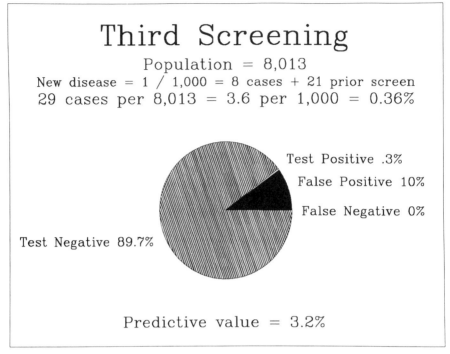

Figure 6–5. Classification of persons by test results after third screening.

not have disease, and the subsequent diagnostic workups should prove that there is no need for treatment.

With cancer screening, there has been concern about the high frequency of false positives resulting from repeated testings. There is occasionally uncertainty about the cancer diagnosis even with extensive workups, which may lead to unnecessary treatment of individuals with false-positive screening tests. This potential for overtreatment may be of less concern in industrial settings than the perception on the part of the industry that the screening program and the test itself may be useless. After the first successful screening round, the test appears unable to distinguish disease from nondisease. When the costs of the program remain relatively constant, management may find it difficult to accept that the lack of true disease among the group who test positive is the result of a successful screening program to prevent disease.

CONCLUSION

Screening and biological monitoring are developing as important future tools for providing health for workers. New tests for measuring individual environmental exposures, early disease, and genetic or predisposing disease traits are appearing in abundance. The use of each test must be carefully evaluated to decide its purpose in ensuring the health of workers. Epidemiological principles regarding detection of disease in populations must be carefully considered when evaluating the impact of such programs in working populations. Occupational medicine as practiced in industries is no longer focused only on the care of the sick. This field is now practicing epidemiology as they provide longitudinal follow-up of populations through many years. The evaluation of the predictive value of these data are important not only to industry but to the general population as well.

REFERENCES

1. Athas, W. F. (1988). *Recombinant methods for screening human DNA excision repair proficiency.* Dissertation for doctor of philosophy, Johns Hopkins University.

2. Blair, A., Stewart, P. A., Hoover, R. N., Fraumeni, J. F. J., Walrath, J., O'Berg, M., & Gaffey, W. (1987). Cancers of the nasopharynx and oropharynx and formaldehyde exposure. *Journal of the National Cancer Institute, 78,* 191.

3. Calabrese, E. J. (1978). *The biologic basis of increased human susceptibility to environmental and occupational pollutants.* New York: Wiley–Interscience.

4. Corn, M., & Esmen, N. A. (1979). Workplace exposure zones for classification of employee exposures to physical and chemical agents. *American Industrial Hygiene Association Journal, 40,* 47–57.

5. Eddy, D. M. *Screening for cancer: theory, analysis and design.* Englewood Cliffs, NJ: Prentice-Hall.

6. Goldstein, B. D. (1977). Hematotoxicity in humans. In S. Laskin and B. D. Goldstein (eds.). *Benzene toxicity* (p. 102). New York: McGraw-Hill.

7. Huang, T. W. (1967). Respiratory system. In N. K. Moffet (ed.). *Environmental pathology* (pp. 212–16). Oxford: Oxford University Press.

8. Hughes, H. B., Biehl, J. P., Jones, A. P., & Schmidt, L. H. (1954). Metabolism of isoniazid in man as related to the occurrence of peripheral neuritis. *American Review of Tuberculosis, 70,* 266.

9. International Agency for Research on Cancer.

(1980). IARC Monographs on the Evaluation of the Carcinogenic Risk of Chemicals to Human. *Some metals and metallic compounds* (Vol. 23). Lyon: International Agency for Research on Cancer.

10. McGill, H. C., Jr., & Stern, M. P. (1979). Sex and atherosclerosis. In R. Paloetti and A. M. Gotto (eds.). *Atherosclerosis reviews* (pp. 157–242). New York: Raven Press.

11. Medical Research Council. (1976). *Questionnaire on respiratory symptoms and instructions for its use.* London: MRC.

12. Office of Technology Assessment. (1983). *The role of genetic testing in the prevention of occupational disease* (Library of Congress 83-600526). Washington, DC: U.S. Government Printing Office.

13. Stewart, W., Gordis, L., Diamond, E., Selnes, O., Gordon, B., Tusa, R., & Celentano, D. (1987–87). *Amateur boxing study.* (Annual Report of The Department of Epidemiology). Baltimore: The Johns Hopkins University, School of Hygiene and Public Health.

14. Troll, W., & Belman, S. (1967). Studies on the nature of the proximal bladder carcinogens. In W. B. Deichman and K. F. Lampe (eds.). *Inter-American conference on toxicology and occupational medicine. Bladder cancer: a symposium.* Birmingham, AL: Aesculapius.

15. Vine, M. F., & McFarland, L. T. (1990). Markers of Susceptibility. In B. S. Hulka, T. C. Wilcosky, and J. D. Griffith (eds.). *Biological markers in epidemiology.* New York: Oxford University Press.

Injury Prevention in the Workplace

Susan P. Baker, Ann H. Myers, and Gordon S. Smith

Since the first decade of this century, when more than 2,500 railway employees and 2,500 coal miners were killed *each year* in the United States (20), work injury death rates have decreased dramatically. Much of the improvement has been due to labor laws, safety acts, compensation requirements, and improved medical care (49,62). Progress is still retarded, however, by continued emphasis on "accident proneness" and by the lack of integrated study of the interaction between characteristics of the worker and characteristics of the work environment (50,52). Tragically, epidemiological methods and principles are seldom applied to the problem of work injuries. As a result, progress is slower than it might have been with systematic, scientifically designed studies (13).

Recent years have witnessed increasing interest in occupational diseases and proportionally less attention to worker injuries on the part of public health researchers and the National Institute for Occupational Safety and Health (NIOSH). Yet injuries account for 98% of all reported occupational injuries and diseases. In the 17- to 64-year age group, one-fourth of all injuries (40) and one-tenth of fatal injuries occur at work. Typically, the work environment offers many opportunities for control of hazards. Although these opportunities are often ignored, the responsibilities of employers for the safety of their employees means that the work environment often is more susceptible to intervention than the home environment.

National statistics on worker injuries are meager and often discrepant. Bureau of Labor Statistics (BLS) estimates of work fatalities place the total at about 3,750 per year but exclude categories with large numbers of deaths: government workers, the self-employed, and employees in companies with fewer than 11 employees. [One study found that in Allegheny County, Pennsylvania, nearly 80% of all work injury fatalities occurred in worksites with fewer than 100 employees and 40% at worksites with fewer than 20 employees (43); other investigators have reported especially high death rates in small companies as well (9,56).] The National Safety Council (NSC), on the other hand, uses a variety of sources and includes all occupational groups in making its estimate of about 11,600 work injury fatalities each year, or 11 per 100,000 workers (42). The National Institute for Occupational Safety and Health receives reports of about 7,000 work injury deaths each year, based on death certificates that include the notation "injury at work." Estimates of annual nonfatal work injuries range from about

2 million "disabling" injuries (National Safety Council) to 11 million injuries requiring medical attention or activity restriction (National Health Interview Survey). Unlike the data presented in Table 7–1, most statistics combine so many industry subcategories the effect is to mask groups of workers having especially high rates. For example, the trucking industry has a lost time injury rate that is more than six times the rate of its parent industry, transportation and public utilities (42).

Exemplifying the many unrealized opportunities for prevention are transportation-related injuries, of special import because of their number and severity in the occupational setting. Cars and trucks are associated with one of three occupational fatalities (42) and a substantial, but largely unmeasured, portion of nonfatal work injuries. Among Baltimore City employees, who represent 8% of all employed people living in Baltimore, one of eight work-related injuries involves the use of motor vehicles. In the Baltimore Police Department, 43% of all injury costs are vehicle-related (48). Nation-

Table 7–1. Injuries of Full-Time Employees Involving Death or Days Away from Work

Industry	Category mean	Exceeds category mean
All industries	1.86	
Mining	1.18	
Metal		1.96
Coal		2.52
Manufacturing	1.59	
Machinery except electrical		1.74
Fabricated structural metal products		2.03
Paper products		2.20
Blast furnace & basic steel products		2.22
Leather		2.29
Cement		2.40
Stone, clay, glass		2.54
Food products		3.10
Paperboard containers		4.00
Meat products		4.18
Lumber, wood products (excludes furniture)		4.18
Ship building and repair		4.20
Railroad equipment		4.74
Sawmills, planing mills		5.02
Wholesale and retail trade	1.85	
Services	2.03	
Transportation	2.45	
Railroad		3.56
Water supply		5.94
Local and suburban transit		8.93
Trucking		17.55
Construction	2.93	
Public administration	3.83	
General government		4.26
State departments of transportation		4.30
Fire protection		5.36

Source: Accident Facts (1989 Ed.). Chicago: National Safety Council. Adapted from Waller (60).

wide, truck drivers are the second largest category of injured workers in the Supplementary Data System (14).

EXAMPLES OF OCCUPATIONAL INJURY PROBLEMS

Two excellent overviews of occupational injury have been written by Waller (60) and Kraus (31). Rather than attempting to duplicate their work, we illustrate points that are of major importance to the study and prevention of occupational injuries by presenting details on (a) work injury deaths in Maryland, (b) back injuries in the workforce, and (c) needlestick injuries in hospital employees.

Work Fatalities in Maryland

Our review of fatal work-related injuries in Maryland in 1978 (7) revealed major gaps in the ability of any given data source to identify the cases. Eventually, using four sources, we found 148 fatalities. (a) A death certificate search that identified all cases coded as "injury at work" missed one-third of the cases, including all homicides and many of the motor vehicle-related deaths. (b) Similarly, a Workers' Compensation list of fatalities omitted about 40% of the deaths, including all of the self-employed. (c) Fewer than one-half of the deaths were reported to Maryland's Occupational Safety and Health Administration (OSHA) officials. (d) A hand search of Medical Examiner (ME) cases initially identified about 90% and eventually was found to contain 96% of the 148 cases despite the fact that the annual ME report for the same year categorized only 72 deaths as work-related. The lack of computer-search capabilities and the difficulty of recognizing and coding many work-related deaths that occur outside the industrial setting make even the ME office an inadequate initial source of data on occupational fatalities. Improved recognition and recording of occupational fatalities would greatly increase the utility of ME data. In general, the cases most likely to be missed by all sources are those involving transportation, as "automobile accident" and "airplane crash" do not suggest a job-related death.

Organized concern with occupational safety, as reflected in regulations, training programs, and the occupational safety literature, generally emphasizes industry, especially the manufacturing industry. Perhaps as a result of this emphasis and the corresponding improvements in the safety of machinery, only one-fifth of all the work injury deaths in Maryland occurred in manufacturing, and only 5% involved fixed machinery (Table 7–2). Transportation vehicles were involved in 41% of all deaths, a matter of special interest because of the dearth of federal regulations that would provide crash protection to truck drivers and pilots. Similarly, the Occupational Safety and Health Act has ignored homicide as an occupational problem, although 11% of the deaths were from firearm homicide; in California and Texas the rates of work-related homicide are 2.2 and 2.1, respectively, per 100,000 male workers (16,17,32). Most commonly, occupational homicides involve robbery attempts at gas stations, liquor stores, convenience stores, and so on, which are not required to protect employees from assault.

Members of the military are often excluded from research using a series of deaths, perhaps because of lack of denominator information. Among the Maryland deaths were

Table 7-2. Occupational Deaths in Maryland, 1978: Fatal Event by Industry

Type of event	No. of fatal events										Total no. (%)[b]
	Manu-facturing	Con-struction	Quarrying/mining	Agriculture/fishing/forestry	Trade	Trans-portation/utilities	Services	Public	Military	Other/unknown	
Road vehicle	8	5	1	0	2	11	4	3	0	3	37 (25)
Boat	0	0	0	3	0	1	1	0	11	0	16 (11)
Airplane	0	0	0	0	1	2	0	1	2	1	7 (5)
Nonroad vehicle	11	2	0	2	1	2	1	4	0	0	23 (16)
Fixed machinery	5	0	0	2	0	0	0	0	0	1	8 (5)
Fall from height	1	9	0	2	0	0	1	0	0	0	13 (9)
Shooting	0	0	0	0	8	3	0	4	0	1	16 (11)
Other	6	5	1	3	1	3	2	3	1	3	28 (19)
Total	31	21	2	12	13	22	9	15	14	9	148 (101)[b]
Rate/100,000[a]	13	21	133	52	3	26	3	4	c	c	7

Source: Baker et al. (7).

[a]Source of denominator data: U.S. Department of Labor, Bureau of Labor Statistics, Report on Employment for 1978, Maryland; and Maryland Department of Human Resources.
[b]Does not add to 100 because of rounding.
[c]Denominator data not available.

two Navy pilots killed when the wing of their T38 jet touched the runway while making touch-and-go landings and 11 men killed when their Coast Guard cutter sank following collision with another ship. Exclusion of such cases is unfortunate because the lessons that can be learned from military tragedies are often applicable in the civilian setting. For example, the cutter sank quickly because its watertight compartments had been left open; escape from rapidly flooding crew quarters was hampered by the lack of emergency lights; and the lifejackets had all been placed in a single bin, which could not be reached because of the damage.

Most work injury deaths in Maryland involved either hazards that are not addressed by OSHA regulations or workers in categories excluded by law from regulation by OSHA: 53% of the workers killed were occupants of transportation vehicles, homicide victims, or self-employed. Clearly, the time has come to redirect the emphasis of occupational safety programs to problems that are not receiving commensurate attention.

The Maryland study is unusual in the degree to which the details of each death were reviewed and analyzed, in contrast to more typical research in which the circumstances of injury are pigeonholed into such uninformative categories as "struck by moving object."

Exemplifying the potential for injury prevention through product design, once the details of circumstances are known, were two deaths in Maryland in 1978 that resulted from the explosion of tires with multipiece wheels. Designed for pressures of 25 and 35 psi, the tires were being inflated by compressors that did not shut off until pressure reached 130 or 150 psi, respectively. Although failsafe inflation systems and single-piece wheels would probably be the most effective countermeasures to address a problem that has killed or injured hundreds of workers, OSHA and most employers have continued to rely on ineffective training and information programs (23).

Back Injuries in the Workforce

Low back injuries are the most common (25%) compensable claim by NSC industrial employees covered by state compensation claims (29,42). Low-back pain affects more than one-half of the working population at some time during their working careers (35,37). The annual rate of low-back pain for industrial workers has been estimated to be approximately 2% (54). The number of low-back injuries per 100 workers per year varies by *industry*, with construction and mining having the highest rates: 1.6 and 1.5, respectively. *Occupations* with the highest rates are miscellaneous laborers and garbage collectors: 12.3 and 11.1, respectively (29). The length of time spent in physically demanding jobs is also important (34).

The physical requirements of their jobs place certain groups of workers at high risk of low-back injury. Included are prolonged postural stress or vibration, as for miners, concrete reinforcement workers, truck and other vehicle drivers, and jackhammer operators (1,3,10,15,18,51,58,61); prolonged sitting or standing (35); and overexertion associated with maximal physical efforts, characterized by unexpectedness (36). Men filed 77 to 80% of the back injury compensation claims in 26 states. The highest rate for men (1.95 claims/100 workers) was observed for ages 20 to 24, whereas the highest female rate (0.87 claims/100 workers) was seen for ages 24 to 34. For both genders, the highest risk of compensable low-back strain/sprain occurred between ages 20 to 44 years (29).

Previous back pain is one of the best predictors of low-back pain (8). Other possible risk factors (generally with inconclusive evidence) include anthropometry (3,63), posture and musculoskeletal disorders (3,61,63), muscle strength and physical fitness (11), psychological factors (63), and social problems (3).

When a group of dockworkers was compared with a control group of clerks, the prevalence of disc changes was higher among the dock workers at all disc levels studied (T12–L5) (12). In a retrospective study, 35% of the sedentary workers and 47% of heavy materials handlers had made visits to physicians for low-back pain within a 10-year period (47). Magora's study comparing eight occupational groups found low-back pain to be more pronounced in the more physically demanding occupations and related to the period of time spent in the same occupation (35).

The costs of low-back injuries underscore the importance of research aimed at reducing these injuries.

- Approximately 1 of 10 compensable medical claims is of low-back origin (36).
- Medical care and claims for low-back sprains/strains in 26 states has been estimated at over $1 billion (29).
- Overexertion injuries associated with manual materials handling jobs account for 12 million lost workdays (41).
- Low-back pain is a major cause of industrial disability, with the work loss equivalent to a loss of wages in the United States of $4 billion per year (15).
- In most industries, low-back disability is the top item in compensation payments and ranks second only to upper respiratory infections in payout for sickness benefits (47).
- The recurrence rate for low-back symptoms during the first year has been reported to be as high as 50 to 60% (57).

Many aspects of the physical act of manually lifting a load have been identified as potentially hazardous to a person's musculoskeletal system. Some aspects have been sufficiently explored in lifting injury research to provide a strong basis for guidance (4,5,11,41). Other factors, such as spatial aspects of the task (distance moved, direction, obstacles, and postural constraints), need further investigation. Studies that include environmental factors such as temperature, humidity, illumination, vibration, and frictional stability of the foot would enhance our knowledge of the injury process so that preventive interventions can be implemented (41). Multidisciplinary research incorporating the above factors as well as worker variables, task components, and system characteristics is rare.

Snook (53) found that changing the lifting task (e.g., the size and shape of the container to be lifted) was more effective in reducing back injury than exercise or training. Other successful measures for preventing back injuries have included wheeled carriers for sanitation workers or containers that are picked up by "arms" on the garbage trucks, and stretchers for paramedics that reduce lifting stresses (33). Despite the difficulty of providing protection in many unstructured work locations, the success of such automatic protection in other settings (19) underscores the potential for progress in reducing back injury among workers. All too often, however, victim-blaming has characterized responses to the problem, and emphasis on training and education have taken precedence over more effective ergonomic and "passive" approaches that do not place the burden of prevention on the workers.

Needlestick Injuries in Hospital Employees

Injuries from needlesticks help to bridge the gap between the study of injury and disease, as the primary concern is the potential for infection, especially with hepatitis or, more rarely, the AIDS virus. Needlesticks cause one-third of all work injuries in hospital employees, and 8 to 9% of hospital employees are stuck by needles annually. Costs are estimated at about $100 per case exclusive of follow-up costs such as vaccination, immune globulin, and human immunodeficiency virus (HIV) testing (38,46).

The problem of needle injuries exemplifies the contrast between approaches that focus on employee "carelessness" in the belief that simple control measures are not followed by employees who engage in potentially dangerous behavior (30) and, on the other hand, more effective approaches that eliminate the task of needle disposal or make it safe and simple. Jagger et al. asked, "Do employees cause needlesticks by their dangerous behavior, or are they victims of inherently dangerous devices which they are required to handle under difficult circumstances?" (25).

Believing the latter to be the case, Jagger and Pearson documented the injury rates per 100,000 needles for various needled devices and the circumstances under which needlesticks occur (24). The circumstances appear to be relatively predictable rather than random, and the hazardous act of recapping needles is sometimes chosen by hospital workers who perceive it to be less hazardous than alternatives, such as carrying an uncapped needle to a disposal box. Needled devices exhibited a fivefold difference in needlestick rates per 100,000 devices; the highest rates are associated with the devices that are most likely to require the worker to move his or her hand and a needle toward one another.

Having found that currently recommended control measures such as the use of needle guards or improved disposal boxes do not effectively prevent most needle injuries among employees, Jagger and colleagues turned to the design of the hazardous devices themselves and invented needled instruments that fulfill the following basic criteria (25,26).

1. Targeted at the specific circumstances under which the injuries occur.
2. Not requiring hands to move toward contaminated needles.
3. Designed to be simple enough to use without special training or additional equipment.
4. So easy to use that workers are not tempted to ignore, circumvent, or disable the protective aspects.

Health facilities must begin to provide employees with devices that meet these recommendations. The urgency of the situation is underscored by a new report by Kelen et al., who found that 5% of all emergency room patients were HIV-positive, and that in four of five cases HIV infection had not been diagnosed (28).

PRODUCTIVITY AND INJURY PREVENTION

An injured worker presents an important drain on a company's productivity. Absence from the job, the costs of medical care and rehabilitation, and adverse effects on morale are among the company's costs.

Many factors in the workplace are common to both injury prevention and a company's productivity.

- Employee selection, training, and job assignment
- Proper record keeping of injuries and near misses
- Feedback systems to correct problems, involving workers in identifying possible solutions
- Alcoholism treatment programs
- Modifications of the physical environment—light, noise, other physical hazards
- Application of ergonomics to the design of the task and the working environment
- Well designed personal protective equipment
- Passive protection that automatically reduces the likelihood that a worker will be injured

These approaches are not always applied, but in general they are now well recognized. Two additional approaches to job safety are important but often ignored.

1. Designing the job so that the quickest way to accomplish anything is also the safest way.
2. Ensuring that productivity pressures do not create incentives or environments that increase the chance of injury.

There can be little question that an injured worker reduces productivity. Less obvious, and with scant research to determine the magnitude of the problem, is the negative effect of productivity pressures on worker safety. In any company where safety is not considered to be as important as production, attempts to increase the ratio of "product" to man-hours and other costs are likely to lead to injury, death, or even disaster. For example:

1. The quickest way to dig a trench is without shoring the sides. Almost all of the 100 trench cave-in fatalities each year in the United States result from failure to shore or slope the sides, as is required by OSHA when the ground is not stable (56).
2. A nurse can move a patient sooner—but at far greater risk to her back—if she does not wait for a second nurse to help her (59).
3. Factory workers can produce more widgets per hour when not hampered by poorly designed machine guards. Therefore guards are sometimes removed, with resulting injuries.
4. The race against weather is an inevitable part of farming. If the hay is ready for harvesting and rain is expected, an 18-hour day may end with an overturned tractor.

5. If the cornpicker jams, the quickest way to break the jam is by leaving the cornpicker's mechanism in gear while the operator gets off and wrestles with cornstalks. But when the jam breaks, the jaws of the cornpicker cannot discriminate between cornstalks and arms, and too often it sucks in both.
6. In contrast, there was a dramatic decrease in injuries among forestry workers in Sweden, when the payment basis for shiftworkers was changed from piece work, with its built-in incentive to work as fast as possible, to an hourly salary (55).

Speed

As the above examples suggest, when the quickest way is not the safest way injuries are a likely product. This result is most obvious on the highway, where the laws of physics dictate that high speed crashes are associated with far more deaths than crashes at lower speeds.

Trucks on major highways generally travel at higher average speeds than cars. One reason is that truck drivers often are paid by the trip rather than by the hour, providing a strong incentive to speed—an incentive that could be removed if they were paid for each hour on duty. Currently under Congressional consideration is a strong disincentive to speed, i.e., a requirement that interstate trucks have "black boxes" for recording speed.

Unsafe Design

Various efforts by the transportation industry to increase ton-miles or passenger miles have had negative results and are of special concern because they affect the public as well as the worker. Until 1982, most states specified a *bumper-to-bumper* maximum legal length of trucks. With the overall length thus fixed, trucking companies "robbed Peter to pay Paul," i.e., they subtracted inches or even feet from the cab or the front of the tractor and added them to the trailer to increase the payload (6). As truck tractors became shorter, truck drivers complained that they would eventually have to stand up as they drove! Indeed, some of the cab-over-engine designs, such as the infamous Ford "Louisville" tractor, had a cab so shortened that a six-foot-tall driver would find his knee against the instrument panel and the brake pedal hard to reach quickly with his foot.

The Surface Transportation Act of 1982 removed the incentives for shortened truck tractors by requiring states to limit the trailer length rather than the overall bumper-to-bumper length. At the same time, however, "doubles" (i.e., two trailers pulled by one tractor) were allowed on all interstate highways. Despite concerns as to the safety of doubles, the trucking industry argued that any increase in crash rates would be minimal and would be more than offset by greater payload. In other words, theoretically there would be fewer crashes per ton-mile.

That argument proved false. Research reported in 1987 shows that when compared to other trucks driven under similar conditions—the same road, the same time of day, and controlling for driver age—doubles have more than twice the crash involvement rate of single-trailer trucks (23). Thus although there no doubt was an increase in productivity in terms of ton-miles in relation to capital investment, there was also a net increase in crashes per ton mile. The resulting losses in lives and injuries affect all highway users, as in a collision between a car and a heavy truck the car occupants are 35 times as likely to be killed as the truck occupants (22). The consequences to the truck drivers are also grave; their occupation has an injury death rate that is even higher than the rate for farming and construction (27).

Death Rates Per Ton-Mile

Regulations that make it cheaper per ton-mile for trucks to transport cargo have an additional adverse effect on safety that goes largely unrecognized; i.e., such regulations give trucking a competitive advantage over safer forms of cargo transport. The number of deaths per ton-mile for cargo shipped by truck is higher than for any other mode of shipment and is more than three times the death rate per ton-mile for goods shipped by rail (45).[1] Thus greater priority to human life would presumably dictate that regulations give a competitive edge to rail transport and, where practical, to marine or pipeline transport. The fact that the reverse has occurred should be a matter of public health concern.

Pressures on Pilots

Air transportation provides further examples of injuries that result from overemphasis on maximizing productivity. In May 1979 the fatal crash of a Downeast Airlines commuter plane called attention to the pressures under which its pilots had been working—pressures, for example, to stick to schedules regardless of unsafe flying conditions; to fly lower than the legal minimum altitude when fog shrouded the runway; to fly aircraft with known, serious mechanical defects; to take off when overweight; to carry dangerously small fuel reserves in order to maximize the payload. In short, the company's president placed productivity and profits ahead of safety, until, almost inevitably, two pilots and fifteen passengers lost their lives (2,39).

Fatigue

The Downeast Airlines crash is probably the most carefully researched example of the pilot stress and ultimately the crashes and deaths that result from company policies aimed at operating with the fewest possible delays for weather or repairs. It is scarcely the only example, however, of unsafe practices induced by pressures to maximize passenger miles while minimizing fuel, wages, and other costs (39). Not uncommon are perfectly legal crew schedules that leave airline crews weary and at times unable to deliver the needed perfect performance. Imagine a 14-hour work day, followed by an 8-hour break and then another long day with six or eight flights in bad weather, plus the stress on pilots of delays that they know may mean substantial losses of revenue for the airline.

Even without such stresses, fatigue may impair the ability of a pilot to process and respond to multiple pieces of information simultaneously at a crucial moment. One airline pilot reported that he sometimes experiences a short-term memory loss when flying at night after two or three long days on duty; as a result, when air traffic control assigns him a new compass heading and altitude, by the time he has reset the heading he may have forgotten the new altitude. Another pilot admitted he had fallen asleep on final approach to a runway one night. He awoke a moment later to find that his copilot had not been aware of the lapse.

For too long pilots have borne the brunt of management decisions and pressures to keep to schedule even when safety may be jeopardized. The captain, after all, has the responsibility of making the proper decision: He or she is expected to give highest priority to the safety of a flight. If it ends in disaster, the decision of a pilot to continue a flight into adverse weather conditions is usually charged entirely to pilot error, regardless of the pressures placed on the pilot to continue the flight. The airline captain who chooses safety over productivity too often may be greeted with "The other planes landed, why did you decide to divert to an alternate airport?" Or, "If you can't fly this trip, I'll find a pilot who can" (44).

NEEDED RESEARCH

Today, an important area of needed research deals with the identification of management-generated or workplace-induced pressures to cut corners, to work when overly fatigued, and to take risks when the consequences can be disastrous or otherwise jeopardize safety. At present, the measurement and quantification of such "human factors" is largely terra incognita.

Beyond the identification of such factors lies their correction or circumvention. It has been too easy to say that a factory worker should have turned off a machine before trying to clean it, or that a farmer should know better than to untangle a jam of cornstalks without making sure that the cornpicker cannot start up suddenly. Better understanding of and greater emphasis on the incentives that cause such behaviors could lead to redesigned tasks and delethalized machinery, making it easier for workers to perform their tasks safely—a cornpicker, for example, that allows the operator to reverse the mechanism so the machine spits out the clotted cornstalks without his even leaving his seat. Unfortunately, cornpickers were always designed so the quickest way to get the job done was hazardous; lawsuits from the numerous amputations of hands, arms, and even legs were common, and the manufacture of cornpickers ceased.

In the long run, therefore, the decision to continue a cornpicker design that made severe injuries inevitable proved to be costly to manufacturers. Similarly, short-term gains in productivity have often yielded substantial long-term losses. The crash of the Downeast Airlines commuter plane not only killed 17 people but also put the airline out of business; in the long run, the short-sighted policy of pushing the pilots to adhere to schedules in the face of bad weather proved to be counterproductive for the company.

Today, many forward-looking companies know that it is good business to prevent injuries. How many, however, specifically try to design every task so that it is just as easy, if not easier, to work safely (e.g., by providing machinery that is so well designed there is no temptation to remove a guard or circumvent a fail-safe mechanism)? Many injuries occur in connection with repairs, but how often are jobs designed so the worker is not tempted to cut a hazardous corner when an unexpected repair is needed?

The other side of this problem is the pressure on workers to produce more, move more, sell more of the company's product. It is time for researchers to include, among the variables they study in the chain of events leading to injury, the incentives and disincentives that often are controlling factors in many aspects of worker behavior. Why did the worker ignore the specified lock-out procedures? What pressures caused him to take a short cut? Why was she driving the forklift so fast? Human factors of this type are crucially important but generally ignored by researchers—and therefore ignored when we seek solutions to work-related injuries.

CONCLUSION

Work-related injuries often receive far less attention from the scientific community than do work-related diseases. Greater consideration must be given to recording and analyzing the details of the circumstances of occupational injuries in order to facilitate their prevention. Emphasis must be placed on injury reduction through measures that automatically decrease the likelihood that workers will be involved in injurious events. Triggered by a desire for greater productivity, workplace pressures often lead to worker injury and consequent reductions in productivity—an important and underresearched aspect of job safety.

NOTE

1. About 4,500 people die each year from injuries in crashes involving trucks (21), which hauled about 950,000 million ton-miles of freight in 1984. About 1,250 deaths are related to trains, which haul more than 920,000 million ton-miles annually.

REFERENCES

1. Afcan, A. S. (1982). Sickness absence due to back lesions in coal miners. *Journal of the Society of Occupational Medicine, 32,* 26–31.
2. Aircraft Accident Report. (1980). *Downeast Airlines, May 1979.* (NTSB-AAR-80-5). Washington, DC: National Transportation Safety Board.
3. Andersson, G. B. J. (1981). Epidemiologic aspects of low-back pain in industry. *Spine, 6,* 53–60.
4. Ayoub, M. A. (1982). Control of manual lifting hazards. I. Training in safe handling. *Journal of Occupational Medicine, 24,* 573–7.
5. Ayoub, M. A. (1982). Control of manual lifting hazards. III. Preemployment screening. *Journal of Occupational Medicine, 24,* 751–61.
6. Baker, S. P., and Members of the Truck and Bus Subcommittee of National Health Statistics Advisory Committee. (1977). *Vehicle length restrictions* (DOT HS 802 377). Report to the Secretary of Transportation by the National Highway Safety Advisory Committee.
7. Baker, S. P., Samkoff, J. S., Fisher, R. S., & Van Buren, C. B. (1982). Fatal occupational injuries. *Journal of the American Medical Association, 248,* 692–7.
8. Buckle, P. W., Kember, P. A., Wood, A. D., & Wood, S. N. (1980). Factors influencing oc-

cupational back pain in Bedfordshire. *Spine, 5,* 254–8.
9. Buskin, S. E., and Paulozzi, L. J. (1987). Fatal injuries in the construction industry in Washington state. *American Journal of Industrial Medicine, 11,* 453–60.
10. Carron, H. (1982). Compensation aspects of low back claims. In H. Carron and R. E. McLaughlin (eds.). *Management of low back pain* (pp. 17–26). Boston: John Wright.
11. Chaffin, D., & Park, K. S. (1973). A longitudinal study of low-back pain as associated with occupational weight lifting factors. *American Industrial Hygiene Association Journal, 34,* 513–25.
12. Chan, O. Y., & Tan, K. A. (1979). Study of lumbar disc pathology among a group of dockworkers. *Annals of the Academy of Medicine, 8*(1), 81–85.
13. Coleman, P. J. (1981). Epidemiologic principles applied to injury prevention. *Scandinavian Journal of Work, Environment, and Health, 7,* 91–96.
14. Coleman, P. J. (1983). Injury surveillance: a review of data sources used by the Division of Safety Research. *Scandinavian Journal of Work, Environment, and Health, 9,* 128–35.
15. Damkot, D. K., Pope, M. H., Lord, J., & Fry-

moyer, J. W. (1984). The relationship between work history, work environment and low-back pain in men. *Spine, 9*(4), 395–9.

16. Davis, H. (1987). Workplace homicides in Texas males. *American Journal of Public Health, 77,* 1290–3.

17. Dietz, P. E., and Baker, S. P. (1987). Murder at work. *American Journal of Public Health, 77,* 1273–4.

18. Frymoyer, J. W., Pope, M. H., Clements, J. H., Wilder, D. G., MacPherson, B., & Ashikaga, T. (1983). Risk factors in low-back pain. *Journal of Bone and Joint Surgery, 65-A,* 213–18.

19. Haddon, W., Jr., & Baker, S. P. (1981). Injury control. In D. Clark and B. MacMahon (eds.). *Preventive and Community Medicine* (pp. 109–40). Boston: Little, Brown.

20. Howard, J. M. (1977). The history of occupational injuries in the United States (1776–1976). *Journal of Trauma, 17,* 411–18.

21. Insurance Institute for Highway Safety. (1980). More deaths, injuries attributed to multipiece rims. *Status Report, 15,* 2–3.

22. Insurance Institute for Highway Safety. (1985). *Big trucks.* Washington, DC: IIHS.

23. Insurance Institute for Highway Safety. (1987). Double-trailer trucks more than double danger on highways. *Status Report, 22*(1), 1–3.

24. Jagger, J., & Pearson, R. D. (1987). A view from the cutting edge. *Infection Control, 8*(2), 51–2.

25. Jagger, J., Pearson, R. D., & Brand, J. J. (1986). Avoiding the hazards of sharp instruments. *Lancet, 1,* 1274.

26. Jagger, J., Hunt, E., Brand-Elnaggar, J. J., & Pearson, R. D. (1988). Rates of needlestick injury caused by various devices in a university hospital. *New England Journal of Medicine, 319,* 284–88.

27. Karlson, T. A., & Baker, S. P. (1978). Fatal occupational injuries associated with motor vehicles. In *Proceedings of the 22nd Conference of the American Association for Automotive Medicine* (Vol. 1, pp. 229–41). Arlington Heights, IL: American Association for Automotive Medicine.

28. Kelen, G. D., Fritz, S., Qaqish, B., et al. (1988). Unrecognized human immunodeficiency virus infection in emergency department patients. *New England Journal of Medicine, 318,* 1645–50.

29. Klein, B. P., Jensen, R. C., & Sanderson, L. M. (1984). Assessment of workers' compensation claims for back strains/sprains. *Journal of Occupational Medicine, 26,* 443–8.

30. Kransinski, K., LaCouture, R., & Holzman, R. S. (1987). Effect of changing needle disposal systems on needle puncture injuries. *Infection Control, 8*(2), 59–62.

31. Kraus, J. F. (1985). Fatal and non-fatal injuries in occupational settings: a review. *Annual Review of Public Health, 6,* 403–18.

32. Kraus, J. F. (1987). Homicide while at work: persons, industries, and occupations at high risk. *American Journal of Public Health, 77,* 1285–9.

33. Leyshon, G. E., & Francis, H. W. S. (1975). Lifting injuries in ambulance crews. *Public Health, 89,* 71–75.

34. Magora, A. (1970). Investigation of the relation between low back pain and occupation. *Industrial Medicine, 39*(12), 28–34.

35. Magora, A. (1972). Investigation of the relation between low back pain and occupation; 3 physical requirements: sitting, standing, and weight lifting. *Industrial Medicine, 41*(12), 5–9.

36. Magora, A. (1973). Investigation of the relation between low back pain and occupation. IV. Physical requirements: bending, rotation, reaching, and sudden maximal effort. *Scandinavian Journal of Rehabilitation Medicine, 5,* 191–6.

37. Maryland Division of Labor and Industry. (1978). *Characteristics of work injuries and illnesses.* Baltimore: Maryland Division of Labor and Industry.

38. McCormick, R. D., & Maki, D. G. (1981). Epidemiology of needlestick injuries in hospital personnel. *American Journal of Medicine, 70,* 928–32.

39. Nance, J. J. (1986). *Blind Trust.* New York: Morrow & Company.

40. National Center for Health Statistics. (1978). *Current estimates from the health interview survey: United States, 1977.* Hyattsville, MD: U.S. Department of Health Education and Welfare.

41. National Institute for Occupational Safety and Health. (1981). *Work practices guide for manual lifting* (No. 81-122) Cincinnati: National Institute for Occupational Safety and Health.

42. National Safety Council. (1986). *Accident facts 1986 edition.* Chicago: National Safety Council.

43. Parkinson, D. K., Gauss, W. F., Perper, J. A., & Elliott, S. A. (1986). Traumatic workplace deaths in Allegheny County, Pennsylvania, 1983 and 1984. *Journal of Occupational Medicine, 28,* 100–2.

44. Power-Waters, B. (1975). *Safety last.* New York: Pinnacle Books.

45. Research and Speed Programs Administration. (1986). *National Transportation Statistics, Annual Report.* Washington, DC: U.S. Department of Transportation.

46. Ribner, B. S., Landry, M. N., Gholson, G. L., & Linden, L. A. (1987). Impact of a rigid, puncture resistant container system upon needlestick injuries. *Infection Control, 8*(2), 63–66.

47. Rowe, M. L. (1969). Preliminary statistical

study of low back pain. *Journal of Occupational Medicine, 11,* 161–9.

48. Runyan, C. W., & Baker, S. P. (1988). Occupational motor vehicle injury mortality among municipal employees. *Journal of Occupational Medicine, 30,* 883–86.

49. Saari, J. (1982). Long-term development of occupational accidents in Finland. *Scandinavian Journal of Work, Environment, and Health, 8,* 85–93.

50. Saari, J., & Lahtela, J. (1981). Work conditions and accidents in three industries. *Scandinavian Journal of Work, Environment, and Health, 7* (suppl. 4), 97–105.

51. Saari, J. T., & Wickstrom, G. (1978). Load on back in concrete reinforcement work. *Scandinavian Journal of Work, Environment, and Health, 4* (suppl. 1), 13–19.

52. Sass, R., & Crook, G. (1981). Accident proneness: science or nonscience? *International Journal of Health Services, 11*(2), 175–90.

53. Snook, S. H. (1978). The design of manual handling tasks. *Ergonomics, 21,* 963–85.

54. Snook, S. H. (1982). Low back pain in industry. In A. A. White and S. L. Gordon (eds.). *Symposium on idiopathic low back pain* (pp. 23–28). St. Louis: Mosby.

55. Sundstrom-Frisk, C. (1984). Behavioral control through piece-rate wages. *Journal of Occupational Accidents, 6,* 49–59.

56. Suruda, A., Smith, G. S., & Baker, S. P. (1988). Trench cave-in fatalities in the construction industry. *Journal of Occupational Medicine, 30,* 552–55.

57. Troup, J. D. G., Martin, J. W., & Lloyd, D. C. E. F. (1981). Back pain in industry: a prospective survey. *Spine, 6*(1), 61–69.

58. Undeutsch, K., Gartner, K. H., Luopajarvi, T., Kupper, R., Karvonen, M. J., Lowenthal, I., & Rutenfranz, J. (1982). Back complaints and findings in transport workers performing physically heavy work. *Scandinavian Journal of Work, Environment, and Health, 8* (suppl. 1), 92–96.

59. Vojtecky, M. A., Harber, P., Sayre, J. W., Billet, E., & Shimozaki, S. (1987). The use of assistance while lifting. *Journal of Safety Research, 18*(2), 49–56.

60. Waller, J. A. (1985). *Injury control.* Lexington, MA: D.C. Heath.

61. Wells, J., Zipp, J. F., Schuette, P. T., & McEleney, J. (1983). Musculoskeletal disorders among letter carriers. *Journal of Occupational Medicine, 25,* 814–20.

62. Wigglesworth, E. C. (1976). Occupational injuries: an exploratory analysis of successful Australian strategies. *Medical Journal of Australia, 1,* 335–9.

63. Yu, T., Roht, L. H., Wise, R. A., Killan, D. J., & Weir, F. (1984). Low-back pain in industry: an old problem revisited. *Journal of Occupational Medicine, 26*(7), 517–24.

8

Biomechanical Basis for Prevention of Overexertion and Impact Trauma in Industry

Don B. Chaffin

Research in biomechanics is beginning to provide a scientific basis for understanding the causes and the means of preventing a great deal of physical trauma in industry. From analyses of workers' compensation data it appears that injuries due to *overexertion* (e.g., from repetitive, sustained, or forceful effort) or *physical impact* (e.g., falls and being struck by equipment) account for more than two-thirds of all serious injuries in industry, disabling about 5 million workers annually. This chapter describes some of the biomechanics research that has helped to identify and evaluate the complex conditions that cause such injuries. Specifically, examples of biomechanics research to prevent occupational low-back pain and industrial slips and falls are presented. Also presented is a three-stage injury prevention model that distinguishes among primary, secondary, and tertiary prevention strategies for such events.

SCOPE OF THE PROBLEM

When a worker slips and falls or is struck by moving equipment in industry, the impact force, often over a short period and applied to a localized tissue, can cause serious injury and even death. Workers' compensation data from Michigan indicate that these "impact trauma" events account for about 37% of all injury and illness claims (16). When a worker is required to perform manual exertion, either occasionally or repetitively (sometimes several thousand times each day), the physical stress of the exertions(s) can cause a wide variety of serious, disabling injuries. Workers' compensation data indicate that such "overexertion trauma" accounts for more than 31% of serious injury and illness claims (16).

In one study (26) the two types of trauma were distinguished physically. With the first type of event, "impact trauma", energy transfer to the body is fast, occurring within milliseconds to minutes at most. With the second type of event, "overexertion trauma", energy transfer can be much slower, with a gradual deterioration of human tissue over weeks and even years. Figure 8–1 distinguishes these two events. Epidemiological studies (11,19,23) yield the type of statistics presented in Figure 8–2,

EVENT:		TRAUMA TYPE:		TYPICAL MEDICAL OUTCOMES
Sudden Force	→	Impact Trauma	→	Contusions, Lacerations, Fractures, Amputations, Joint Subluxations, Concussion
Volitional Activity	→	Overexertion Trauma	→	Tendinitis, Tenosynovitis, Myofascial Disorders, Nerve Entrapment Disorders (CTS) Low-Back Pain

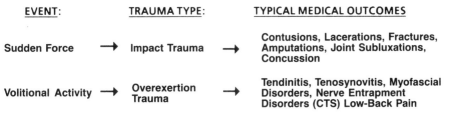

Figure 8–1. Two biomechanical injury mechanisms common in industry. From Chaffin and Redfern (7).

which demonstrate that overexertion injuries cause the most disability and associated costs in occupational health, whereas impact trauma causes most occupational deaths.

With both impact and exertion-related trauma, knowledge of biomechanics is essential to understand the mechanism of injury as well as to devise scientifically valid strategies for controlling the risk factors so identified. In the latter regard, a major traditional goal of ergonomics has been to design work conditions that are compatible with human capabilities and needs. Knowledge of biomechanics becomes essential to establish scientifically valid job design guides that prevent injury inducing physical trauma and allow workers to perform at or near their capability for their entire working lives.

Unlike biomechanical research on vehicle-related injuries, it has been only during the last couple of decades that serious scientific research on biomechanics has produced findings directly applicable to worker protection (6). When organizing and conducting such research, one is soon confronted with the multiplicative nature of the risk factors involved.

For instance, it has been shown that lifting, pushing, or pulling on objects in certain ways is associated with back problems related to overexertion (17). The *load*

Overexertion Injuries Account For Approximately

- 31% of workers compensation claims
- 60% of lower back pain
- Permanent disability of 60,000 workers/year and temporary disability of 4,300,000/year
- Costs estimated between $20 billion to $50 billion/year, or as much as $400/worker

Impact Injuries Account For Approximately

- 37% of workers compensation claims
- 600,000 disabling workplace injuries annually
- 8,000 worker deaths annually
- Injury costs estimated at $5 billion to $7 billion/year

Figure 8–2. Some overexertion and impact trauma statistics.

being handled and the specific *postures* that are involved combine to raise the risk of injury. It has also been shown that the *time duration of awkward postures* and highly *repetitive hand/arm exertions* are major risk factors in various types of overexertion-related trauma (20,22,23). In particular, many inflammatory musculoskeletal disorders are classified now as "cumulative trauma disorders" (CTDs) caused by overexertion (22). In any manual work situation it is not a single risk factor that causes musculoskeletal injury; rather, several combine to increase the probability of harm. A 1978 National Institute of Occupational Safety and Health (NIOSH)-sponsored review of the literature regarding the cause of occupational low-back pain emphasized this point. The NIOSH review listed 17 potential risk factors (both personal and workplace-related) associated with occupational low-back pain. An expert panel assembled by NIOSH (17) two years later recommended that five workplace risk factors be considered major causes of occupational low back pain: (a) the weight of the load being lifted; (b) the horizontal distance away from the person; (c) the location of the load from the floor at the beginning of the lift; (d) the distance the load is moved upward; and (e) the frequency of the lifting. The panel's analysis resulted in a widely used document referred to as the *NIOSH Work Practices Guideline for Manual Lifting*.

It is interesting to note that in July 1988 the Occupational Safety and Health Administration (OSHA) requested additional information from the public to determine if a federal safety regulation for manual lifting is justified. Based on the responses, OSHA requested that NIOSH undertake a thorough evaluation of the NIOSH Guideline, which is still under way. Clearly, any such regulation must be a comprehensive statement due to the multiplicative nature of the risk processes involved in such manual exertions. The basis for such a standard is being slowly developed through biomechanics research.

BIOMECHANICS RESEARCH ON MUSCULOSKELETAL SYSTEM

Because of the complex etiology of many overexertion- and impact-related injuries in industry, much fundamental research in biomechanics is needed to understand the underlying cause of the injuries. Figure 8–3 shows how some of this research is being structured. Beginning at the top of Figure 8–3, research is under way to better measure the types of force to which workers are subjected in various job situations, along with postural and motion description data in jobs suspected of causing an excessive number of injuries. Advances in portable video and force measurement systems make it possible often to acquire such data on the job and to classify the kinesiological (movement) aspects of manual labor in many industries (6,12). Also, population studies of human size, shape, flexibility, and strength are slowly being undertaken with the detail necessary to represent the large variations that exist in different ethnic, gender, and age groups.

Despite the limitations of the existing data on worker populations and job characteristics, some human kinetic models have been devised to predict the forces and torques within various joints while performing common industrial tasks (6). The torques (or moments) are important to know because muscles and ligaments at joints are positioned to respond to them. If their magnitude is large, the bending or twisting at the joint causes the tissue to tear (i.e., become overstrained or sprained). These models

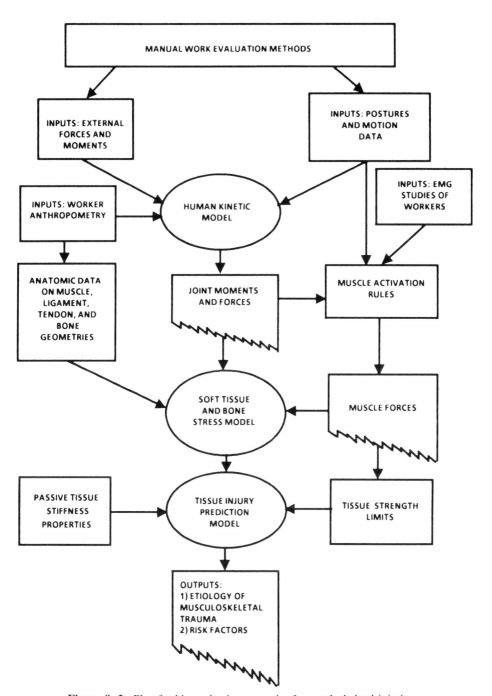

Figure 8–3. Plan for biomechanics research of musculoskeletal injuries.

of the musculoskeletal system have been developed to allow a job analyst to input (a) specific postural data (angles of the body during an exertion), (b) anthropometry of the population (body weight and stature), and (c) load magnitude and direction operating on one or two hands. A model developed by Chaffin is typical of these approaches (6). It assumes that the human body is a kinetic chain comprised of body segments joined at the joints. Torques or moments (i.e., the tendency of a body segment to rotate at a joint) caused by any load in the hands acting at the end of the kinetic chain and the body segment weights are computed at each major joint of the body for a given task. These joint moments are systematically compared to the strength moments demonstrated by worker populations who have been isometrically strength-tested to produce these limits. In addition, a gross estimate of the compression force acting on the L5/S1 disc is predicted and compared to the NIOSH strength limits for spinal compression force failure. The NIOSH limits are 770 lb for an *action limit,* wherein about 3× the risk of low-back pain would exist, and 1,430 lb for the *maximum permissible limit* (about 10× risk).

The practical implementation of this strength prediction method has been facilitated by the wide-scale use and computational power of the personal computer. As an example, consider the act of lifting an object from the floor as shown in Figure 8–4 using the data listed in Table 8–1.

The 2D Static Strength Prediction Program™ used for this analysis was developed by the Center for Ergonomics at The University of Michigan. The above data are entered from the keyboard and displayed on the screen as indicated in Figure 8–5. In this particular lifting situation, the 44-lb reel would be difficult for almost one-half of the female workforce because of the large amount of muscle strength required at the hip joints; i.e., the model predicts that only 58% of women could perform the lift in this position. The results of the analysis indicate that the L5/S1 compression forces are also high because they exceed the NIOSH Action Limit basis for compression forces. When these values exceed 770 lb (which is the NIOSH Action Limit), special action is recommended by the NIOSH *Guide* either to reduce the load (use a hoist) or to select and train people to handle the load in a manner that would minimize such forces.

This case is one example of how biomechanical concepts can be used to evaluate gross physical stress on the human musculoskeletal system when performing heavy manual labor. Because it is executed on a personal computer, it provides a means to easily simulate the effects of alternative workplace designs and mechanical handling aids. In this way the model assists in developing sound engineering changes.

One of the biggest limitations of existing biomechanical models meant to predict stress on specific tissues is the lack of knowledge regarding the neurological motor control strategies (referred to as "muscle activation rules" in Figure 8–3) used to activate various muscles during a given work situation. With the advent of multiple electrode electromyographic measuring systems combined with computerized data acquisition and processing systems, such muscle activation rules are slowly being revealed (14). Also, the precise anatomical shape and relative positions of distinct musculoskeletal components are beginning to be documented with the wider use of computed tomography and magnetic resonance imaging.

Finally, it must be conceded that the existing biomechanical models are limited in that the failure strain parameters for various relevant musculoskeletal tissues are only now being estimated in laboratory studies. Ultimately, these tissue failure data will

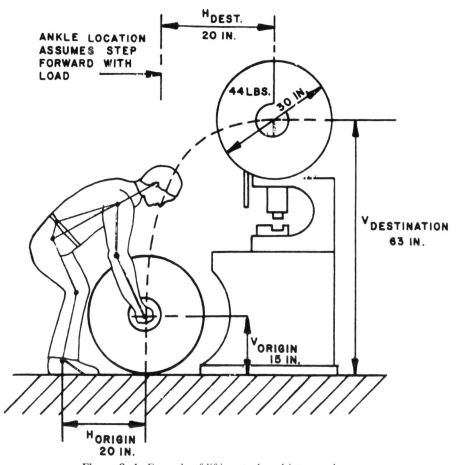

ANKLE LOCATION
ASSUMES STEP
FORWARD WITH
LOAD

H_DEST.
20 IN.

44LBS.

30 IN

V_DESTINATION
63 IN.

V_ORIGIN
15 IN.

H_ORIGIN
20 IN.

Figure 8–4. Example of lifting stock reel into punch press.

Table 8–1. Data for the Biomechanical Strength Model Used to Analyze Initial Posture When Lifting Stock Reel in Fig. 8–4

Parameter	Data
Load	44 lb in magnitude acting vertically down (−90° from horizontal) and lifted with both hands.
Posture	Angles (relative to horizontal) measured from a stopped-frame video or photograph of a person performing the lift are as follows at origin of lift task.
Lower arm	−68° (below horizontal)
Upper arm	−87° (below horizontal)
Torso	+32° (above horizontal)
Upper leg	+116° (above horizontal)
Lower leg	+78° (above horizontal)
Anthropometry	Depends on worker population, but an average-sized man and woman are assumed for this example.

105

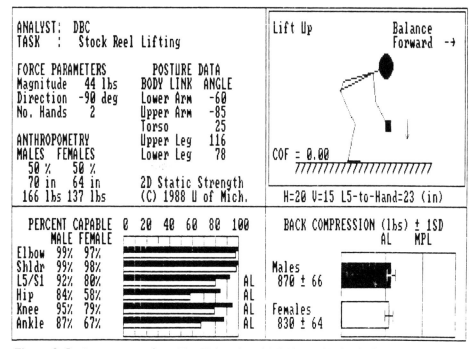

Figure 8–5. Output screen from The University of Michigan, 2D Static Strength Prediction Program™ depicting an evaluation of lifting a stock reel as shown in Figure 8–4.

provide the means to predict how tissue is injured in specific manual activities. Once biomechanical models of tissue failures are available, they must be validated by well controlled occupational epidemiological studies.

Biomechanics research is progressing at each step of the plan described in Figure 8–3. Research results have already made it possible to better understand how risk factors in the workplace combine to cause over exertion-related low-back pain and sciatica, carpal tunnel syndrome, and finger flexor tendinitis and tenosynovitis (1,3,4). In addition, studies have disclosed how fibers are destroyed by certain types of stretching and repetitive exertions at physiological loads (15). Studies also have disclosed that spinal discs fail at relatively low loads when stressed repeatedly over a short period(5). Finally, human gait analysis studies have documented how important appropriate shoes and walking surfaces are to the prevention of certain types of lower-extremity injuries (18).

BIOMECHANICAL ISSUES REGARDING IMPACT TRAUMA IN INDUSTRY

Industrial traumatic impact injuries are also important. One of the major causes of impact trauma is foot slippage while walking. It is estimated that 20% of workers' compensation claims in the United States are from foot-slip or fall events (25), and 11% of occupational injuries in Sweden are due to foot-slip events(24).

In the simplest biomechanical terms, foot-slip occurs either shortly after the heel first strikes the walking surface or immediately before the toe lifts off the walking surface. It is during these two periods when the required coefficient-of-friction (μ^* as the ratio of the foot shear force divided by the contacting force normal to the ground) is highest. Figure 8–6 illustrates the concept and the resulting μ^* values during normal walking on both high traction (without slip) and lower traction (with some slip) surfaces. The values of the required coefficient-of-friction depend mainly on the task (e.g., walking, running, pushing), the slope of the floor, and the stride length and posture. As shown in Figure 8–6, during normal walking the required μ^* values most often are less than 0.3. If a person is pushing a cart, walking down a ramp, or running, however, values for μ^* can approach or even exceed 1.0 (13).

For comparison, one study tested what can be expected for the static and dynamic coefficient-of-friction of 31 types of industrial flooring systems under dry and wet conditions (7) (Table 8–2). Another report described the general procedures for testing each sample (2).

The static and dynamic coefficients-of-friction were measured with sled devices (Bigfoot device, Safety Sciences, Inc.; Tortus Slipometer, Idos Instruments, Ltd.). The resulting coefficient-of-friction values for both static and dynamic tests and for dry and wet floors are plotted in Figure 8–7, for leather shoe material. The tests disclosed a large variability in the traction of the different floor materials. Dynamic μ values tended to be slightly higher or equal to static μ values, except for wood block floors, where the dynamic tests were lower. A wet wood block floor, possibly because the wood is oil-soaked, is particularly hazardous in general, with dynamic μ values in the range of μ^* values shown earlier for normal walking. The conclusion of the analysis is that aisles where fast walking and turning occurs and where carts are often pushed and pulled should not be of a wood block material but, rather, of some type of flooring system that presents much higher traction values.

It is also clear from the above data that floor traction is only one risk factor for foot-slip-related injuries. In fact, if workers are aware of reduced floor traction, often they can slow the speed of walking and shorten stride lengths to maintain balance. Such a reaction, however requires more metabolic energy expenditure in the low-back muscles, thus possibly causing leg and torso muscle fatigue if a person has to walk on slippery surfaces for a long period. Also in some jobs it may not be possible to modify one's walking speed, as the tasks to be performed and pace of the work require fast motions, turning, and manipulative, whole-body exertions. In these types of job special care in the selection of appropriate high traction shoes and flooring systems is necessary.

Complicating the slip problem is the realization that with age not only is a person more vulnerable to serious injury in a fall but the muscle coordination necessary to arrest a fall once foot-slip occurs is compromised (10,21). If an older work force is involved, even greater care is needed to ensure well designed flooring.

From the preceding discussion it can be recognized that biomechanics research has been and should continue to be a major contributor to the prevention of overexertion and impact-related injuries in industry. When determining the cause of industrial impact injuries, much like the biomechanics research on vehicle design, it is important to understand the physical effects of various floors and shoes during tasks that are known to cause slips, falls, and lower-extremity impact trauma. Understanding the kinetic resulting effects and neuromuscular reactions during a slip or trip event should assist also in the selection and training of workers for specific tasks.

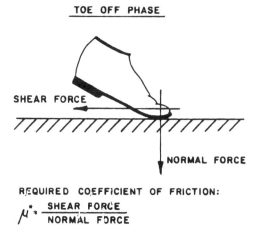

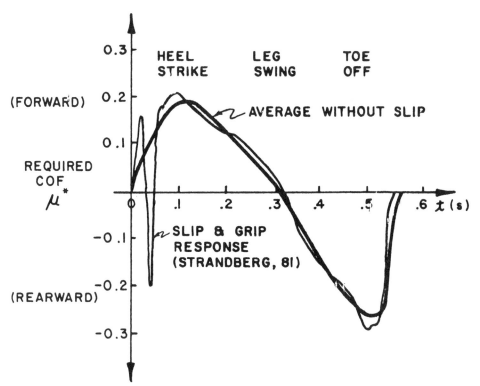

Figure 8–6. Required coefficients-of-friction during walking with and without small foot slippage.

Table 8–2. Industrial Flooring Systems

Mats (3)[a]
Coatings (11)
Gratings (1)
Panels/plates (5)
Films (2)
Woodblocks (3)
Cinderblock (1)
Wax on tile (5)

[a]The number of samples are shown in parentheses.

Similarly, we now have limited guidelines based on biomechanical findings for specifying personal protective clothing, e.g., wire mesh gloves to protect against hand lacerations, tie-off lanyards to protect against falling from heights, and hard hats and face shields to protect against falling objects and projectiles. Biomechanical knowledge must be developed and applied in these systems to ensure their effectiveness under a variety of work conditions.

PREVENTION OF OVEREXERTION AND IMPACT TRAUMA

Prevention of overexertion and impact trauma in industry requires a multidisciplinary team approach to understand some of the basic injury mechanisms discussed earlier. Such an approach must deal with potential problems at primary, secondary, and tertiary

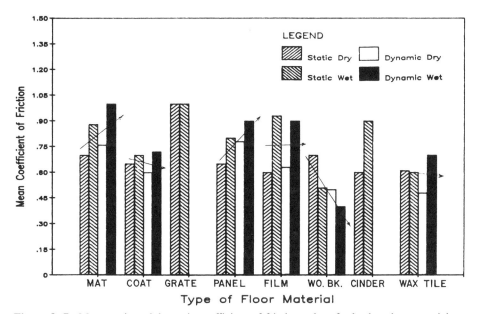

Figure 8–7. Mean static and dynamic coefficient-of-friction values for leather shoe material on various floor materials.

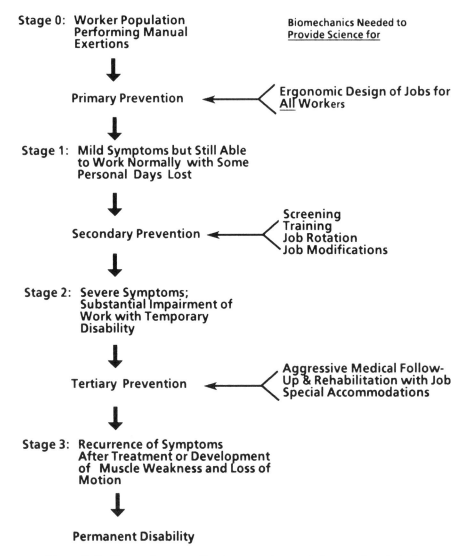

Figure 8–8. Stages of overexertion trauma and suggested prevention strategies.

levels of prevention. This point is particularly true when attempting to prevent overexertion trauma. Figure 8–8 illustrates various prevention concepts, each of which requires fundamental knowledge of occupational biomechanics.

If *primary prevention* is the intent, knowledge of biomechanics becomes critical for defining the manual requirements of the job (e.g., postures, forces, repetitions) and the engineering guidelines necessary to redesign the jobs. In this context, biomechanics becomes the foundation discipline for the ergonomic job improvements mentioned earlier. With *secondary prevention,* knowledge of biomechanics can provide the means to fairly evaluate people who wish to engage in certain types of hazardous manual work, e.g., providing job-related muscle strength testing parameters (9). Biomechanics becomes important also when prescribing certain types of manual training, e.g., lifting methods (8), and under what conditions job rotation should be considered to prevent recurrence of an injury. For *tertiary prevention,* if a person is impaired it is vital to know precisely the person's performance capability related to specific manual job requirements. This knowledge ensures that any disability is fairly and objectively determined and that job-related rehabilitation can be effectively undertaken.

SUMMARY

Overexertion and impact trauma are the major causes of occupational injury and death. These injuries result from a lack of knowledge of biomechanics combined with the ineffective dissemination and use of existing principles of occupational biomechanics. There is no single cause of these injuries, and hence research and prevention strategies must be comprehensive and multidisciplined.

ACKNOWLEDGMENT

The preparation of this chapter was partially supported by NIOSH ERC Training Grant OHO7207.

REFERENCES

1. Anderson, C. Chaffin, D., Herrin, G., & Matthews, L. (1985). Biomechanical model of the lumbosacral joint during lifting. *Journal of Biomechanics, 18,* 571–84.

2. Andres, R., & Chaffin, D. (1985). Ergonomic analysis of slip-resistant measurement devices. *Ergonomics, 28,* 1065–79.

3. Armstrong, T., & Chaffin, D. (1979). Some biomechanical aspects of carpal tunnel. *Journal of Biomechanics, 12,* 567–70.

4. Armstrong, T., Radwin, R., Hansen, D., & Kennedy, K. (1986). Repetitive trauma disorders: job evaluation and design. *Human Factors, 28,* 325–36.

5. Brinckmann, P., & Johannleweling, N. (1986). *Fatigue fracture of human lumbar vertebrae* (No. 32).Münster: Orthopadische Universtatisklinik Münster.

6. Chaffin, D. B., & Andersson, G. B. J. (1984). *Occupational biomechanics.* New York: Wiley.

7. Chaffin, D. B., & Redfern, M. S. (1987). Slip resistance measurements of industrial flooring. In. S. S. Asfour (ed). *Trends in ergonomics/ human factors IV* (pp. 453–6. Amsterdam: North Holland/Elsevier.

8. Chaffin, D., Gallay, L., Woolley, W., & Kuciemba, S. (1986). An evaluation of the effect of a training program on worker lifting pos-

tures. *International Journal of Industrial Ergonomics, 1,* 127–36.

9. Chaffin, D., Herrin, G, & Keyserling W. (1978). Preemployment strength testing: an updated position. *Journal of Occupational Medicine, 20,* 403–8.

10. Greenwood, R., & Hopkins, A. (1976). Muscle responses during sudden falls in man. *Journal of Physiology, 254,* 507–18.

11. Kelsey, J., & White, A. (1980). Epidemiology and impact on low back pain. *Spine, 5,* 133–42.

12. Keyserling, W. M. (1986). A computer-aided system to evaluate postural stress in the workplace. *American Industrial Hygiene Association Journal, 47,* 641–9.

13. Lee, K., Chaffin, D., & Herrin, G. (1986). Simulation of cart pushing and pulling. In *Proceedings of 31st Annual Factors Society,* Santa Monica, CA.

14. McCulley, K., & Faulkner, J. (1986). Characteristics of lengthening contractions associated with injury to skeletal muscle fibers. *Journal of Applied Physiology, 61,* 293–9.

15. McMahon, T. (1984). *Muscles, reflexes and locomotion.* Princeton, NJ: Princeton University Press.

16. Michigan Department of Labor. (1985). *Com-*

pensable Occupational Injury and Illness Report. Lansing, MI: Michigan Department of Labor.

17. National Institute of Occupational Safety and Health. (1981). *Work practices guide for manual lifting*. DHHS Publication (NIOSH) 81-122. Cincinnati: NIOSH.

18. Nigg, B. (1986). *Biomechanics of running shoes*. Champaign, IL: Human Kinetics.

19. Pope, M., Frymoyer, J., & Andersson, G. (1984). *Occupational low back pain*. Westport, CT: Praeger Publishing.

20. Punnett, L., Robins, J. M., Wegman, D. H., & Keyserling, W. M. (1985). Soft tissue disorders in the upper limbs of female garment workers. *Scand. J. Work Envir. Health, 11,* 417–25.

21. Romick-Allen, R., & Schultz, A. (1988). Biomechanics of reactions to impending falls. *Journal of Biomechanics, 21,* 591–600.

22. Silverstein, B., & Armstrong T. (1986). Hand wrist cumulative trauma disorders in industry. *British Journal of Industrial Medicine, 43,* 779–84.

23. Snook, S., & Jensen, R. (1984). Cost. In M. Pope, J. Frymoyer, & G. Andersson (eds.). *Occupational low back pain*. Westport, CT: Praeger Publishing.

24. Strandberg, L. (1983). On accident analysis and slip-resistance measurement. *Ergonomics, 26,* 11–32.

25. Szymusiac, S. M., & Ryan, J. P. (1982). Prevention of slip and fall injuries. In *Professional Safety*. Des Plaines, IL: American Society of Safety Engineers.

26. Waller, J. A. (1987). Injury: conceptual shifts and preventive implications. *Annual Review of Public Health, 8,* 21–49.

III

CHANGES IN THE WORKPLACE: RESULTS OF THE POSTINDUSTRIAL REVOLUTION

The main aim of this book is to explore the extent to which the changing nature of the workplace will have a different (more favorable or less favorable) impact on health and productivity, as well as the relation between the two. This section deals with changes in the design and technology of productive work, changes in workplace hazards of both physical/chemical and psychosocial origin, and the potential effects of personal characteristics of gender and personality type.

In an examination of office workers, a rapidly expanding segment of the workforce, Celentano (Chapter 10) notes the changing physical and chemical nature of the office workplace, e.g., the tight building syndrome, as well as changes in the physical and psychosocial environment associated with the new technologies of communication and information. The new physical/chemical agents, requiring characterization and control, fall basically in the industrial hygienist's domain of traditional workplace exposures. Changes in the psychosocial conditions associated with advanced information and data-processing technology are closely related to such issues as the following.

1. Increased power and versatility of the individual worker armed with the sophistication of computer control and the operation of a family of related machines.
2. Psychological stress caused by the loss of control over one's workspace due to the greater interconnectedness of these technologies.
3. Increased demands of learning new information-processing systems and other technologies.

Hirschhorn (Chapter 9) describes "operators working at a single work station . . . doing a large variety of operations (that is, milling, grinding, and drilling) at a single work station," which can be compared to a modern secretary communicating through a network of phones and computer-linked word processors and data banks. It simply becomes more efficient to have one person or team complete a work product while it is being processed by powerful technology than to pass it around to narrow specialists for bits and pieces of processing. Again, the office worker shares with Hirschhorn's description of the manufacturing processor the need to "be more vigilant and understand the manufacturing process . . . the operators focusing on machine (word processor) output making sure that the machine is functioning and monitoring output." Additionally, "the operator plays a role . . . when the machine fails. His or her ability to identify why the process has failed (e.g., the photocopying machine) . . . is as important as manning the machine in its steady state." The office worker as well as the manufacturing worker needs to know how and why things go wrong rather than simply that it is happening.

As Hirschhorn points out, any office supervisor can see the change in the modern office, as the staff members spend a much greater proportion of their time learning computer programs and new office systems compared to their predecessors, who learned typing and dictation and used these same skills throughout their careers. The potential for stress and stress-related health effects is substantial, as the power of the technology magnifies the inefficiency as well as the efficiency of the worker, both of which should be clearly detectable in output measures of productivity.

On reading Chapter 11 by Morell and her colleagues one is reminded that, in addition to changes in workplace designs, purposes, and technologies and in environmental and psychosocial hazards, the agents of disease and the pattern of illness and disease have altered markedly over the last several decades from a predominant concern with acute infectious diseases with early mortality to a concern with chronic disease with long morbidity. These chronic diseases cost more in medical care and disability, have greater impact on productivity, have multiple causes, and are aggravated by lifestyle and behavioral factors.

The lifestyle element of many chronic diseases forces us to consider lifestyle factors away from work as well as in the work environment if intervention is to be effective. Morell and colleagues present the early results of an original study on the effects of gender and personality type on subjective (job satisfaction) and objective (heart rate and blood pressure) measures. This study indicates that gender, personality type, and job fit may be relevant to both health and productivity. This point introduces more lifestyle considerations in the effort to determine an individual's suitability for work placement and prospects for health and productivity.

If there is a shift in the postindustrial world away from highly specialized, multicompartmental, assembly-line production to a more complex, interconnected, multipotential role for workers, psychosocial factors may be as relevant to workers' health and productivity as physical trauma, chemical toxins, and airborne dusts in the traditional industrial workplace of the past.

9
Stresses and Patterns of Adjustment in the Postindustrial Factory

Larry Hirschhorn

New sources of stress are emerging in the postindustrial factory. The new technologies reduce the time and material buffers that once separated units, divisions, and people from one another: Workers are asked to become more accountable for and to feel more psychologically linked to the entire workflow; and the rate of technical and product change burdens people's ability to learn new process and techniques.

This chapter is divided into three sections. The first, using case studies of two factories, highlights the new sources of stress. The second examines the impact of these stressors on felt stress. The third examines the links between older patterns of adjustment to stress and the new tasks of the postindustrial factory. It argues that the new tasks undermine the coping behaviors of the old factory, suggesting that we need to develop new coping systems based on social cooperation rather than individual strengths to create a new social/emotional balance in the factory. The chapter is based on field visits and interviews at an engine factory, an electronics assembly factory, and the repair division of an elevator factory; and its ideas are buttressed by the author's prior site visits to other factories and offices.

NEW FACTORIES AND NEW STRESSORS
From Job Shop to Continuous Process

Investing in computers, factories throughout the United States are transforming their production methods radically. Workers who once performed semiskilled work, were responsible for rote tasks, and paid attention to the flow of materials at their work stations alone find instead that they must frequently learn new tasks, perform skilled monitoring work, and understand how their work contributes to the production process as a whole. Although these changes are welcomed because they upgrade work, they also paradoxically impose new and difficult stresses.

Consider the following. Engine, Inc. is a world class factory producing engine parts and complete engines for a wide range of heavy industrial and commercial uses. Walking through its cavernous rooms and halls, one is struck by the extraordinarily large numbers of semifinished parts, tagged and marked, that are placed to the side of the myriad work stations and sections of the factory. Forklift trucks abound, moving quickly down a two-lane internal "highway," picking up and transporting parts between sections according to the process plan that accompanies each part on its long and extended journey from inception to completion. The variety of machines is staggering. Operators work with computer numerical control machines, drill presses that almost touch the factory ceiling, classic lathes to produce new parts and developmental tools, and large tank stations filled with chemicals used to coat metals that must withstand high pressures and temperatures. In effect, the factory is a gargantuan job shop, heavily capitalized with modern equipment but still organized according to materials flow and machine layout principles inherited from the machine shops of a half-century ago. However, facing competition, demands for quality products, a labor force that is barely growing, and new technology, it is a factory in transition. One trainer noted:

> We used to organize just functionally by machines, and we found that the parts simply hopped back and forth. Some of the parts are in process for months, and we would like to reduce that to days. We once used a layout in which similar machines were in one part of the factory, but now we are going to a system where we will put different machines together that make similar parts in the same place. We once tracked an engine casing: In 7 months it traveled 22 miles around the shop floor from grinding, to cleaning, to milling; and most of the time it was sitting around. In one study we found that different sites in the factory were producing the same parts in different ways. We need a more systematic approach.

As the trainer suggested, factory managers are rationalizing the flow of materials and the organization of machines so that the production process more nearly resembles a continuous, sustained flow of raw materials to finished parts without disruptions, discontinuities, and gaps. Using the engineering concept of "group technology" in which different machines are grouped together to make a family of similar parts, engineers and factory managers hope to reduce inventory while standardizing methods for producing a particular engine part. "We are in transition—the whole philosophy is changing; we are now grouping by similar parts and are getting flow lines for them," another trainer noted.

Sustained and intense competition is pushing Engine, Inc. to transform its operations and the role of its operators. The variety of parts produced is increasing, and costs must be kept low despite the increased variety because buyers can purchase parts from factories around the globe. A trainer, reflecting on the changing product profile in the production of engineered parts noted, "Within our company we are now talking about a large variety of parts, and we are often producing eight or ten models of the same engine at the same time. We really need more understanding of the manufacturing processes, and the worker has to be more vigilant overall." In other words, because the factory must become flexible and responsive to a varied and changing demand for its products, it must make the production process itself more rational and systematic (2). By enabling operators to keep track of parts and supervise whole operations, the new factory organization helps the operator sustain his or her vigilance despite the growth in the variety of products. Otherwise, the inherited job shop culture could lead to increasing numbers of lost parts, mistaken operations, and delayed production schedules.

Workers and Vigilance

It may appear at first glance that Engine, Inc. is simply rationalizing its operations in the same way that assembly operations were reorganized into assembly lines more than a half-century ago. The computer, however, introduces a difference. The operator becomes a generalist rather than a specialist and no longer focuses on a single machine and a narrow task. With computer control, machine tools are multifunctional rather than unifunctional. Operators working at a single work station can cut, mill, grind, and drill. "In the past," noted a trainer, "operators would operate a single bank of machines such as grinders or milling machines, but now they operate a family of machines and are doing a large variety of operations at a single work station." Indeed, as another noted, in the "old days," up to about 20 years ago, basic or "vestibule training" helped a novice operator become an expert on a single machine. "We would put the operator through a 4 to 8-week course, and he would learn one machine thoroughly. But now we don't do that. In those days we were organized by a functional layout, so that all machines of the same type were together." Factory managers are transforming the basic character of its inherited job shop culture. Workers once identified with machines rather than parts, and the different machining stations were buffered from one another by large stocks of inventory and loose schedules. In the new settings, departments are more interdependent, and workers identify with products rather than processes. They become more aware of the production process as a whole; and to operate multifunctional machines they have to understand a wider array of operations.

Managers and trainers consequently argue that workers must now be more vigilant, must understand how machines work and why they fail, and must be able to relate technical information to engineers and managers. Because operators no longer actively manipulate tools and materials, they are primarily responsible for the integrity of the process as a whole. "They need to be more vigilant and understand the manufacturing process," noted one trainer. "The operator is focusing on machine output, making sure that the machine is functioning and monitoring output using Statistical Process Control techniques [SPC]." Another noted, "I think the CNC [Computer Numerical Control] machine tool requires a conceptual understanding more than the regular machine tools because everything is happening so fast and so much is happening. You are taking bigger cuts and running at higher RPMs [rotations per minute]. Most of the operators don't fully know what is taking place, and some are afraid of the equipment." Moreover, because the machines are automatic, the operator plays a role largely when the machine fails. His or her ability to identify why the process has failed (e.g., why it is producing parts out of tolerance) is as important as manning the machine in its steady state.

Thus the operator must increasingly ask "why" something is happening rather than "what" is happening. "Hand-me-down" training, as one trainer noted, may prove inadequate. "If you think of hand-me-down training," noted one trainer, "you see, for example, that the foremen could teach all the welding, but he addresses only a functional concept of the task, like how you hold the torch, how you watch the backup materials. He ignores how things go wrong, why things go wrong, what to do and what to watch out for if you don't want to get burn-back. Without such training in the 'whys' you start to get a high number of rejects."

Because the operator focuses increasingly on failures and discontinuities he or she interacts increasingly with a wider range of roles in the plant. As production at Engine, Inc. is rationalized, workers are more sensitized to errors. Process planners, who specify the basic steps or building blocks for producing a part, and engineers, who write programs to guide a particular machining operation, are more frequently consulted to assess how a production process can be corrected. Instead of relying on extra inventory, people, or time, managers want workers and engineers to solve problems together rather than skirt them with extra resources. As one trainer noted, "The mechanical engineer has to spend more time out on the shop floor to check if the SPC is working, so there is now a closer relationship between the engineer and the shop floor person." It means that the operator must be able to talk with intelligence and conviction about the operation he or she supervises and must understand the point of view and interest of the mechanical engineer. One trainer noted, "If there is a mistake in one of the operator's programs—for example, something may be wrong in the CAD-CAM design—the engineer then comes down to the shop floor to find out what is happening. If the operator has a feel for what is taking place, the two can solve the problem, and they can immediately address it and correct it. On a five-axis machine the operator can say 'I noticed a little zig in the Y axis that shouldn't have been there.'" Thus operators can no longer psychologically be confined to their own role or job. Instead they must be prepared to interact with other workers, engineers, and process planners as the implicit factory team is mobilized to solve problems.

New Autonomy

Finally, just as the operators must be more vigilant, they are more interdependent with workers and managers in other departments, units, and divisions. As parts are more carefully tagged and tracked, machines are regrouped, and inventory is minimized, workers, foremen, and department chiefs lose control over the pace and timing of work in their own units. Unable to buffer the demands on their own capacity to produce a required volume of products within a certain time to a specified tolerance by using inventory, they must be more alert to broader scheduling changes in the shop while increasing their own efficiency and competence. Thus *the margin for error falls.* It does not mean, however, that units and divisions lose their integrity and semi-autonomous status. Rather, the source of their autonomy changes. On the one side such units have more integrity and identity because they are based on the production of whole parts or a family of parts. *Operators are psychologically and practically linked to a less fragmented task system.* On the other hand, because they can no longer control their boundary with inventory or scheduling delays they must be more responsive to the planning system of the plant as a whole. In this sense each individual unit loses some of its autonomy as the plant as a whole becomes more effective and responsive to customer demands. The older division of labor based on fragmented tasks and a segmented factory gives way to a more complex division of labor based on whole tasks and an integrated factory. Consequently, the sense of participation, accountability, and vulnerability grows.

Learning

Stress also increases because operators face new equipment designs and new parts more frequently. Taking the learning role more often, they must acknowledge their own temporary incompetence and loss of control.

Consider Control, Inc., which produces control circuits for engines used in industrial processes. Entering its shop floor one sees a relatively unified office-manufacturing setting in which engineers in offices walk freely between their desks and the circuit assembly and testing areas. The environment is clean and quiet, and each assembler works at his or her own bench following written assembly instructions and diagrams to build a circuit. The flow of materials, however, is still loosely organized. Assemblers retrieve operations sheets or instructions from baskets placed atop the cabinets that divide the technicians' work space from the assemblers' benches; and they go to a storeroom to get the material and tools they need. Management has just installed a new material retrieval system to replace the storeroom so that assemblers will be able (as soon as all the materials are appropriately tagged and stored) to press a computer console to request a particular part. Knowing where every part or tool is stored, the computer then calls up a particular bin or cabinet, which moves like an elevator along rollers to the place where the assembler is standing. Such a system will simplify storing and retrieving, as workers in the stock room can randomly place a part in a bin, and so long as it is appropriately tagged and coded the computer finds it and sends it to the worker requesting it.

The manager in charge of plant modernization believes that this setup is only the beginning of a program for rationalizing the flow of materials and circuits. For example, plant engineers are experimenting with placing assembly and wiring instructions on computers that can generate three-dimensional pictures. Instead of retrieving operations sheets from a basket, assemblers will be able to call them up on terminal work stations, thereby minimizing lost work time. Moreover, because the terminals can be hooked into the engineering work stations on the other side of the wall dividing the shop floor from the engineering offices, operators can more easily call for assistance from an engineer if they cannot understand the diagram. The diagrams themselves will be easily updated, and the picture in three dimensions will be clearer.

Technical and market forces are at work here. First, engineers are designing increasingly complicated and packed circuits as the demand for the sophisticated controls increases in all industries. "The circuit boards are complex," the modernization manager noted, "and the designers are trying to make a smaller and smaller package, which is making the assembly complicated." Moreover, as the factory produces an increasing range of controls to meet the competition, assemblers have to become familiar with a broader range of operations and cannot rely simply on memory or routine when assembling a particular circuit. Until recently, noted one trainer at Control, Inc., "the procedures for assembly were frequently locked in the head of the general foreman, and the way in which work was done was informally passed on from senior to junior workers." Because the range of circuits produced was relatively stable workers did not have to rely on their own ability to learn how to assemble new circuits. Today, however, to cope with the growing variety of parts, increasing circuit density, and faster changes in circuit technology, workers can no longer depend on the experienced foreman. Instead, they must learn to read the operations sheets and decipher new instructions themselves. Moreover, this learning ability becomes increasingly important as customers demand the highest quality circuits and plant managers expect the highest yields.

Learning ability is becoming a more important and more manifest dimension of the operator's job at Engine, Inc. as well. As was noted managers have introduced statistical process control (SPC) techniques to improve quality. Workers are trained to understand the basic statistical concepts of deviations and trends, are introduced to the concept of feedback as an instrument of control, and are taught how to fill out statistical control sheets. By observing deviations from the required length, width, or thickness of a particular part and tracking their notations on a control sheet, they can either stop or adjust the machine when parts that violate "tolerances" or standards are produced. The skills and concepts are not difficult, but their application increases the operator's attention to the results of an operation and helps him or her acquire statistical and experiential data on when and why a particular operation seems to go wrong.

Though manifestly an element of the total job design, SPC functions as a learning tool. Operators always learned from their experience, but SPC speeds up the learning process while sensitizing the operator to a broader range of variances. As one trainer noted, "We used to inspect at the tailgate—we found mistakes and then would go back and do the rework. But operators are now doing their own inspection and entering their own data as parts are being produced, and they are certifying that the parts have been produced to specification."

Abstract Technologies

The case of Control, Inc. highlights the stresses that emerge when workers face novel situations and problems more frequently. The case of Elevator, Inc. highlights the special burden that learning poses when workers must learn and master increasingly abstract tasks, in which symbol manipulation replaces physical contact with machines and tools (5). In such situations, not only must workers increasingly take the learner role, figuring out something new, but the nature of the learning process changes. Facing increasingly electronic systems, manipulated with controls, the worker can no longer rely on just his or her physical senses—the smell, feel, and look of a machine— to understand the apparatus. The capacity to imagine, to think abstractly and cognitively, becomes increasingly important. However, lacking the help of the five senses, the learning process itself becomes more difficult and taxing.

Consider the apparently straightforward problems of maintaining and repairing elevators. Elevator technology was generally stable until the mid-1980s, when the advent of microprocessor technology transformed and complicated the elevator control system, enabling building owners to provide a more responsive elevator service. For example, in big office buildings, a central computer can integrate the controls of all the elevators and, by discerning patterns of use over time, minimize waiting time at any particular floor. These "smart" elevator systems possess computer systems that can learn and can therefore adapt to the conditions of use in any particular building. Such complicated controls have transformed the repair and maintenance task itself, while creating a greater variety of elevators and elevator services. "We have moved from the electromechanical systems to microelectronics," noted one elevator mechanic and trainer. "If you consider that we have been in business for a long time and that 100-year-old elevators must be maintained, the technology gap between the old and the new is widening."

The impact of microelectronics has transformed the nature of the repairman's skills. The mechanic described his own experience in adapting to the new technology. "In the early days elevator control systems resembled the arrangements of simple house wiring. A controller had 120 relays and switches and a selector that enabled the elevator to know where it was. Every relay had a coil and contacts that controlled a different circuit, so that the wiring diagram told you which circuits are controlled by which contacts. Generally, it was a one-to-one relation."

The shift from electrical to microelectronic systems changes both the nature of the technology and the way in which the repairmen solve problems. Abstract thinking, thinking in terms of functions and relations, replaces visual, auditory, and sensual methods of pattern detection. The elevator mechanic/trainer went on:

> The approach today is much different. In the past when you opened the door of the control system you could see the problem. Now when you open it you see only a black box. You must be trained in the systems to follow a routine. Instead of using a wiring diagram you would use a flow chart. The input function goes to the circuit board, which then goes to the microprocessor that controls the output and in turn drives the motor. The flow chart would take you through it. The visual things are gone. You can no longer look at it and say you can see the problem. You used to be able to hear a certain sequence of sounds with the electromechanical system, but with the solid state there is no noise. You have to imagine more things than you did before. . . . I am a pretty old guy, and when the transition was made from the conventional to the microprocessor control I thought it was the end of the world for me. You can compare it to riding a bike all your life and then switching to a 747.

Working with "abstract" technology, the workers need to have a more fundamental grasp of the total system of relations underlying an apparatus or machine. With mechanical technology the worker can more readily and sensibly learn incrementally, e.g., first learning about the elevator motor, then the circuits that drive it, and then mastering the control system, the selector, and the governor. The more transparent division of function within the machine system enables workers to master the machine piecemeal so that their systems understanding is itself implicit and often rooted in a primarily tacit and sensual feel for the machine. They can diagnose it but cannot explain it. Abstract technology, shaped by integration of functions, reinforces, by contrast, a systems view.

In sum, new sources of stress are emerging in the postindustrial factory: (a) the creation of integrated production systems, the use of computer-based tools, and the declining margin for error; (b) the growing variety of products and the pressure for high quality; and (c) the greater importance of learning—without the aid of the five senses. Each of these factors creates new stresses in the workplace.

STRESS

Felt stress is the product of situational demands and the individuals' capacity to cope. Three new situational demands, i.e., the demand characteristics of the factory's sociotechnical system, are emerging that undermine inherited methods for coping with work stress.

First, in the old job shop and factory, situational demands were limited paradoxically *by the narrow scope and fragmented nature of the work flow*. Units and divisions were protected from one another by inventory, scheduling slips, and loose quality standards. If machinery in one unit broke, it could continue to meet its production quota by drawing down inventory (Indeed, it is why "just-in-time" production methods, which promise to force inventory levels down, are so difficult for factory managers to implement (4). Moreover, when U.S. companies faced less competition from foreign manufacturers, factory managers, facing slipping schedules due to excessive downtime could often put off customers anxious for timely delivery. Disappointed customers could not turn to alternative suppliers. Working within oligopolistic markets, factories could produce inferior products and so pay less attention to production failures.

Similarly, because operators lacked a relation to a whole product and were accountable for only a narrow portion of the factory task, they did not have to consider the broadest features of the work environment. They could narrow the focus of their attention. Indeed, critics of the factory once focused on the operator's narrow and monotonous job and neglected the hidden benefit of monotony—the operators' right to daydream, to work without paying attention to the activities and events beyond the work station. The workers could exercise psychological control over their work space just as they had no political or economic control over the broader features of the factory environment.

Today, however, as we saw in the case of Engine, Inc., workers must relate to the widest possible features of the factory setting, to a whole product or family of parts, to a large number of role holders and actors, and to plant-wide production schedules. They must psychologically take in a broader system of relations and can no longer restrict their attention to their own immediate situation. Their capacity to attend, therefore, to pay attention, is stressed.

Second, these new demands on attention are matched by the decline in the familiar and psychologically containing rhythms of work. Early research in industrial psychology highlighted the central role that traction played in tying the worker to his or her job (1). Workers feel less tired despite the monotony of the job because it can be matched with a comfortable rhythm of work that pulls the workers along without conscious effort on their part. Traction frees their attention, and they perform their work without conscious awareness. Paradoxically, when broken or unavailable tools and machines disrupted work, workers resented the interruption even if it afforded them unexpected time off because they had to work to regain the feeling of traction. As we saw in the case of Engine, Inc., however, operators no longer work to straightforward production rhythms, but, instead, monitor machines. In such settings workers find it difficult to establish feelings of traction, as they rarely intervene in the production process. Work becomes monotonous on the one hand (which is why operators "fall asleep" at the controls) but exceedingly demanding when workers must act quickly to control a failing production process. Because the rhythms of work are discontinuous, the worker can no longer rely on the subconsciously organized rhythms of action to contain the stress of work.

Third, the worker is faced with the stress of learning. In both the traditional craft setting and the setting of the older job shop or assembly line, traction was matched by the pleasure that comes with competence, by the sense of mastery that enables one to successfully anticipate and control contingencies. In the craft setting, competence and traction were linked by the "feel" of the tool; in the factory setting, traction was linked to the pull of the line and competence to the "tricks of the trade," e.g., how to get the tools you need, to bank inventory, and to "make out." As was seen in the case of Control, Inc. and Engine, Inc., however, the operators must more frequently acknowledge their incompetence in order to effectively take the learner role and master a new machine, design, or technique.

Because novelty can promote anxiety, workers may nonetheless resist the learner role. This point is why, for example, workers in a control room, may deny the existence of production anomalies, preferring to believe that an emergency indicator light on the control panel, for example, is broken rather than that an emergency is about to ensue. Studies of control room failures suggest that workers prefer to link control room events to occurrences they have experienced before, rather than to believe that they are facing a genuinely new problem.

Moreover, as we also saw in the case of the elevator repair, learning is burdened by the task of abstraction. Like the boxer who has one hand tied behind his back, the worker must rely increasingly on the mind's capacity to imagine, stimulate, and abstract rather than on the interaction of mind and senses. The human body is designed to function as a simulator, so that, for example, when learning to drive we integrate the feelings we obtain from the resistance of the clutch, the pull of the steering wheel, the noise of the motor, and the data in our field of vision to create a total visuusensual image of our situation on the road. The body maps the situation onto its sensory apparatus. Working with abstract technologies, however, where the operator relies only on visually coded data, he or she must compensate for the lack of a "natural" simulator by more consciously constructing a strictly cognitive model or map in the mind.

TOWARD A BALANCE

The postindustrial factory thus produces new stresses of attention. Managers want to extract the worker's "surplus" attention once inhibited by narrow tasks and displaced by daydreaming and social posturing. No longer focusing on effort and muscle power, managers want workers to deploy their attention and vigilance in productive ways. The question is: Are these new claims on attention producing a more stressful factory environment? Was not the old factory, with its monotony, fatigue, fragmented division of labor, and class divisions that infantalized workers, also a stressful setting?

Clearly, the old factory posed its own stressors. However, workers and managers together created an unconsciously organized system of adjustments that helped integrate the worker into the job. They created an equilibrium of forces and stressors in which stressors and their corresponding patterns of adjustment produced a stable sociotechnical system. By moving to a new postindustrial factory we not only produce new sources of stress but also lose the established pattern of adjustments. Thus as Table 9–1 suggests, we are faced with the peculiar dialectic in which stressors in the new factory undermine the patterns of adaptation in the old one. Behaviors that once helped establish an equilibrium between situational demands and the capacity to cope now interfere with the new situational demands.

This argument suggests that if workers and managers are to create a new steady state that fits the new situational demands they must design new patterns of social adjustment. Let me briefly outline one possible set here.

First, as we have seen, workers face broader tasks and are more interdependent. Felt stress and uncertainty in this new setting may be reduced, however, if workers are able to participate in the policy process that shapes the context for all departments, units, and divisions. In other words, if tighter schedules reduce each unit's freedom of maneuver, workers may nonetheless regain a sense of control if they participate actively in setting the production schedules themselves. They can then anticipate and plan for the impacts of particular schedules. Integration on the operational level is matched by the participation at the policy level.

Second, the burdens of learning can be matched by tools for learning and learning communities. With learning tools such as simulators, ergonomically designed control rooms, and feed-forward and feedback computer systems that help the operator "review and preview" production runs, the operator can support his or her potentially overburdened imagination with learning aids. Similarly, if workers take the learning role as a learning group, e.g., participating in simulation exercises as a team, attending training classes on a regular basis, and participating in group processes that facilitate learning (quality circles, for example), an individual's feelings of incompetence are reduced by the presence and support of other similarly "incompetent" colleagues.

Third, the workers' loss of traction can be matched by their participation in broader planning cycles. Instead of staying fixed on rhythms and discontinuities shaped by individual machines or a particular production line, they can participate in the wider time cycles of planning a production run, purchasing materials on a seasonal basis, and developing and implementing a maintenance schedule. The loss of rhythms on the factory floor is then matched by their participation in the broader, more all

Table 9–1. Stressors and Adjustments

Stressors ⟶ in old factory	Adjustments ⟶ in old factory	Undermining stressors ⟶ in new factory	Proposed adjustments in new factory
Monotony	Daydreaming	Novelty	Learning tools and communities
Fatigue	Traction	Discontinuity	Participation in broader or higher level rhythms
Narrow tasks	No responsibility	Broad task	Participation in policy making

encompassing rhythms that shape both the steady state and developmental tendencies of the plant as a total organization.

As Table 9–1 suggests, these three innovations would help shape a new sociotechnical system in which new stressors and their adjustments created a new socioemotional balance at work. Indeed, advanced team designs in certain North American plants do provide workers with new and expanded roles. For example, members of semiautonomous teams have the right to reject purchased materials, control their own vacation schedules, sit on policy boards that review broad plant-wide issues, and participate in "pay for learning" schemes through which they learn new trades and skills on a continuing basis. Rankin's detailed description of one such plant suggested that participation in all facets of plant life is broad and deep. Indeed, attendance at local union meetings in the new plant is paradoxically far higher than attendance in traditional plant settings. People are connected to one another, and the potential stress that comes with high involvement and commitment is balanced by the psychological sense of community (3).

Finally, as Table 9–1 suggests and as these examples indicate, the new patterns of adjustment require more cooperation among workers and between workers and managers. Whereas in the past each individual worker could adjust to the stressors based on his or her own individual capacities and temperament, the stresses of the postindustrial factory require social inventions and the development of new cooperative institutions. We can no longer leave the individual alone to cope as best as he or she can. Instead, we need to embed his capacity to cope in wider social institutions that amplify his coping responses. Stress and its vicissitudes become irrevocably tied to the politics of roles and relationships in the factory.

SUMMARY

New sources of stress are emerging in the postindustrial factory. The new technologies reduce the time and material buffers that once separated units, divisions, and people from one another. Workers are asked to become more accountable for, and to feel more psychologically linked to, the entire workflow; and the rate of technical and product change burdens the worker's ability to learn new processes and techniques.

Whereas the old industrial factory posed its own stressors in the form of monotony, narrow tasks, and infantile roles, a century of development enabled workers and managers to create a system of adjustment based on traction, daydreaming, and the gains to not feeling responsible. The adjustments limited felt stress while confirming the factory's basic role system. The new sources of stress, however, undermine these old patterns of adjustment so that stress grows not only because new tasks emerge but because old coping behaviors prove dysfunctional. We need a new system of adjustments to balance the new sources of stress that derive from the development of learning tools and learning communities, as well as participation in the strategic decisions and operations of the plant. In contrast to the old system of adjustments, the new one is based on social inventions and group coordination, rather than on the individual strengths or weaknesses of each worker. Stress and politics are intertwined.

REFERENCES

1. Emery, F. (1972). Characteristics of sociotechnical systems. In L. E. Davis and J. C. Taylor (eds.). *Design of jobs*. London: Penguin.
2. Hirschhorn, L. (1984). *Beyond mechanization.* Cambridge: MIT Press.
3. Rankin, T. (1986). *Unions and the emerging paradigm of organization—the case of E.C.W.U.,*

local 800. Ph.D. dissertation, University of Pennsylvania.
4. Schonberger, R. (1984). *World class manufacturing.* New York: Free Press.
5. Zuboff, S. (1988). *In the age of the smart machine: the future of work.* New York: Basic Books.

10
Health Issues in Office Work

David D. Celentano

There is general agreement that the contemporary office is being transformed by automation and computerization (16,19). Traditional tasks and duties are being altered, jobs redesigned, and job skills and requirements upgraded. As industrialized nations become information societies to an even greater degree, the impact on workers will be felt in a variety of ways, including increased demands for productivity, the need for developing new skills and the "deskilling" of former jobs, increased as well as diminished access to occupational advancement and personal development, and altered physical and mental demands. Underlying the emergence of new technology is the belief that it contributes to organizational effectiveness through improved efficiency, reduced employee turnover, and reduced labor costs (4,32). Weighing the benefits and costs associated with this large-scale social change is an issue demanding attention from the business and health communities.

The investigation of health issues in office work is important for several reasons. First, offices are increasingly becoming the principal physical worksite for workers in modern societies. What we learn about contemporary problems with office work will be directly applicable to a growing sector of the economy in the years to come. Second, we are currently witnessing a "natural experiment": Traditional office work is in the midst of a transformation in which new technologies are being thrust on an existing structure. The outcomes of this technological and social process have implications for the future structure of our workplaces, for workplace and workstation design, and, perhaps, as important, for the demand and availability of health services.

This chapter considers the issues surrounding health and office work. First, the magnitude of office work, projections for the future, and the potential impacts of technology are reviewed. Next, a framework is given to better understand the health and illness of workers by considering the man–machine–workplace interface (commonly referred to as ergonomics in the engineering profession) from a public health (epidemiological) perspective. The illness-producing capacity of the office environment is then assessed, including physical and psychosocial aspects. The literature on health consequences of visual display terminal (VDT) exposures, and musculoskeletal and visual disturbances associated with office work as well as mental health and psychosomatic illness is reviewed. Finally, the challenge to engineering, social science, and industrial organization of the double-edged sword of increased productivity

127

and health consequences of advancing technological development in the work environment is raised.

OFFICE WORKERS: CURRENT WORKFORCE AND FUTURE PROJECTIONS

The Department of Commerce, Bureau of the Census, reported in 1984 that 16.7 million Americans were employed in clerical jobs, representing approximately 16% of the total labor force (41). When considering the occupational titles most frequently subsumed under the rubric "office work," we include professional, technical, and related occupations and managers, officials, and proprietors in addition to the traditional job title "clerical workers." We find that slightly under one-half of the total workforce is found in these "office worker" categories. Table 10–1 shows the distribution of office workers in the United States in 1982 by industry sector (42). It is evident that the financial, insurance, and real estate (FIRE) sector is the most common locus for office workers, with the services, health services, and transportation/communications/utilities sectors following, each with slightly over one-half of their workforce being office-based.

The Bureau of Labor Statistics (34) in 1984 projected an increase in office-based workers of 28% by 1995, or nearly three-fourths of all jobs to be added to the economy. The largest sector accumulating new jobs is projected to be in "other services," which includes a variety of occupations ranging from business consultants to janitorial services (40). Clearly, occupational growth is linked to industry growth, and the role of technology must be incorporated into projections. When discussing scenarios for growth in the office field, the Bureau of Labor Statistics stated:

> Most office clerical occupations are expected to grow more slowly during 1982–1995 than in the 1970s because of office automation. . . . Secretaries will increasingly use advanced office equipment in the future, thereby becoming more productive. This in turn will dampen demand for the occupation [34, p. 44].

Leontief and Duchin (25) prepared an economic forecast regarding the impact of automation on employment from 1963 to 2000 for the National Science Foundation. They developed a number of scenarios in which economic growth, technological developments, and computerization were varied, and the impact on growth in various employment sectors were assessed. With anticipated developments in technology and their rapid adoption, the number of clerical jobs, as a percentage of total employment, is projected to drop from 17.8% to 11.4%, partially offset by an increase in professional employment from 15.6% to 19.8% by the year 2000 (25). In a discussion of the results of their analyses, the Office of Technology Assessment (40, p. 42) summarized the implications of these forecasts for the job title "secretary."

- Thirty percent of secretaries will not be affected by word processing.
- Twenty percent of a secretary's time is spent in tasks not affected by word processing.
- Word processing saves 80% of the time required for conventional typing.
- Thirty-five percent of secretaries are affected by other office technologies.

Table 10–1. Distribution of "Office Workers" in Selected Industry Sectors, 1982

Industry sector	Total (%)	Employment level (%)		
		Professionals[a]	Managers[b]	Clerical
Financial, insurance,				
real estate	90.0	9.5	17.1	63.4
Services	59.6	33.7	6.8	19.1
Health services	55.9	34.5	4.4	17.0
Transportation,				
communications,				
utilities	50.2	7.9	9.0	33.3
Trade	33.8	3.8	9.3	20.7
Manufacturing	28.8	10.3	6.7	11.8
All industries	46.2	16.4	9.4	20.4

Source: U.S. Department of Labor, Bureau of Labor Statistics, 1983. After (40).

[a] Includes professional, technical, and related occupations.
[b] Includes managers, officials, and proprietors.

- Forty-five percent of their time is affected by other office technologies.
- Seventy-five percent of secretaries' time is saved by new technology relative to old technology.

Clearly, the work of this specific job title is undergoing fundamental change; the health impact experienced by this group is of public health concern, not only because of their large number but because their jobs are being altered so dramatically.

It is acknowledged that although professionals comprise a large part of the work force (approximately 16%) and are located in all industry sectors, a large proportion are not located in offices per se. However, their tasks frequently require administrative and clerical/secretarial support, and they may use office automation directly (e.g., a personal computer) or indirectly (through word processing or information processing using mainframe computers). The Office of Technology Assessment (40) estimated that approximately one-half of all professionals are found in "office-oriented" occupations.

In essence, the argument can be made that office workers comprise one of the largest sectors of employment. As such, occupational health attention to their special needs and health problems is warranted (perhaps to a greater extent than we have seen to date).

TECHNOLOGICAL CHANGES IN OFFICE WORK

The Office of Technology Assessment in 1985 published an important report entitled "Automation of America's Offices." (40) The study, requested by the Senate Committee on Education and Labor, addressed the issues of the effects of the continuing introduction of information and telecommunications technologies in offices. To understand the extent of change that has recently been experienced in the nation's offices, they provided a synopsis of the history of technology used in offices (summarized in Table 10–2). As is evident, the major strides in office automation came after World War

Table 10–2. History of Technology Used in Office Work

Mechanical era
    1810   Fountain pen
    1835   Babbage computing machine
    1868   Carbon paper
    1875   Telephone; typewriter
    1880   Cash register; adding machine
    1900   Addressograph
    1902   Hollerith machines (key punch and sorter)
    1911   Power statistical accounting machine
Electrification era
    1920   Ditto machines (gelatin duplicating)
    1927   Adding/subtracting calculating machines
    1935   Bank check sorting/proofing machines
    1940   Dictating/stenographic machines with plastic belt
    1950   Data processing: computypers, telewriters
    1955   Xerographic duplication
    1958   Data processing: paper tape or cards
Office automation
    Phase 1
        1955   Electronic digital computers: vacuum tubes
        1958   Electronic digital computers: transistors
        1960   Computer magnetic tape; microcomputers
        1965   Computer tape "selectric" typewriters
        1970   Electronic (solid state) calculating machines; facsimile transmission; video display
                terminals
    Phase 2
        1970   Optical scanning and recognition equipment; microcomputers
        1980   Software packages: word processing, databased management; nonimpact printers
    Phase 3
        1980   Local area networks, integrated systems

Source: U.S. Congress, Office of Technology Assessment (40).

II, with more rapid developments seen during the 1970s, reflecting the advent of microchip computers, facsimile transmission, and more recently microcomputers and local area networks. Approximately 15 million microcomputers are now found in America's businesses; it is apparent that the number of offices with computer capabilities has skyrocketed during the 1980s, and the rate of growth continues; for example, a total of 3.15 million personal computers were shipped by the major vendors to the U.S. business and professional markets in 1986 (33).

Addressing the technology of office automation, a number of trends have been projected, including: (a) continuation of the introducing of microcomputers and distributed data handling; (b) linkages and networking between personal computers, mainframes, and peripheral systems; (c) more capture of data at the point of origin (thereby eliminating repeated data entry); and (d) improved communication across sites of data and devices (40). These anticipated trends will have direct and indirect impacts on office work and workers. The consequences may be felt and measured along the lines of productivity, employment, job opportunities, and health. It is the latter factor we address herein.

HEALTH AND ILLNESS IN OFFICE WORKERS

Framework of Human Factors: Epidemiology

In one of the first volumes on technological impacts of office automation (9), published in 1984, the notion of "human factors epidemiology" was proposed as a model to understand how technological transformations affect changes in the nature of work and the health consequences of adaptation to the new environment (1). This approach integrates human factors, "the application of information about human beings and their capabilities and limitations to the design of equipment which people use and to the environments within which people live and work" and the epidemiological method— the investigation of the influences and patterns of health and illness in human populations (23). Whereas ergonomists relate the task and design of the working environment to productivity, satisfaction, and (sometimes) symptoms or illness, the epidemiologist seeks to relate factors in the environment (be they physical, social, or psychological) to acute and chronic health problems. Their integration into one approach allows simultaneous consideration of the physical configuration of the man–machine interface with the nature of the work process in its human dimension.

With office work, for example, the individual is constrained, in a physical sense, by the characteristics of the work setting. These constraints are several: (a) the physical architecture of the work area, including the ambient lighting and the size and configuration of the setting (e.g., whether the layout is open space or cubicles separated by partitions); (b) the technological elements and their placement (e.g., the existence of a VDT and its location, height, and distance in relation to the chair of the worker); (c) the nature of the task itself; and (d) the social interaction possibilities of the worker (i.e., Is the individual isolated from human contact by virtue of the physical architecture of the work area or technologically by the man-machine bond?). The National Academy of Sciences presented a poignant example of the interaction of these elements in their presentation of the needs for updated workstation designs for computer-mediated work; they found that in most offices in which automation has been introduced the physical environment commonly had not been redesigned. Rather, the technology was simply changed without consideration of the human needs or concerns.

As technology is introduced into the work process, a variety of adaptations are required. This point has been especially observable in the case of office work. As workers use technologies to perform their tasks, the physical design of their workstation places limits on their capabilities. These constraints can range from the minimal annoyance of familiar objects being moved, to minor muscle fatigue or temporary blurred vision produced by improperly oriented computer components, to severe somatic reactions to noxious elements in the environment, as is reported in the case of "tight" buildings. The human factors epidemiological approach, then, "describes the complexity of the worker–environment interaction, allowing specific relationships to be established between the physical and structural work environment, worker behavior, and health" (1).

Physical and Psychosocial Environment of Office Work

Until recently, office work was considered one of the "safer" worksites with respect to occupational safety and health concerns, especially compared to the manufacturing and agricultural sectors. However, rapid change has altered this situation. For example, new materials, such as formaldehyde-containing desk tops, chemicals used for duplicating and printing, and carbonless paper are found in abundance in offices (27). Advances in construction have led to the introduction of office environments with reduced air circulation, and sealed portals of entry have resulted in poor air quality and exceedingly low levels of ambient humidity. The focus on the "tight building" or "sealed building" has been precipitated, in part, by the large number of complaints registered by office workers with federal health agencies. For example, approximately 30% of complaints to the National Institute for Occupational Safety and Health (NIOSH) concerning requests for health hazard evaluations have come from office workers (15,43).

The incidence of health effects of "indoor air pollution" has reached such a level that the "tight building syndrome" has been identified (18), characterized by nonspecific complaints of headache and dizziness and accompanied by upper respiratory infections, rashes, and fatigue (28). Principally, the causes of such complaints are traced to toxic levels of a variety of contaminants found in the office environment, including elevated levels of carbon dioxide, nitrogen dioxide, formaldehyde, and solvents, among others (18).

A recent review by NIOSH of more than 80 indoor air quality Health Hazard Evaluations lists three general routes of air contamination: (a) external sources drawn into office buildings through air intake units; (b) reentrainment of exhausted contaminants that are recaptured through air intake units; and (c) internal sources, such as photocopying machines, furniture, cigarette smoking, and building materials (26). The problems of the first two routes can generally be solved through appropriate engineering controls; internal sources require more attention.

Internal air contamination may arise for a variety of reasons. First, point source emissions may be associated with the use of specific work tasks that directly expose workers to noxious agents. For example, work involving the use of telephone facsimile records (butyl methacrylate), carbonless paper (formaldehyde), and photocopying (ozone and carbon black) may be corrected by local ventilation. Less easily solved are nonspecific sources, such as building materials (urea formaldehyde-insulated walls, fibrous glass duct insulation) and bacterial, fungal, and viral agents found in heat pump water condensate pans or outdoor air intake units (26).

Laubli et al. (24) have reported that one of the principal issues related to the physical environment design of offices resulting in health complaints is the level of ambient lighting. Lighting levels typically achieve needed levels, but glare and improper contrasts in luminance are common. Stammerjohn et al. (38) reported that in an evaluation of lighting in a workplace where VDT work was frequent, 85% of operators reported screen glare, 70% character brightness, 68% screen flicker, and 62% screen brightness. Significantly, these complaints have been registered worldwide, wherever VDTs have been put into use and evaluated (35).

The issues and problems of the environmental design of offices reflect both generic heath issues associated with new building designs (as reflected in health concerns of new residential housing as well) and the special needs of workers to meet the requirements of the technology with which they work. Extensive interchange between architects, engineers, and environmental health scientists is essential for such problems to be solved.

HEALTH HAZARDS OF OFFICE WORK

In general, clerical workers and white collar professionals have low injury rates and comparatively high levels of health compared to other workers. However, in some respects this generalization minimizes some important findings from the literature: Although clerical women have good health status, men in clerical occupations have the worst health among white-collar workers. Furthermore, clerical men are more likely to report chronic conditions that affect the type and amount of work they can do, and they are more likely to report recent hospitalizations. Thus it is important to consider the environment of office work and its impact on health status.

Vision

Visual fatigue (or asthenopia) is a common complaint among office workers, especially among workers who use VDTs extensively; design problems in VDT workstations are associated with eye strain (38). The major causal factors include improper illumination, glare, contrast, and computer setup (37). The results of an investigation conducted by NIOSH staff is shown in Figure 10–1. In a comparison of 250 VDT operators with 150 nonoperators, visual system health complaints can be seen to vary systematically between the two groups. These findings have been corroborated by a number of other investigations (14); for example, Cakir et al. (5) found that more than one-half of all VDT operators in some 30 companies investigated reported eye strain and visual problems. Chapnik and Gross (8) summarized the evidence that VDT operators and office workers who use computers report significantly more visual problems (including irritation, fatigue, blurred vision, and headaches) than persons who do not use this technology.

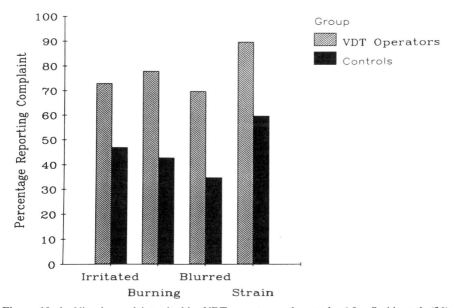

Figure 10–1. Visual complaints cited by VDT operators and controls. After Smith et al. (36).

There remains a significant concern about lighting in workplaces, especially given the apparent lack of attention paid to the need for proper illumination in offices when new technologies are introduced. As Cushman (13) stated, "Lighting that is suitable for general office work, such as typing, filing, reading, and handwriting, is not necessarily suitable for workplaces with visual display terminals. . . . A different approach to lighting is necessary because information is displayed differently." The difference in orientation (traditional office work is horizontal with vision directed downward, VDT work is oriented vertically, thereby increasing the likelihood of glare) is rarely appreciated until significant worker complaints are voiced.

Musculoskeletal Problems

Acute musculoskeletal complaints are commonly reported by workers. This point is significant because of the limitation of activity produced by such disorders; musculoskeletal problems are the leading cause of disability among workers and a leading cause of claims for workers' compensation (22). Factors associated with the work environment include ergonomic issues, such as workstation/user fit (body/keyboard, body/chair, eye/focus element) and physical constraints, as well as the physical aspects of the task performed. Much of office work is repetitive; that dependent on technology may have the capability of producing significant physical trauma and eventual harm (2). For example, improper keyboard height and placement can prove painful for the word processor or data entry worker who spends an entire 8-hour workday at the workstation.

As an example of the consistency of the findings on increased rates of musculoskeletal complaints among office workers, especially among those who frequently use VDTs, Figure 10–2 summarizes the previously cited NIOSH study (36). It is evident that these complaints are frequent and real. Others have reported similar results comparing data entry operators and traditional office workers and have found rates of "almost daily pains" to be significantly higher among the former group. Repetitive strain injuries, e.g., carpal tunnel syndrome and tendonitis, are much more common among office workers who perform repetitive tasks than other workers; the costs borne by industry and the health care sector in treating these largely preventable disorders should not be minimized (24).

Reproductive Risks of Working with VDTs

There has been widespread concern over the observation that women working with VDTs were suffering from an inordinately high incidence of poor pregnancy outcomes (29). These clusters occurred in a variety of settings, but most were observed in relatively large firms in which a high proportion of their labor force used VDTs. Two explanations have been offered to account for these occurrences: radiation emissions and stress. Although there is no evidence for the latter cause, there has been much interest and observation with respect to ionizing radiation. The Office of Technology Assessment (40, pp. 146), after reviewing the evidence, concluded that "no long-term risk is associated with very low frequency radiation emitted from the visual display

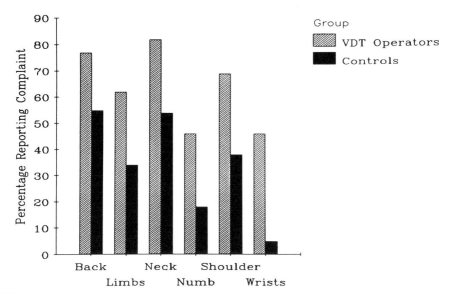

Figure 10–2. Musculoskeletal complaints cited by VDT operators and controls. After Smith et al. (36).

terminal, but continuing evaluation is warranted in light of the large number of people exposed, to see if modified or new standards need to be developed."

NIOSH has investigated the potential threats posed by VDT use on operators, specifically addressing the radiation effects of various VDTs (30). Responding to requests from labor unions, NIOSH performed measurements of both ionizing (x-ray) and nonionizing (ultraviolet, visible, and radiofrequency) radiation on a wide variety of VDTs. The results indicated that no workers were exposed to hazardous levels of radiation.

Despite the current lack of evidence associating VDT work with spontaneous abortions and other adverse pregnancy outcomes, the International Labor Organization recommended that pregnant workers be permitted to transfer jobs during the period of pregnancy. Sweden has extended this right to all pregnant women. The reduction in fear is viewed as a chief outcome of these actions. This literature was reviewed by Stein and Hatch (39).

Psychosocial Disorders

A major issue associated with office work is the matter of "stress." One of the central adjectives associated with the study of office work and its physical health consequences is that it is inherently "stressful." Demands for increased productivity, time urgency, a high degree of competition, and the need for accuracy are seen in the contemporary office, whether it is in the secretarial pool or the board room. Although it is argued that perhaps the level of stress may not differ dramatically across occupations, a consistent finding emerges in studies of white-collar workers: Physical health disorders attributed to stress are common. Studies ranging from harried executives, to air traffic controllers, and to computer operators systematically demonstrate elevated rates of disorders commonly viewed as "psychosomatic," or stress-related. These problems range from elevated blood pressure, ulcers, and sleep disturbances, to anxiety and depression, and ultimately to premature death.

A recent analysis of the effects of stress on the health and functioning of one class of workers, health care professionals, may serve as a framework for understanding the dynamics and outcomes of stress at work (7). There are two contemporary approaches to understanding how the stress process develops. One, called the Person-Environment Fit model (17), states that when there is a discrepancy between the demands of the job and the capabilities of the individual to meet the demands, strains develop that may ultimately culminate in physiological manifestations. The alternative perspective, called the Job Demands/Control model (20), suggests that when the job demands exceed the control of the worker to meet the demands, unreleased strain overtaxes the individual. The crucial distinction in these models has been shown by Baker (3): The Person-Environment Fit approach places the emphasis on the individual's needs and abilities, whereas the Demand/Control model focuses on environmental constraints (i.e., the structural characteristics of work). From an occupational safety and health perspective, the latter allows more opportunities for intervention and prevention strategies.

The study of stress-related health outcomes has frequently been the study of white collar illness. The outcomes of stress are frequently subsumed under three broad headings: physiological effects, psychological outcomes, and behavioral manifestations (3).

Physiological Outcomes. By physiological impacts, we mean acute (short-term) changes in normal functioning, e.g., in heart rate and pulse. These strains are important because of their longer-term effects; coronary artery disease and hypertension are the ultimate outcomes of uncontrolled heart rate or blood pressure. Clearly, these disorders occur more frequently in white-collar workers, although the effect of lesser physical demands on the job may account in part for why blue-collar workers are less often affected by these problems (21).

Psychological Outcomes. Psychological outcomes attributable to stress at work have been widely cited and demonstrate consistent findings: Occupational stress (both objective and perceived) has direct and important impacts on mental health. In an important investigation on the variation in health and well-being across occupations conducted by NIOSH (6), psychological status was determined to be higher among certain job classes. It was concluded that the greatest psychological impact of work was experienced by clerical and low-level blue collar workers, based in part on perceived stressors by the workers as well as the accumulation of risk factors confronting these workers: high demands, little individual control over the work and its conduct, repetitive tasks with little opportunity for self-expression, little challenge and few rewards, and poor overall working conditions. Short-term psychological impacts include boredom and low job satisfaction, anxiety, and depression, as well as somatic conditions (19).

Behavioral Outcomes. The behavioral outcomes attributable to stress at work are those most obvious to managers. They include employee tardiness, absenteeism, and turnover (31) as well as drinking and drug use at work (11) and their negative impact on performance and productivity (12). It has been well established in industrial settings that work-related morbidity and mortality frequently have their roots in lack of attentiveness, alcohol and drug use, and refusal to follow company policy and directions. In the office setting we have been far less attentive to similar situations, with the exception of job monitoring for productivity. Other, less direct results of stress can be seen to affect the health (and consequent productivity) of workers in nonindustrial settings (10).

Introduction of a New Technology: Case Study

The opportunity to systematically assess the effects of introducing a new technology into the work environment was presented in 1985, when an office of 15 persons made the decision to computerize the workplace. The worksetting, a white collar service establishment, had traditionally been physically arranged in a "decentralized" fashion, such that the secretarial support was provided to individual professionals in clusters. The secretarial functions consisted largely in typing using electric, and in a few cases, electronic typewriters. Additional clerical functions included a heavy volume of filing and duplicating, as well as more traditional secretarial functions, such as handling incoming telephone calls.

The secretarial personnel were of varied backgrounds, ranging from a recent high school graduate who had some limited introduction to computing and word processing as part of her education to a competent, experienced woman who was approaching retirement age. The professional staff all had experience with computing, although predominantly geared toward statistical computing using mainframe computers. Almost none had had any prior experience with minicomputers or personal computers.

The office was computerized in two "waves": The first step consisted in providing a separate office in which two personal computers were located, and the second step was provision of personal computers for all staff. The first method, that of creating a "word processing center," was met initially with significant resistance by the secretarial staff. In-depth interviews with the staff yielded the following: (1) There was significant variation among the secretaries in the amount of apprehension and fear associated with learning the system; (2) there was little if any training or support in learning the relatively sophisticated word processing system; and (3) the long learning curve in attaining sufficient skill to create text led to a long lag in productivity. The workplace was generally characterized by tension and anxiety among the secretarial staff compounded by the problem that the computing equipment itself was from a new vendor with new software, for which there was insufficient experience or support locally.

Within 1 month of the introduction of this system, there was a dramatic alteration in the office environment. There was a division among the secretaries with respect to social interaction drawn along the lines of their relative abilities to do their work on the computers. The accommodation to this split was that those workers who felt comfortable with the new technology began to spend a large part of their time working with the computers, which served only to increase the rift between the two groups: It also demonstrated in a public forum one group's relative productivity and shifted the burden of tasks between the groups (i.e., the less able group spent more time answering telephones, copying manuscripts, and so on). Furthermore, time spent in the "word processing center" was time where there was little supervision or accountability, except that the final product was expected to be produced within a reasonable time.

With respect to physical complaints associated with the introduction of the VDTs in this workplace, there were the usual reports of eye strain, difficulty focusing, and other visual complaints. Muscle fatigue and sore backs were also reported. Typically, these problems resulted from spending a prolonged period at the VDT without taking a break, as well as from the improper ergonomic arrangement of the office environment. After these factors were assessed, the second phase developed.

At this time, the "word processing center" approach was scrapped, primarily because of the friction among the personnel. Personal computers were then purchased, with a unit given to each of the secretaries. A standard national vendor was selected and a widely available word processing package selected. At this time most of the professional staff also began using personal computers, with common software selected. Some care was taken to redesign the office environment such that ergonomic considerations were taken into account (e.g., ambient lighting needs and availability were assessed, as was desk height and type of chair). This change led to significantly greater self-reported productivity on the part of personnel, although at some initially increased expense. Furthermore, as the technology became a greater part of the environment, with its widespread availability and greater utilization, complaints and concerns diminished. In some respect, the learning curve had been reached.

CONTEMPORARY ISSUES REGARDING THE HEALTH OF OFFICE WORKERS

It is clear that the changes taking place in modern offices reflect broad social changes. The ultimate policy concerns associated with technological development are several.

1. *What does "automation" of office work mean with respect to productivity?* First, consideration must be given to the evaluation of productivity, with the development of clear and comprehensive measures. Productivity in terms of the "bottom line" can certainly be assessed, though it is clear that there are numerous trade-offs between output per unit of time and other factors, such as employee morale, fatigue, and job satisfaction. Automation introduced with the participation of workers seems to lead to increased productivity, but this transformation of the work process may have other implications.

2. *How will the transformation of the office affect well-being?* It is clear that the introduction of technology into the office environment can have a variety of psychosocial outcomes. Computerization is usually met initially with apprehension and anxiety. Then, depending on the extent of training and support, workers accommodate to the new work process. The extent to which their well-being is affected by new technology reflects an organic process. Furthermore, new cohorts of office workers will be different from the present workforce, as they will be more computer-literate and technologically focused. However, new technologies will continue to be introduced into the work environment, requiring alteration of behavior.

3. *What will be the financial implications of a possibly reduced labor force in the office?* It is apparent that technology in the office setting can reduce costs, primarily by

reducing the number of personnel required to conduct office tasks. For the individual firm, it may mean increased income. For society, however, such reductions in personnel lead to growth in the underemployed or unemployed population. This situation clearly has policy implications that can be addressed only at a state or national level. Although the service sector itself is growing, the loss of skilled positions will lead to a large workforce of individuals requiring retraining for different skills.

4. *How will computerization change the skills needed for white-collar jobs?* This review has focused mainly on clerical and secretarial personnel. Yet the introduction of new technology into the office is having a major impact on professionals as well. Though computers were seen at first as a mark of prestige in the professional's office, the rapid growth in the use of personal computers has made them commonplace. Clearly, older cohorts of professionals have experienced the same psychological problems in adapting to the use of computers for performing their work. Initially, learning how to type may be the principal stumbling block for the older executive. Future cohorts who have been educated in the use of computers in school will hopefully not suffer this problem. For certain occupations, computer knowledge has become a requisite component of the job, e.g., drafting, architecture, design, accounting, and business management. An inability to master computer-aided design or statistical spreadsheets renders the executive or professional nonproductive.

A variety of additional concerns has been raised with respect to office automation and the future health problems we may anticipate. Many of these issues are beyond the scope of this discussion, yet they remain important policy concerns for society, business, and the health sector. Some require major alterations in the way we consider the work environment as well as the extent to which considerations about the responsibility for the health status of workers are viewed. Among such concerns are the following.

1. Are we educating and training our future office workers appropriately?
2. What types of health problems should we anticipate as a larger proportion of the workforce is found in offices?
3. How must we implement or restructure our contemporary employee health services and employee assistance programs?
4. What may be the impact of technological development on the need and demand for health services?
5. How much contemporary "office work" may soon be translated into "home office" work?
6. Is "telecommuting" a positive vanguard of the future or a form of entrapment?
7. Will advances in automation increase the loss of jobs to "off-shore work"?
8. Will small businesses and their workers be affected by the information revolution as has large business?

REFERENCES

1. Amick, B. C., & Celentano, D. D. (1984). Human factors epidemiology: an integrated approach to the study of health issues in office work. In B. G. F. Cohen (ed.). *Human aspects* *in office automation* (pp. 153–66). New York: Elsevier.

2. Arndt, R. (1983). Body posture. In *Health and ergonomic considerations of visual display*

units (pp. 29–44). Akron: American Industrial Hygiene Association.

3. Baker, D. (1985). The study of stress at work. *Annual Review of Public Health, 6,* 367–81.

4. Becker, F. D. (1981). *Workspace: creating environments in organizations.* New York: Praeger.

5. Cakir, A., Hart, D. J., & Stewart, T. F. M (1982). *Visual display terminals.* Norwich: Page Brothers.

6. Caplan, R. D., Cobb, S., French, J. R. P., Van Harrison, R., & Pinneau, S. R. (1975). *Job demands and worker health.* DHHS publication (NIOSH) 75-160. Washington, DC: U.S. Department of Health, Education and Welfare.

7. Celentano, D. D., & Johnson, J. V. (1987). Stress in health care workers. *Occupational Medicine, 2,* 593–608.

8. Chapnik, E-B., & Gross, C. M. (1987). Evaluation, office improvements can reduce VDT operator problems. *Occupational Health & Safety, 56,* 34–37.

9. Cohen, B. G. F. (ed.). (1984). *Human aspects in office automation.* New York: Elsevier.

10. Communications Workers of America (1986). *Occupational Stress: The hazard and the challenge.* Washington, DC: Communications Workers of America.

11. Conway, T. L., Ward, H. W., Vickers, R. R., & Rahe, R. H. (1981). Occupational stress and variation in cigarette, coffee and alcohol consumption. *Journal of Health and Social Behavior, 22,* 155–65.

12. Cummings, T. G., & Molloy, E. S. (1977). *Improving productivity and the quality of work life.* New York: Praeger.

13. Cushman, W. H. (1983). Lighting for workplaces with visual display terminals. In *Health and ergonomic considerations of visual display Units* (pp. 73–86). Akron: American Industrial Hygiene Association.

14. Dainoff, M. (1983). VDU work task categories. In *Health and ergonomic considerations of visual display units* (pp. 103–18). Akron: American Industrial Hygiene Association.

15. Ferrand E. F., & Moriates, S. (1981). Health aspects of indoor air pollution: social, legislative and economic considerations. *Bulletin of the New York Academy of Medicine, 57,* 1061–6.

16. Francis, A. (1986). *New technology at work.* New York: Oxford.

17. French, J. R. P., Caplan, R. D., & Van Harrison, R. (1982). *The mechanisms of job stress and strain.* New York: Wiley.

18. Hollowell, C. D., & Miksch, R. R. (1981). Sources and concentrations of compounds in indoor environments. *Bulletin of the New York Academy of Medicine, 57,* 962–77.

19. Kalimo, R., El-Batawi, M. A., & Cooper, C. L. (1987). *Psychosocial factors at work and*

their relationship to health. Geneva: World Health Organization.

20. Karasek, R. A., Baker, D., Marxer, F., Ahlbom, A., & Theorell, T. (1981). Job decision latitude, job demands, and cardiovascular disease: a prospective study of Swedish men. *American Journal of Public Health, 71,* 694–705.

21. Kasl, S. V. (1978). Epidemiological contributions to the study of work stress. In C. L. Cooper and R. Payne (eds.). *Stress at work.* Chichester: Wiley.

22. Kelsey, J. L. (1982). *Epidemiology of musculoskeletal disorders.* New York: Oxford.

23. Kleinbaum, D., Kupper, L., & Morgenstern, H. (1982). *Epidemiologic research & principles and quantitative methods.* Belmont, CA: Lifetime Learning.

24. Laubli, T., Hunting, W., & Grandjean, E. (1980). Visual impairments related to environmental conditions in VDU operators. In E. Grandjean and E. Viliani (eds.). *Economic aspects of visual display terminals* (pp. 85–94). London: Taylor & Francis.

25. Leontief, W., & Duchin, F. (1984). *The impacts of automation on employment, 1963–2000.* Washington, DC: Institute for Economic Analysis for the National Science Foundation.

26. McGlothlin, J. D. (1984). Field design and solutions to office worker illness: an industrial hygiene perspective. In B. G. G. Cohen (ed.). *Human aspects in office automation* (pp. 23–31). New York: Elsevier.

27. Messite, J., & Baker, D. F. (1984). Occupational health problems in offices—a mixed bag. In B. G. F. Cohen (ed.). *Human aspects in office automation* (pp. 7–14). New York: Elsevier.

28. Michaels, D. (1984). Tackling tight building syndrome: what can workers do? In B. G. F. Cohen (ed.). *Human aspects in office automation* (pp. 15–22). New York: Elsevier.

29. Murray, W. E. (1983). Is there a radiation risk? *Health and ergonomic considerations of visual display units* (pp. 87–102). Akron: American Industrial Hygiene Association.

30. Murray, W. E., Moss, C. E., Parr, W. H., & Cox, C. (1981). A radiation and industrial hygiene survey of video display terminal operations. *Human Factors, 23,* 413–20.

31. Porter, L. W., & Steers, R. M. (1973). Organizational, work, and personal factors in employee turnover and absenteeism. *Psychological Bulletin, 80,* 151–76.

32. Rubin, A. (1983). *The automated office—an environment for productive work, or an information factory? A report on the state-of-the-art.* Washington, DC: U.S. Department of Commerce, National Bureau of Standards.

33. Schlender, B. R. (1987). The electronic storm. In *The Wall Street Journal,* June 12.

34. Silvestri, G. T., Lukasiewicz, J. M., & Einstein, M. E. (1984). *Occupational employment projections through 1995: employment projections for 1995* (bulletin 2197). U.S. Department of Labor, Bureau of Labor Statistics.
35. Smith, M. J. (1984). Ergonomic aspects of health problems in VDT operators. In B. G. F. Cohen (ed.). *Human aspects in office automation* (pp. 97–114). New York: Elsevier.
36. Smith, M. J., Cohen, B. G. F., Stammerjohn, L., & Happ, A. (1981). An investigation of health complaints and job stress in video display operations. *Human Factors, 23*, 387–400.
37. Snyder, H. (1983). Vision and the VDU. In *Health and ergonomic considerations of visual display units* (pp. 12–20). Akron: American Industrial Hygiene Association.
38. Stammerjohn, L., Smith, M. J., & Cohen, B. G. F. (1981). Evaluation of work station design factors in VDT operations. *Human Factors, 23*, 401–12.

39. Stein, Z. A., & Hatch, M. C. (eds.) (1986). Reproductive problems in the workplace. *Occupational Medicine, 1*, 361–539.
40. U.S. Congress, Office of Technology Assessment. (1985). *Automation of America's offices.* OTA-CIT publication 287. Washington, DC: U.S. Government Printing Office.
41. U.S. Department of Commerce, Bureau of Labor Statistics. (1984). *Current population survey annual averages, 1984.* Washington, DC: U.S. Department of Commerce.
42. U.S. Department of Labor, Bureau of Labor Statistics. (1983). *Employment and earnings* (Vol. 30, No. 1). Washington, DC: U.S. Department of Labor.
43. U.S. General Accounting Office. (1980). *Indoor air pollution: an emerging health problem.* Washington, DC: U.S. General Accounting Office.

11
Stress in the Work and Home Environments as Related to Ischemic Heart Disease Risk Factors

Marie A. Morell, Megan E. Sullaway,
and Vicki S. Helgeson

Ischemic heart disease (IHD) is the leading cause of death in the United States, accounting for the loss of nearly one million lives annually (69–71). Overall IHD prevalence and incidence rates are at least twice as great for men as for women, and the difference is even greater during the fifth and sixth decades of life (69). In addition to the considerable emotional and physical distress experienced by IHD patients and their families, societal costs are substantial. For example, in 1986 impaired health due to IHD cost business and industry the equivalent of 6.5 million days' wages (68).

Known medical risk factors such as high serum cholesterol and hypertension account for less than 50% of the variance in IHD rates (9,34), and the best combinations of risk factors fail to identify most new cases (33). In recognition of these limitations, investigators increasingly have utilized biopsychosocial research paradigms in efforts to identify the factors responsible for individual differences in IHD.

TYPE A BEHAVIOR AND IHD

During the 1950s cardiologists Ray Rosenman and Meyer Friedman, emphasizing the assessment of *specific behaviors* possibly related to IHD, established the concept of the Type A Behavior Pattern (TABP). Type A behavior encompasses a cluster of cognitive, affective, physiologic, and behavioral factors that are elicited in "characterologically predisposed" individuals with high achievement goals, competitiveness, time urgency, and productivity. Type A individuals demonstrate excesses in drive, job involvement, upward striving, time urgency, impatience, hostility, tense musculature, explosive speech patterns, and alertness (35,62). In contrast, Type B persons, with the antithetical pattern, generally appear relaxed, easygoing, and cooperative.

Among individuals considered to be predisposed to TABP by the combination of biological and psychological factors, the behavior is elicited by environments that emphasize competitiveness, high productivity, and deadline pressures, i.e., many work environments (10,39). Research has shown that more objective rewards are accorded to Type A than to Type B individuals, e.g., higher occupational status, prestige, income, and more rapid career advancement (44). Type A behavior also has been positively correlated with self-esteem, enhanced job involvement, higher skill utilization, along with greater feelings of work efficacy and work satisfaction (13).

Nonetheless, concern has been expressed about the interpersonal satisfaction (or dissatisfaction) Type As receive from their work. Type A behavior is negatively related to satisfaction with coworkers (10). Compared to Type Bs, Type As report more problems related to the disruptive effects of long work hours on activities with family, friends, and pursuit of avocational interests. Nonetheless, Type As report greater *overall* life satisfaction compared to Type Bs, suggesting that the positive effects of work outweigh its negative consequences on home life and interpersonal relationships (10).

What is it about Type A behavior that might lead to greater IHD risk in the work environment? Some studies here suggested that the *combined* interactive effects of poor "fit" between person, the type of work she does, and the work environment trigger physical and emotional stress (49) and hence increase the risk of IHD. For example, the independent Type A person may find a job with little autonomy stressful, whereas the Type B person may feel stressed by a job that *requires* autonomy (13).

There has been extensive research on the relation between TABP and IHD. Studies conducted during the 1960s and 1970s generally indicated that IHD incidence risk was at least *twice* as great for Type A as for Type B individuals, even when traditional risk factors were statistically controlled (9,28). Because TABP prevalence is higher among persons working in the competitive labor market and fewer women are employed than men, Type A prevalence is estimated to be lower in women than in men (27,48). Overall IHD rates are comparable in Type A men and women, although women are more likely to have the less serious angina pectoris than the myocardial infarction found in men (26,28).

In 1981 the Coronary Heart Disease Review Panel concluded that TABP constitutes a significant IHD risk factor of magnitude similar to that of elevated systolic blood pressure and serum cholesterol (17). Some more recent reviews, however, have summarized a growing body of negative findings (26,58). Haynes and Matthews (26) concluded that these findings may reflect (a) an increase in positive health behaviors, such as smoking cessation; (b) implementation of an exercise program and related reduction in TABP; (c) variability in the assessment of Type A behavior that produced different outcomes; and (d) secular trends whereby IHD decreased markedly between 1970 and 1983, thereby leaving a different, lower risk population than was included in early studies.

The current status of Type A research is characterized by a shift in focus away from the global behavior type and toward efforts to identify those *components* of the behavior type that may be pathogenic for IHD, such as anger and time urgency. The more broadly defined behavior type now often serves as the focus of research that investigates factors associated with interpersonal distress or satisfaction in work and home environments. In addition, investigators have begun to study women and minority groups within each of these areas, although the bulk of the prior data are on white men. Overall, the evidence indicates that Type A behavior remains a significant risk factor in IHD incidence and possibly angina prevalence among men, particularly when behavior type is assessed by the Structured Interview (7). However, the broader claims made from the early research (e.g., the relation between TABP and extent of coronary atherosclerosis) appear to be no longer warranted.

EMPLOYMENT, GENDER, AND STRESS

Demographic Changes in Employment Rates for Women

Dramatic changes have occurred in women's employment in the United States over the last several decades that have affected men as well as women. Whereas 40.8% of women ages 20 to 43 were employed outside the home in 1970, this rate increased to 65% in 1980 (62). In 1985 women constituted 50% of the national labor force (63) and by 1988 73.3% of women between the ages of 25 and 59 years were in the labor force (24). The greatest increase in women working outside the home has been among those married with children under 6 years of age; 17% in 1960, 30% in 1970, and 54% in 1988 (20). Marked changes also have occurred in *types* of employment available to both women and men (55,56): however, women are proportionately overrepresented in lower paying positions, often despite having advanced degrees (67).

Employment, Multiple Roles, and Health

For individuals who have household, child care, or elder care responsibilities, the number and the diversity of roles necessary to perform is greater than for persons who do not have comparable responsibilities (2,15,66). Interestingly, employed women who hold multiple roles report *better* health and general well-being than women who engage in fewer roles, typically having higher self-esteem, greater job satisfaction, and less depression (1,8,53). It has been suggested that multiple roles offer greater access to privileges and resources that can be used to buffer problems arising from any one role (3,53). Thus the role of paid worker may buffer, rather than exacerbate, stress in the home, and the positive aspects of home life may buffer work stress. However, multiple roles do not always lead to positive outcomes, particularly when they produce *role strain,* i.e., role overload (time and task constraints) and role conflict (incompatible demands among roles). Women generally suffer greater role strain than men, especially when they are married and have children (15,37,50,54) or are a single parent (55,56). Men who are actively involved in family life also may experience role strain when they perceive that they have insufficient time or energy for their careers and complain that family responsibilities interfere with employment activities and potential for career advancement (1,57). Obviously, for both women and men, stresses and strains at work may carry over into home life and vice versa (21,29,30,60). A negative outcome does not necessarily result, however. Research suggests that negative effects of multiple roles occur at high levels of stress but have comparatively small impact at moderate or low stress levels (52). Furthermore, absence of social support under high stress circumstances is associated with increased psychological and physiological symptomatology although it appears to have little effect at low stress levels (52). Additional investigations in this area promise to provide information regarding how work environments might be structured to decrease the occurrence of negative effects on health and well-being.

Carryover Effects of Stress in the Work and Home Environments

The erroneous belief that work and family activities are unrelated in their psychological and physiological impact has been discussed as the "myth of separate worlds" (38). Clearly, when a stressful event occurs in the workplace or the home (e.g., death of a loved one, serious job injury), the initial impact of carryover effects is recognized by family, friends, and coworkers in both the work and the home domains. However, when the effects of major life stressors are more subtle (e.g., chronic marital dissatisfaction, job dissatisfaction) and long-lasting (e.g., bereavement), carryover effects between settings frequently are underestimated or unrecognized. Conversely, work-related stressors may exert unrecognized deleterious effects on family relationships (72). Although few studies have been conducted in this area, available data document this effect (25,59,61).

Socioeconomic Status

A potent mediator of the interrelation between work and home experience is socioeconomic status. Among low socioeconomic status families, more negative effects (e.g., lower marital quality) have been observed when the wife is employed outside the home than when she is not (59). Not surprisingly, women in low-prestige, low-paying jobs generally report more symptoms of depression than do those in high-prestige, better-paying positions (61). This finding may reflect more than the influence of limited financial resources and may occur because low-paying jobs often are more noxious (e.g., poor work environment, repetitive tasks, exposure to hazardous materials) and are held because of economic necessity rather than personal preference (61). Furthermore, employed women of low socioeconomic status are more likely to be burdened by role overload. They may lack access to many household conveniences and services as well as interpersonal activities. For such individuals, long work hours at home and in their paid employment position interfere with family life and create scheduling problems (14,54).

Compared to men, women generally complain much more of time shortage (65), apparently because women maintain primary responsibility for housework and childcare, regardless of their employment status and whether or not they have a husband living at home (49,53). This is especially true for women who are married to blue-collar workers because these men are less likely to share family and household responsibilities. Lower income families also have greater difficulty arranging childcare when women are employed and the ease of arranging childcare affects women's mental health. Research has shown that egalitarian role relations constitute a significant predictor of women's, but not men's, marital adjustment (for a review, see 18), and that employment is only associated with *better* mental health among women whose husbands share family responsibilities (34). Data also suggest that when men help with tasks at home marital satisfaction is increased for women, but decreased for men (44).

Intuitively, it appears that the negative effects associated with multiple roles and role overload would interfere with work performance. However, no data have been published on this issue, and employers seldom look beyond the workplace as a possible cause of poor employee behavior, negative attitude, or low productivity. Studies are needed in order to develop a more comprehensive understanding of how stress at work and home exert direct and interactive effects on health, job satisfaction, marital and family functioning, and overall well-being.

MARRIAGE, STRESS, TYPE A BEHAVIOR, AND IHD

The quality and number of interpersonal relationships (particularly marriage) may affect emotional adjustment and overall health status (including cardiac health) both positively and negatively (19,51). Data suggest that marital happiness contributes more to global happiness than does any other variable, including satisfaction with work and friends (8,22,74). Generally, happiness or "well-being" is more prevalent among married than unmarried individuals; however, the positive effects of marriage are greater for men than for women (40). Some epidemiological research has reported that satisfaction with marriage and other social relationships is associated with lower mortality (5,51) although other studies have not found health-related effects (3,31).

One potential psychologic mediator of health and marital status or satisfaction is vulnerability to stress. Men rely heavily on their wives as buffers against stress and "hassles in living" (45,46) and as their *exclusive* source of social support. In contrast, women generally have a broader support network that includes friends and extended family members, as well as their spouses. This network may provide women with greater opportunity to buffer or directly decrease stress that arises from any one relationship.

Regarding the effects of these interpersonal styles, husbands are more likely than wives to perceive that their spouses are affectionate and positively affirming; however, men also are more apt to experience depression if their wives are unaffectionate, especially when men fail to receive personal satisfaction from their work. Depression itself has been linked with a small, albeit significant, increased risk for IHD (7,33) suggesting that men who are depressed because of marital or work distress may be more susceptible to heart disease than are those with greater work or marital satisfaction. Further study appears to be warranted in this area.

Behavior Type, Marital Satisfaction, and IHD

Investigators report that marital distress is greater among Type A than Type B women (8,64), although findings are inconsistent (39). In part this is because of the different measures of assessing behavior type, different socioeconomic status of the samples, and the variable presence or absence of children. The Framingham Heart Study and other research have revealed that Type A men were more emotionally labile, ambitious, anger-prone, and likely to be involved in marital disagreements than Type B men (18) and display more behavior indicative of hostility and disgust (12). Wives of Type A men have reported less marital satisfaction than wives of Type B men, but they also complained more that their husbands' jobs had negative effects on personal, home, and family life (10,39).

Regarding the associations between behavior type and disease, the highest overall IHD rates in the Framingham cohort occurred among *Type A men married to Type B women* (18). Specifically, Type A blue-collar men developed IHD six times as often as Type B blue-collar men who were married to Type B women. Among white-collar male employees, however, the wife's behavior type was unrelated to the husband's IHD status. Furthermore, there were no differences in IHD rates between Type A and Type B men when they were married to Type A women (incidence rates of 15.4% and 16.4%, respectively). Eaker and colleagues (18) speculated that Type A blue-collar husbands with Type B wives had greater IHD risk because their ambition and desire to increase their occupational status was not supported by their wives, thereby leading to conflict. However, other investigations have provided mixed support for this interpretation. For example, in a study of professional couples, Type A husbands with Type B wives showed the *lowest* marital adjustment and, presumably, the greatest IHD risk (4). In our own research, among middle- to upper-middle-class couples, marital satisfaction was lowest when the wife was Type A (as assessed by the Framingham Type A Scale and the Jenkins Activity Schedule) regardless of whether the husband was Type A or B (64).

Spouse Characteristics and IHD Risk

A variety of additional spousal characteristics have been implicated in IHD risk. For example, men married to women with 13 or more years of education had increased IHD risk, even when biological risk factors were controlled (11,28). Western Collaborative Group Study data reported that wives of men with IHD also reported greater accomplishments (11) and were more dominant than wives of men without IHD (65). However, data on the wives were collected post hoc, making it uncertain whether wives' characteristics existed prior to their husbands' disease or were a response to it.

The physiologic mechanisms by which the marital relationship ultimately becomes associated with IHD mortality and morbidity are unknown. One possibility is that the marital relationship affects cardiovascular health indirectly by influencing health behaviors such as eating habits, exercise, and cigarette smoking (41). Some studies have shown that personal qualities of the spouse are related to IHD *independent* of other risk factors (45). Emotional support and intimacy may have a beneficial impact on physiological reactivity (36). Perhaps individual characteristics associated with IHD risk also affect marital satisfaction, tension, and conflict in ways that have pathophysiological consequences (16).

Stress Reactivity Models of IHD

Biopsychosocial theorists have hypothesized that individual differences in IHD risk may be associated with variability in cardiovascular reactivity to stress. Stress reactivity is evaluated as elevations in cardiovascular system activity (e.g., heart rate, blood pressure) and concomitant biochemical changes (e.g., elevations in catecholamines). In persons with atherosclerosis, heightened physiological arousal also can be associated with clearly pathologic responses, such as mycardial ischemia (and possibly anginal pain), coronary wall motion abnormalities, and possibly myocardial infarction and death.

Summarizing research on the stress reactivity theory, Manuck and colleagues (43) have noted that heightened blood pressure and neuroendocrine responses lead to coronary artery endothelium injury and increased cell turnover. Plasma lipoproteins then infiltrate the intima and release mitogenic substances that promote intimal smooth muscle cell proliferation and disrupt cellular lipid metabolism. Theoretically, such a response pattern is associated with rapid or extensive development of atherosclerosis and may lead to clinical coronary disease events (43).

Results of animal studies of both acute and long-term stress have consistently documented the presence of individual differences in propensity to respond to stress with heightened physiological reactions and the associations between such reactivity with the development of atherosclerosis-like conditions. This effect has been more extreme when the animals were fed a lipid-rich diet, but it also was observed (albeit to a lesser extent) when the animals were treated with a "prudent" (i.e., low fat, low cholesterol) diet (43).

Individual differences in stress reactivity have been observed in children and heightened reactivity typically is maintained on repeated testing over many years, suggesting that it may be a trait. However, it would not be accurate to assume that persons who experience heightened reactivity to stress inevitably are more likely to develop IHD than their less reactive peers, as the *frequency* of exposure to relevant stressors also is important (42).

Research findings indicate that Type A men typically respond to laboratory stress with greater increases in cardiovascular (particularly β-adrenergic) activity than do Type B men (42). From the few investigations that have included women, findings have varied from no significant differences in Type As and Bs to results that parallel outcomes from studies of men (32,42). Overall, findings indicate that women show *less* reactivity than men, an effect that has been interpreted as suggesting that women's lower stress reactivity may partially account for their lower IHD rates. It may be that the *combination* of relatively lower women's TABP prevalence and less stress reactivity may influence their IHD rates compared to men.

Research examining the relation between marital factors and stress reactivity or the relation between work factors and stress reactivity is sparse and has yielded inconsistent results. Investigations of the specific physiological reactions associated with particular marital interactions or types of work rarely have been investigated in vivo.

UCLA MARRIAGE AND HEALTH PROJECT; PRELIMINARY FINDINGS

Description of the Study

The overall goal of the UCLA Marriage and Health Project was to examine gender differences in stress reactivity across a number of biopsychosocial factors that potentially are associated with gender differences in IHD rates. In this chapter we specifically discuss variability in stress reactivity associated with differences in biological sex, perceived work environment support, and marital satisfaction. Although it was our intention to also examine the interactive or crossover effects of stress at work and stress at home, our sample size was insufficient to permit such analysis.

For the overall investigation, participants were involved in three research sessions. In the first, the Structured Interview (SI) was administered and videotaped for later assessment of behavior type. Questionnaire measures of Type A behavior included the Jenkins Activity Survey (JAS) (35) and the Framingham Type A Scale (FTAS) (28). (Unless otherwise indicated, all results reported concern behavior type classified by the

SI.) For the second session, subjects participated in an individual assessment of stress reactivity, as determined by respiration, heart rate as measured by continuous electrocardiography, and systolic and diastolic blood pressures (SBP, DBP), measured continuously through an automated system (63). Subjects were monitored during a 15-minute resting baseline, four stress tasks (in a fixed order), and a final 15-minute "recovery" (rest) period. The stressors were mental arithmetic, public speaking, forced choice reaction time (23), and autonomic habituation (bursts of white noise presented at random intervals). During the third session, physiologic measures were recorded while husband and wife concurrently went through baseline, stress tasks, intertask rest periods, and a final recovery period. Findings from this session are not presented.

Research participants were solicited via newspaper advertisements. Not all data were collected at the time this report was prepared, so findings presented here are based on 81 heterosexual couples 39 to 60 years of age. Education level ranged from less than seventh grade to postgraduate professional degrees. Average total family income was between $50,000 and $75,000.

Demographically, our sample was skewed toward the upper end of the distributions of income, education, and occupational status. Nevertheless, gender differences emerged that were consistent with previous research: women had completed less education and earned lower incomes than men. Although women were just as likely as men to be classified as professionals, there were more male managerial workers and more female sales/clerical workers. On an overall measure of status, women scored lower than men.

The prevalence of Type A and Type B behaviors was comparable for men and women. This finding contrasts with previous research findings of a higher Type A prevalence in men, but it is consistent with our sample characteristics, as almost all of the women in our investigation held paid employment positions. Neither income nor status was related to behavior type, a finding that contrasts with previous research that has found that Type As achieve higher status than Type Bs, but it confirms Friedman and Rosenman's claim that Type A behavior is not necessarily associated with higher levels of success at work; i.e., it depends on the nature of the job.

Work Environment Factors

A number of variables associated with work were assessed. *Objective work characteristics* included number of days worked per week, number of hours worked per day, job flexibility, and number of hours spent doing housework per week. *Subjective work characteristics* were measures of the individual's perception of the work environment as assessed by Moos's Work Environment Scales (Job Autonomy, Task Orientation, and Work Pressure scales). The *emotional environment* at work was evaluated by self-reports on job and family involvement measures. Also, environmental support was evaluated with the Institute of Survey Research's questionnaire. Among those employed outside the home, men reported spending more hours at work than did women, but working women indicated working more hours at home than did men. In addition, men claimed higher job involvement compared to home involvement, whereas women scored higher on family involvement. These results are consistent with previous research on gender differences.

From one perspective, findings for overall status paralleled those for gender: low status respondents (defined through a combined index that incorporated education, income, and occupational status) reported working more unpaid hours at home and scored higher on family involvement than high status respondents. In addition, women were more likely than men to hold low status positions.

Among all persons employed outside the home, more women than men indicated that their jobs lacked flexibility. When evaluated by status groups, however, low status participants were more likely than those of high status to report that their jobs had high flexibility. That is, although low status was associated with high job flexibility and female sex, women still were more likely than men to report that their jobs lacked flexibility. It is unclear whether different flexibility needs were related to *actual* job differences or only to *perceptions* of job flexibility: women may require high job flexibility so that they can arrange their schedules to accommodate both work and family responsibilities. Supporting this speculation is evidence that, for women only, job flexibility was associated with self-reported greater job autonomy and lower work pressure.

TABP interacted with gender and status on various occasions, which underscores the importance of considering Type A in the context of other variables. Among men Type As reported greater job involvement than Type Bs, whereas among women Type Bs reported greater job involvement than Type As. High status Type As reported working more hours than did low status Type As; conversely, low status Type Bs worked more hours than did high status Type Bs. These results suggest that high status positions may be beneficial for Type As and detrimental for Type Bs in terms of support at work and job autonomy. High status Type As work more hours than low status Type As; conversely, low status Type Bs work more hours than high status Type Bs.

Gender differences on the self-reported work environment support suggest that men perceive more autonomy and women perceive more task orientation in their work environment. Autonomy may be valued in higher status positions, where taking initiative is rewarded and is more central to the traditional male sex role than the traditional female sex role. In contrast, autonomy may be detrimental to success in low status positions where the worker is not expected to challenge decisions of their superiors. Instead, an orientation toward task completion may have fewer deleterious consequences for persons in low status positions, which are more likely to be held by women than men.

Type A Behavior, Employment, and Marital Satisfaction

At the time this report was prepared, data from the Marital Satisfaction Inventory (MSI) were available for a subset of the entire sample, 43 couples ($n = 85$; data for one woman were unusable, and the "unpaired" man's data were used only for analyses that did not require data from the couple). Demographic analyses of this subset indicated results comparable to those for the total sample. Results summarized here were reported in greater detail by Sullaway and Morell (64).

The MSI consists of 11 subscales, including Conventionalization (distorting appraisal of marriage in a socially desirable direction), Global Distress, Affective Communication, Problem Solving Communication, and Time Together. Other subscales include Disagreement about Finances, Sexual Dissatisfaction, Conflict over Childrearing, Dissatisfaction with Children, Role Orientation (traditional versus nontraditional gender role values), and Family History of Distress (conflict in the family of origin). Other marital measures used included the Communication Patterns Questionnaire (73), a measure of couples' interaction patterns during conflict, and the Areas of Change Questionnaire (14), a measure of couples' desired change in a relationship and the degree to which partners agree on desired changes.

Behavior Type and Marital Satisfaction. Results indicated that Type A men and women did *not* differ in Global Distress, although *all* men were significantly more distressed about their marriages than were Type B women as indicated by the Global Distress measure and several other MSI subscales. Overall, Type B women exhibited the least Global Marital Distress of any group. These results differ from previous research that has shown women typically report more marital distress than men. The multiple roles held by many of our female participants may have buffered them against marital distress.

Surprisingly, men in our study endorsed slightly *less* traditional gender role values than did women. We expected that husbands would have similar or more traditional gender role values than wives. This unexpected finding may reflect accommodation to the changes in family structure associated with being married to a working woman. However, the demand characteristics of our experiment also may account for these data: The research team included 8 women and only 1 man.

Because of sample size limitations, analyses comparing behavior type pairing combinations must be considered tentative. Individuals were categorized into one of four husband–wife type pairs: AA, AB, BA, or BB. Examining the effects of couples' behavior type and scores on the MSI subscales' results suggested that type AA couples experienced significantly more marital distress than did AB couples, particularly in regard to problem-solving communication.

Analyses of the relation between behavior type and marital distress showed that TABP in women was associated with increased marital distress and communication difficulties (as indicated on MSI Global Distress and Problem Solving Communication scales) for both men and women. Furthermore, when women were Type A, both members of the couple reported more blaming and hostile communication patterns on the Communication Interaction Pattern Questionnaire and desired increased changes in the relationship, as indicated on the Areas of Change Questionnaire. However, these effects held *only* when behavior type was assessed using the JAS and FTAS questionnaire measures. There were virtually no significant results based on the SI classification of behavior type. These findings are consistent with previous research showing a negative association between women's TABP and marital satisfaction (64). Based on the multiple measures of marital distress used in this study, information suggests that women's TABP was associated with both overall marital distress and problems in specific areas of communication.

The relation between women's TABP and marital distress may be influenced by different roles filled by husbands and wives in marriage as well as to the relation between TABP and high work involvement. Blumstein and Schwartz's 1983 study of 12,000 couples (6) indicated that in most couples one partner, usually the wife, is the more "relationship oriented"; perhaps Type A wives are less likely to fulfill this traditional role. Also, research suggests that husbands of working wives report lower life and job satisfaction than husbands with wives who do not work. Perhaps employed Type A wives are least likely to fill the traditional marital role of maintaining responsibility and focus on the marriage itself. Clearly, this hypothesis requires further research.

Our findings raise the issue of technique used to assess Type A. The FTAS was most strongly related to marital distress, perhaps owing to the fact that of the three measures of behavior type the FTAS is most strongly related to psychological distress and the SI the least strongly related (see ref. 64 for further discussion). It is not surprising that a measure that assesses negative affect associated with TABP also demonstrates a strong relation to negative effect within a marriage.

Marital Satisfaction and Work Environment Associations. We had predicted that certain aspects of the work environment would be related to marital distress (particularly those that might be relevant to Type A behavior, e.g., self-reported Work Pressure and Task Autonomy), and that these relations would differ between men and women. To test these hypotheses, MSI subscales were correlated with measures of the work environment.

For both women and men, increased Task Orientation at work was related to decreased Global Marital Distress and decreased Affective Communication Problems at home. However, for men only, decreased Work Autonomy was related to increased Marital Distress and Marital Communication Problems (which may be related to our earlier report that men with more prestigious jobs and higher salaries had greater work autonomy). By contrast, work autonomy was relatively unimportant to Global Marital Satisfaction among women but was linked to increased Work Flexibility and decreased Work Pressure. The latter relations did not hold for men.

For both women and men, a greater number of hours spent doing housework was positively related to greater Global Marital Distress and Communication Problems. The men in our study were no different from national samples: All performed fewer hours of housework relative to their working wives. However, in our sample, men who performed more housework reported greater marital distress than men who spent less time on housework. This result is consistent with Blumstein and Schwartz's (6) finding that "married men's aversion to housework is so intense it can sour their relationship. The more housework they do . . . the more they fight about it." For women, increased hours spent doing housework was associated with Communication Distress, Dissatisfaction with Children, and a Gender Orientation that was traditional. Thus for women in our sample, hours spent doing housework had negative effects on home life.

For men only, a Conflictual Family of Origin was associated with more work pressure and greater involvement in work versus family life. Speculatively, men from conflictual families of origin may have a more sensitized response to stress and may more readily experience and report pressure. An alternative explanation suggests that men from high conflict families "bury" themselves in their work to avoid interpersonal distress. This finding may be interpreted in several ways, and more data are required for a definitive conclusion.

Gender differences also were noted in the relation between Environmental Support and marital satisfaction. Women who described their workplaces as supportive were more optimistic and less distressed about their marriages and were less likely to be distressed about a lack of time together with their spouse. In contrast, support at work was not related to marital satisfaction among men. These findings are consistent with previous research that suggests work influences home life among women, and that men compartmentalize their relationships more than women.

Men who worked more days per week reported greater marital problems, especially with communicating affection and intimacy. On the other hand, the number of hours worked per day was not related to MSI distress scales, suggesting that added days at work was more detrimental to the marital relationship than added hours per day. Women who worked more days per week also reported greater global marital distress. In addition, it was only for women that a significant relation was observed between the number of work days and Conflict Over Childrearing. Because child care-taking has traditionally been the task of women, women may feel more conflicted than men when spending time at work rather than at home.

Cardiovascular Stress Reactivity

Gender and Stress Task Effects on Cardiovascular Reactivity. A detailed presentation of our stress reactivity methodology and findings is available elsewhere (47). The information described here summarizes only the major findings.

Results revealed that during the baseline period men had significantly higher SBP than women (123.19 versus 108.86 mm Hg respectively) and marginally higher resting DBP than women (74.31 versus 68.86 mm Hg, respectively). The heart rate was not different between the sexes. These resting baseline sex differences have been reported by other investigators and appear to reflect predominantly biological differences. For example, substantial evidence indicates that blood pressure in premenopausal women is substantially lower than that in comparably aged men. Men also have a greater incidence and prevalence of hypertension than women at these ages. Although younger women typically have higher heart rates than comparably aged men, heart rates decrease with increasing age, which may account for the absence of a sex difference in this parameter.

After statistically controlling for the baseline effects, results showed that men had significantly greater DBP than women during the mental arithmetic task (82.72 versus 78.32 mm Hg, respectively). However, there were no sex differences on the speech, reaction time, or habituation tasks as measured by *any* of the dependent variables. Findings further revealed that for each of the stress tasks there were significant increases over baseline levels for SBP, DBP, and heart rate. For example, on the most potent stressor, the speech task, the SBP elevation was almost 40 mm Hg and DBP about 15 mm Hg. The lack of sex differences on stress reactivity is not attributable to the inadequacy of the tasks. During the mental arithmetic and reaction time tasks SBP levels rose almost 20 mm Hg and DBP levels increased about 10 mm Hg compared to the baseline.

Several factors may account for the absence of sex differences. First, the middle-aged status of our participants may have contributed: increasing age is associated with less psychological gender differentiation (e.g., adherence to "traditional" sex role stereotyped review on what "men" or "women" are like and *should* like and how they *should* behave), that may be related to greater similarity in physiologic response.

The second and probably more important factor appears to be related to our failure to consider the potential gender differences in reactivity as a function of menopausal status. In subsequent analyses, stress reactivity was evaluated in women who were premenopausal, postmenopausal due to complete hysterectomy, and postmenopausal for natural reasons compared with age-matched men. Findings revealed that there were strong sex differences in cardiovascular reactivity between premenopausal women and age-matched men, but there were no significant effects between women who had a complete hysterectomy and age-matched men. These results highlight the importance of considering menopausal status as an independent variable in stress reactivity research with both women and men.

Gender and Environmental Support Effects. We conceptualized environmental support as representing a type of social support that was relevant in the workplace. We investigated the possible relation between environmental work support and cardiovascular reactivity, expecting that, irrespective of gender, women and men with high support would exhibit lower physiological reactivity than would persons with comparatively less support. To evaluate the potential differential effects of environmental support, a median split was conducted for scores within each sex group: participants then were designated as having low or high environmental support.

Analysis of variance for sex (male, female) × environmental support (low, high) revealed significant interactions of sex × environmental support for both heart rate and SBP. Specifically, the baseline heart rate (HR) in beats per minute (bpm) and SBP were significantly lower for men with low environmental support (HR = 56.51 bpm; SBP = 117.38 mm Hg) compared to those with high environmental support (HR = 71.47 bpm; SBP = 128.52 mm Hg). By contrast, women with low environmental support had significantly higher resting SBP levels than did those with high environmental support (111.17 versus 103.82 mm Hg, respectively).

After controlling for the baseline effects, analyses were conducted for gender × environmental support separately for each of the stress tasks. Results showed that DBP levels were significantly higher for men than for women during mental arithmetic (82.80 versus 78.08 mm Hg, respectively). Environmental support was unrelated to reactivity on this task. Findings further revealed that, regardless of gender, heart rates during the speech task were significantly higher in those with high environmental support than in those with low support (84.6 versus 71.14 bpm, respectively). Specifically, women with low environmental support had greater physiological reactivity than did those with high environmental support. No other findings were significant. The only notable stress task response that was affected by environmental support was reactivity to the speech task. Persons with high environmental support had significantly greater heart rates than did those with low environment support, regardless of gender. As suggested previously, perhaps participants who have high environmental support may be characterized by an increased need for social desirability or positive self-presentation or receive more support because they request it from others (or are perceived by others to need such assistance).

Gender and Marital Satisfaction. Subjects were categorized into high and low marital satisfaction groups based on a median split of their scores on the Global Marital Distress MSI subscale. Analyses of variance then were conducted for sex (male, female) × marital satisfaction (low, high) for the stress reactivity session baseline and individual stress tasks periods.

Findings revealed that baseline heart rates were significantly higher in men with high marital satisfaction than in those with low satisfaction (67.48 versus 55.50 bpm, respectively). In contrast, women with low marital satisfaction had significantly *higher* heart rates than those with high marital satisfaction (68.16 versus 59.49 bpm, respectively). SBP was significantly greater overall in men than women, but this effect was qualified by a marginal interaction between gender and marital satisfaction. Men with high marital satisfaction had more elevated SBP than did those with low marital satisfaction (125.97 versus 120.58 mm Hg, respectively); conversely, women with low marital satisfaction had higher SBP than those with high marital satisfaction (113.79 versus 104.37 mm Hg, respectively). Nonetheless, there were no main effects for marital satisfaction or interactions between gender and marital satisfaction on any of the stress tasks.

The finding that men who were in less happy marriages were *less* reactive is puzzling though consistent with the findings for work support noted above. Perhaps such men simply are more emotionally detached and hence less reactive. Analysis of additional data collected for this study is necessary to understand this finding. After covarying the baseline effects, analyses were conducted for sex (male, female) × marital satisfaction (low, high) separately for each of the stress tasks. Results indicated that men had greater DBP levels than women during the mental arithmetic task. However, there were no other sex differences, nor were there any marital satisfaction or sex × marital satisfaction interactions on any of the tasks.

It is unclear why marital dissatisfaction was not associated with greater differences in stress reactivity, particularly as such effects were observed for work support. In part, the nature of the experimental tasks may be responsible. That is, the tasks used in the experimental session discussed here involve those that bear some similarity to the work activities in which many persons engage, from the cognitive demands of the mental arithmetic task, to the personal performance pressure of the simulated public speaking task, to the competitiveness and time pressure of the reaction time task, to the ability to withstand the passive stress imposed by the intermittent stressor of the habituation task noise. Thus it may be that a certain specificity exists between particular psychosocial variables and their ability to buffer (or exacerbate) various types of stress. Such issues are addressed as we analyze other aspects of the data collected in our investigation.

Evaluated from another perspective, however, if the baseline effects were not covaried, data show that these higher physiological levels persist across the stress tasks. Thus men may be at greater risk for cardiovascular disorders (particularly IHD and hypertension) than women according to the prevailing state model of stress reactivity. Of course, further clarification of the present results is necessary, along with additional research that examines the impact of support in the work environment and marital satisfaction on cardiovascular reactivity to stress.

Practical and Theoretical Implications.

Results from the present research indicate that a wide array of variables must be considered when examining the effects of satisfaction and distress at work and at home, along with the relation of these factors to health. Variables to be considered include gender, Type A behavior, support at work, marital satisfaction, and socioeconomic status. Because these factors are interrelated, considering each in isolation may lead to distortions of the overall picture. Our research suggests that if the fit between work and behavior type is poor, employees' perceptions of adequate support and autonomy at work suffer. For example, a Type A person in a slow-paced nondemanding job may ultimately suffer more negative health consequences than would a Type A person in a "Type A environment." The opposite patterns most likely would be distressing for Type Bs. Furthermore, research suggests that under some circumstances the Type A individual is particularly vulnerable to increased marital distress, which in turn has implications for job performance and health.

Gender differences in stress reactivity as a function of tasks must be examined in real work settings in addition to laboratory settings. Thus our findings showing differential effects of support on stress reactivity as a function of gender need to be replicated and extended before they are accepted as valid and generalizable to other populations. The theoretical implications of this type of biopsychosocial research lie in the possibility that such findings will help us increase the currently low specificity of Type A as a predictor of IHD and allow us to illuminate the roles played by biological and psychosocial sex differences in IHD risk.

In many ways, the research presented here is a "snapshot" of a fairly unique transitional and historical period. The age range of the research participants studied, 40- to 60-year-olds, is that of a generation that has witnessed tremendous changes in the traditional roles of men and women. Many of the women in our sample began their married life as traditional but well educated homemakers, only later to enter the workforce as paid employees, small business owners, district attorneys, and so on. Current and subsequent generations of women and men more likely will be accustomed to women working outside the home. It seems appropriate to predict that the interactions among behavior type, gender, work stress, and home stress will change as the workforce and its values change; the effect of such changes on health remain to be seen.

ACKNOWLEDGMENTS

Our deep gratitude is expressed to the married couples who participated in the research investigation summarized in this review. Robin Apple, Meg Cho, Noelle Griffin, Anja Leppin, Lisa Rapport, Anna Ruef, and Robert Twillman of the UCLA Marriage and Health Project research team are commended for their extensive contributions to the execution of this investigation. We also thank Mei Jung Wu Hsu, Hsu-Lin Yang, and Ivan Yeung for programming data analysis assistance. Jeff Hanson provided valuable help in preparing this manuscript.

This research was supported by a grant from the National Heart, Lung, and Blood Institute, Behavioral Medicine Division (HL34642), and by a Biomedical Support Grant (RRO7009) from the University of California, Los Angeles, awarded to M.A.M.

REFERENCES

1. Baruch, G. K., & Barnett, R. (1986). Consequences of fathers' participation in family work: parents' role strain and well-being. *Journal of Personality and Social Psychology, 51,* 983–92.

2. Beckman, L. J., & Houser, B. B. (1979). The more you have, the more you do: the relationship between wife's employment, sex-role attitudes, and household behavior. *Psychology of Women Quarterly, 4,* 160–74.

3. Berkman, L., & Breslow, L. (1983). *Health and ways of living: findings from the Alameda County study.* New York: Oxford University Press.

4. Blaney, N. T., Brown, P., & Blaney, P. H. (1986). Type A, marital adjustment, and life stress. *Journal of Behavioral Medicine, 9,* 491–502.

5. Blazer, D. (1982). Social support and mortality in an elderly community population. *American Journal of Epidemiology, 115,* 684–94.

6. Blumstein, P., & Schwartz, P. (1983). *American couples: money, work, sex.* New York: Pocket Books.

7. Booth-Kewley, S., & Friedman, H. S. (1987). Psychological predictors of heart disease: a quantitative review. *Psychological Bulletin, 101,* 343–62.

8. Bradburn, N. (1969). *The structure of psychological well-being.* Chicago: Aldine.

9. Brand, R. J., Rosenman, R. H., Sholtz, R. I., & Friedman, M. (1976). Multivariate predictions of coronary heart disease in the Western Collaborative Group Study compared to the Framingham study. *Circulation, 53,* 348–55.

10. Burke, R. J., & Weir, T. (1980). The Type A experience: occupational and life demands, satisfaction and well-being. *Journal of Human Stress, 6,* 28–38.

11. Carmelli, D., Swan, G. E., & Rosenman, R. H. (1986). The relationship between wives' social and psychological status and their husbands' coronary heart disease. *American Journal of Epidemiology, 122,* 90–100.

12. Chesney, M. A., Ekman, P., Friesen, W. V., Black, G. W., & Hecker, M. H. L. (1990). Type A behavior pattern: facial behavior and speech components. *Psychosomatic Medicine, 53,* 307–19.

13. Chesney, M. A., Sevelius, G., Black, G. W., Ward, M. M., Swann, G. E., & Rosenman, R. H. (1981). Work environment, Type A behavior, and coronary heart disease risk factors. *Journal of Occupational Medicine, 23,* 551–55.

14. Christensen, A. (in press). Dysfunctional interaction pattern in couples. In P. Nobler & M. A. Fitzpatrick (eds.). *Perspective on marital interactions.* Clevedon & Philadelphia: Multilingual Matters.

15. Clark, R., Hye, F., & Gecas, V. (1978). Husbands work involvement and marital role performance. *Journal of Marriage and the Family, 40,* 9–21.

16. Connell, C. M., & D'Augelli, A. R. (1990). The contribution of personality characteristics to the relationship between social support and perceived physical health. *Health Psychology, 9,* 175–94.

17. Cooper, T., Detre, T., & Weiss, S. M. (1981). Coronary-prone behavior and coronary heart disease: a critical review. *Circulation, 55,* 135–54.

18. Eaker, E. D., Haynes, S. G., & Feinleib, M. (1983). Spouse behavior and coronary heart disease in men: prospective results from the Framingham Heart Study (II). *American Journal of Epidemiology, 118,* 23–41.

19. Fontana, A. F., Kerns, R. D., Rosenberg, R. L., & Colonese, K. L. (1990). Support, stress and recovery from coronary heart disease: a longitudinal causal model. *Health Psychology, 8,* 175–94.

20. Foster, C. D., Siegel, M. A., & Jacobs, N. R. (eds.) (1988). *Women's changing roles.* Wylie, TX: Information Aids.

21. Gilbert, L. A., & Rachlin, V. (1987). Mental health and psychological functioning of dual-career families. *The Counseling Psychologist, 15,* 7–49.

22. Glenn, N. D., & Weaver, C. N. (1982). A multivariate, multisurvey study of marital happiness. *Journal of Marriage and the Family, 40,* 269–82.

23. Goldband, S. (1980). Stimulus specificity of physiological responses to stress and the Type A coronary-prone behavior pattern. *Journal of Personality and Social Psychology, 6,* 670–9.

24. Green, G. P., & Epstein, R. T. (eds.) (1988). *Employment and earnings.* Vol. 35 (2). Washington, DC: U.S. Department of Labor, Bureau of Labor Statistics.

25. Gutek, B. A., Repetti, R. L., & Silver, D. L. (1988). Nonwork roles and stress at work. In C. L. Cooper & R. Payne (eds.). *Causes, coping and consequences of stress at work* (pp. 141–74). New York: Wiley.

26. Haynes, S. G., & Matthews, K. A. (1988). Area review: coronary-prone behavior: continuing evolution of the concept. *Annals of Behavioral Medicine, 10,* 47–59.

27. Haynes, S. G., Feinleib, M., & Kannel, W. B. (1980). The relationship of psychosocial factors to coronary heart disease in the Framingham Study. III: eight-year incidence of coronary heart disease. *American Journal of Epidemiology, 111,* 37–58.

28. Haynes, S. G., Levine, S., Scotch, N., Feinleib, M., & Kannel, W. B. (1988). The relationship of psychological factors to coronary heart disease in the Framingham Study. I: methods and risk factors. *American Journal of Epidemiology, 107,* 362–83.

29. Hirsch, B. J., & Rapkin, B. D. (1986). Multiple roles, social networks, and women's well-being. *Journal of Personality and Social Psychology, 51,* 1237–47.

30. Hirsch, B. J., & Rapkin, B. D. (1986). Social networks and adult social identities: profiles and correlates of support and rejection. *American Journal of Community Psychology, 14,* 395–412.

31. House, J., Robbins, C., & Metzner, H. (1982). The association of social relationships and activities with mortality: prospective evidence

from the Tecumseh Community Health Study. *American Journal of Epidemiology, 116,* 123–40.

32. Houston, B. K. (1988). Cardiovascular and neuroendocrine reactivity, global Type A, and components of type A behavior. In B. K. Houston & C. R. Snyder (eds.). *Type A behavior patterns: research theory and intervention.* New York: Wiley.

33. Jenkins, C. D. (1976). Recent evidence supporting psychologic and social risk factors for coronary disease (Part I). *New England Journal of Medicine, 29,* 987–1038.

34. Jenkins, C. D. (1988). Epidemiology of cardiovascular diseases. *Journal of Consulting and Clinical Psychology, 56,* 324–32.

35. Jenkins, C. D., & Zyzanski, S. J., & Rosenman, R. H. (1979). *Jenkins Activity Survey manual.* Los Angeles: The Psychological Corporation.

36. Kamarck, T. W., Manuck, S. B., & Jennings, J. R. (1990). Social support reduces cardiovascular reactivity to psychological challenge. *Psychosomatic Medicine, 52,* 42–58.

37. Kanter, R. M. (1977). *Men and women of the corporation.* New York: Basic Books.

38. Kanter, R. M. (1977). *Work and family in the United States: a critical review and agenda for research and policy.* New York: Russell Sage.

39. Kelly, K. E., & Houston, B. K. (1985). Type A behavior in employed women: relation to work, marital, and leisure variables, social support, stress, tension, and health. *Journal of Personality and Social Psychology, 48,* 1067–79.

40. Kessler, R. C., & McRae, (1982). The effect of wife's employment on the mental health of married men and women. *American Sociological Review, 47,* 216–27.

41. Koskenvuo, M., Kaprio, J., Kesaniemi, A., & Sarna, S. (1980). Differences in mortality from ischemic heart disease by marital status and social class. *Journal of Chronic Diseases, 33,* 95–106.

42. Krantz, D. S., & Manuck, S. B. (1984). Acute psychophysiologic reactivity and risk of cardiovascular disease: a review and methodologic critique. *Psychological Bulletin, 96,* 435–64.

43. Manuck, S. B., Kaplan, J. R., & Matthews, K. A. (1986). Behavioral antecedents of coronary heart disease and atherosclerosis. *Atherosclerosis, 6,* 2–14.

44. Matthews, K. A., Helmreich, R. L., Beanne, W. E., & Locker, G. W. (1980). Pattern A, achievement-striving, and scientific merit: does pattern A help or hinder? *Journal of Personality and Social Psychology, 39,* 962–7.

45. Medalie, J. H., & Goldbourt, U. (1976). Angina pectoris among 10,000 men. II: Psychosocial and other risk factors as evidenced by a multivariate analyses of a five year incidence study. *The American Journal of Medicine, 60,* 910–21.

46. Moos, R. H., & Mitchell, R. E. (1982). Social network resources and adaptation: a conceptual framework. In T. A. Wills (ed.). *Basic processes in helping relationships* (pp. 213–32). New York: Academic Press.

47. Morell, M. A. (1990). Sex differences in stress reactivity in age-matched premenopausal versus postmenopausal women and men. Manuscript in preparation.

48. Morell, M. A., & Katkin, E. S. (1982). Jenkins Activity Survey scores among women of different occupations. *Journal of Consulting and Clinical Psychology, 50,* 588–9.

49. Mount, M. K., & Muchinsky, P. M. (1978). Person-environment congruence and employee job satisfaction: a test of Holland's theory. *Journal of Vocational Behavior, 13,* 84–100.

50. Nickols, S. Y., & Metzen, E. J. (1982). Impact of wives' employment upon husband's housework. *Journal of Family Issues, 3,* 199–216.

51. Orth-Gomer, K., & Unden, A. L. (1990). Type A behavior, social support, and coronary risk: interaction and significance for mortality in cardiac patients. *Psychosomatic Medicine, 52,* 59–72.

52. Parry, G. (1986). Paid employment, life events, social support, and mental health in working-class mothers. *Journal of Health and Social Behavior, 27,* 193–208.

53. Pietromoaco, P. R., Manis, J., & Frohardt-Lane, K. (1986). Psychological consequences of multiple social roles. *Psychology of Women Quarterly, 10,* 373–81.

54. Piotrkowski, C. S. (1979). *Work and the family system.* New York: Free Press.

55. Pleck, J. H. (1977). The work-family role system. *Social Problems, 24,* 417–27.

56. Pleck, J. H. (1985). *Working wives/working husbands.* Beverly Hills, CA: Sage.

57. Pleck, J. H., & Rustad, M. (1980). Husbands' and wives' time in family work and paid work in the 1975–76 study of time use. Working paper, Wellesley College, Center for Research on women.

58. Powell, L. H. (1984). Area review: stress, Type A behavior, and cardiovascular disease. *Behavioral Medicine Update, 6,* 7–10.

59. Repetti, R. L. (1987). Linkages between work and family roles. In S. Oskamp (ed.). *Applied social psychology annual, vol. 7: Family process and problems* (pp. 98–127). Beverly Hills, CA: Sage.

60. Repetti, R. L. (1989). Effects of daily workload on subsequent behavior during marital interaction: the role of social withdrawal and spouse support. *Journal of Personality and Social Psychology, 57,* 651–659.

61. Repetti, R. L., & Crosby, F. 91984). Gender and depression: exploring the adult-role explanation. *Journal of Consulting and Clinical Psychology, 2,* 57–70.

62. Rosenman, R. H. (1978). The interview meth-

od of assessment of the coronary-prone behavior pattern. In Dembroski, T. M., Weiss, Shields, Haynes, & Feinleib (eds.). *Coronaryprone behavior*. New York: Springer.

63. Shapiro, D., Greenstadt, L., Lane, J. D., & Rubenstein, L. (1981). Tracking-cuff system for beat-to-beat recording of blood pressure. *Psychophysiology, 18*, 129–36.

64. Sullaway, M. E., & Morell, M. A. (1990). Marital relationships and Type A—B behavior assessed by the Structured Interview Jenkins Activity Survey and Framingham Type A scale. *Journal of Behavioral Medicine, 13*, 419–36.

65. Swan, G. E., Carmelli, D., & Rosenman, R. H. (1986). Spouse-pair similarity on the California Psychological Inventory with reference to husband's coronary heart disease. *Psychosomatic Medicine, 48*, 172–86.

66. Szinovacz, M. (1977). Role allocation, family structure and female employment. *Journal of Marriage and the Family, 39*, 781–91.

67. U.S. Department of Labor, Bureau of Labor Statistics (1985). *Employment and earnings*. Vol. 32, p. 18. Washington, DC: U.S. Government Printing Office.

68. U.S. Department of Labor, Bureau of Labor Statistics (1986). *Labor force statistics derived from the current populations survey: a databook*. Washington, DC: U.S. Government Printing Office.

69. *Vital and Health Statistics of the United States* (1986). National Health Survey, (Vol. (A): Mortality. Series 10, No. 160.) U.S. Department of Health & Human Services and Public Health Service, National Center for Health Statistics.

70. *Vital and Health Statistics of the United States* (1986). National Health Survey, Series 10, No. 160. U.S. Dept. of Health & Human Services and Public Health Service, National Center for Health Statistics.

71. *Vital and Health Statistics of the United States* (1987). Series 10, No. 14. Washington, DC: National Center for Health Statistics.

72. Voydanoff, P., & Kelly, R. F. (1984). Determinants of work-related family problems among employed parents. *Journal of Marriage and the Family. 46*, 881–92.

73. Weiss, R. L., Hops, H., & Patterson, G. R. (1973). A framework for conceptualizing marital conflict: a technology for altering it, some data for evaluating it. In L. A. Hamerlynk, L. C. Handy, & E. J. Marsh (eds.). *Behavior changes: methodology, concepts, & practice*. Champaign, IL: Research Press.

74. Wills, T. A. (1985). Supportive functions of interpersonal relationships. In S. Cohen & S. L. Syme (eds.). *Social support and health* (pp. 61–81). Orlando: Academic Press.

IV
STRESS, HEALTH, AND PRODUCTIVITY IN VARIOUS WORK ENVIRONMENTS

Stress at work is generally viewed by researchers to result from an imbalance between the environment and the person; two major etiological models have been offered. One is the Person-Environment Fit Model, which states that "strain develops when there is a discrepancy between the motives of the person and the supplies of the environment (job) or between the demand of the job and the abilities of the person to meet those demands" (1). The other is the Job Demands-Control Model, which holds that "strain results from the joint effects of the work situation (stressors) and environmental moderators of stress, particularly the range of decision-making freedom (control) available to the worker facing those demands" (3). In both models the concept of strain refers to individual responses, which may be physical, psychological, or behavioral and are indicators of individual ill health or poor well-being (2).

In both direct and indirect ways, the adverse effects of stress can be costly to business organizations. Both management and labor have vested interests in improving the understanding and control of stress in work environments. Stress and health are global concerns, and various countries have taken an interest in stress-related threats to health in the workplace. The chapters that make up Part IV provide viewpoints on this issue from different cultural and national perspectives.

Part IV begins with chapters that deal with stress-producing aspects of the work environment and their effects on health and productivity in Scandinavia and Japan. It concludes with a chapter by an American researcher who points out the importance of differing values in different countries and cultures as they affect the employee's interaction with the work organization.

In Chapter 12 Kubota suggests that, like humans, workplaces can be regarded as passing through various states of health and ill health; and like individuals, organizations must acknowledge the importance of maintaining and improving health. He emphasizes the importance of having a reliable and valid database that can serve as a foundation for assessing the health status and needs of the organization and its workers. Kubota describes such a data system, the Japan Productivity Center (JPC) Mental Health Inventory, which is designed to determine both the physical and mental health of employees and the overall condition of the entire work organization. For sheer size and scope of commitment to the importance of health in relation to industrial productivity, it would be difficult to match the efforts of the JPC. The JPC has been collecting data for a decade on the physical and mental health of thousands of employees and feeding it back to them and their work organizations in dozens of large and medium-sized industrial firms in Japan. Kubota, director of Research and Development, describes the Japanese health inventory and its uses. This chapter represents one of the first English-language reports on this pioneering effort; and although it is incomplete in terms of what one might like from a scientific point of view, it provides a useful example of the extent to which one of the leading industrial nations is convinced that employee health is a vital factor in maintaining industrial productivity and leadership.

Johansson and Aronsson (Chapter 13) provide a broad overview of Scandinavian research dealing with psychological and sociological factors as they relate to the development of health problems in the workplace. They support the observations made in the previous section by Hirschhorn (Chapter 9), Celentano (Chapter 10), and Morell et al. (Chapter 11) concerning changes that appear to be increasing the stress experienced by workers in the postindustrial workplace. Central to this increased stress appears to be an increase in demands on workers as a result of the introduction of new technologies and concomitant changes in the environment and organization of work. At the same time, employees are experiencing increasing loss of control over their lives at work and elsewhere. Such situations of high demand and low control are viewed by researchers as increasing the likelihood of worker stress.

Cross-cultural comparisons of types and patterns of work organization as they affect health can be informative. Johannson and Aronsson underscore the fact that they approach these issues from a uniquely Scandinavian perspective with its emphasis on unionization and an ideology of mutual understanding; it is natural for them to emphasize work reform programs as the means to attain both health and productivity. Hunt (Chapter 14) shows that such comparisons also allow examination of how differences in workers' orientation and values moderate the relations between workplace factors and human health and well-being and also affect performance and productivity. This chapter relates to the discussion in Chapter 1 of current theory that views stress in work organizations as resulting from the interaction of the person and environmental factors. The individual orientations and values described by Hunt as varying in relation to cultural differences are important variables in person–environment interactions that determine if workers in different situations will develop stress-related illness.

Values are not only relevant to the etiological models proposed to explain the development of stress but also to the assumptions on which stress management is based. Individual responsibility for one's health is emphasized in the United States and Canada, and there has been considerable development of wellness- and health-promotion programs focused on getting individuals to change their health-related behavior in both countries. However, organization managers and researchers in some other countries take a different point of view. Johannson and Aronsson exemplify the Scandinavian approach to improving worker health that emphasizes improvement in the social environment of work. Hunt describes the Scandinavian approach as oriented to "making it easier to put up with the job." Although American firms have experimented with changing the structure of work in order to increase productivity, they have tended not to use such an environmental approach for improving worker health. In Part V of this book, Fielding (Chapter 17) describes the individual-focused approach of educating workers to practice health-promoting and risk-reducing behaviors as is now widely used in American corporations.

REFERENCES

1. Baker, D. B. (1985). The study of stress at work. *Annual Review of Public Health, 6,* 367–81.
2. Beehr, T. A., & Franz, T. M. (1986). The current debate about the meaning of job stress. *Journal of Organizational Behavior Management, 8,* 5–18.
3. Karasek, R. A., Baker, D., Marxer, F., Albom, A., & Theorell, T. (1981). Job decision latitude, job demands, and cardiovascular disease: a prospective study of Swedish men. *American Journal of Public Health, 71,* 694–705.

12
Health, Stress, and Productivity in the Japanese Workforce

If one hypothesizes that productivity is the result of activities carried out by healthy humans, one can say that high productivity can be realized by people who are both physically and mentally healthy. A workplace comprised of people who are both physically and mentally healthy ought to be cheerful and lively, and the workers' morale should be high. On the other hand, in a workplace comprised of people who are in poor physical and mental condition, the activities carried out there tend to stagnate and lack vigor, and the atmosphere is gloomy and depressing. Thus in a sense, a workplace is a living being. Human health is on a continuum from satisfactory health to serious illness. Assuming that workplaces and organizations are also living beings, their states of health pass through the same levels, from very good to very bad. As the maintenance of good health is desirable for both humans and organizations, they should be aware of the need to improve their health when it begins to deteriorate.

To develop an awareness of the need to improve and maintain health, reliable and objective data are required. In Japan, any company that employs more than a certain number of workers is obliged to conduct periodic health examinations of its staff. Workers are promptly informed of the results of these examinations, which include blood pressure, leukocyte count, cholesterol, hematocrit, neutral facts, gamma-GTP, uric acid, glyco-A1C, blood glucose, vision, and electrocardiograms. The physician advises workers with poor test results and recommends, for example, that they decrease their intake of salt, eat more roughage, follow a regular exercise program, or get more sleep. Those who follow the physician's advice usually are rewarded with better results on subsequent health examinations.

This series of activities—periodic health examinations, advice, individual recognition and awareness, and improvement efforts—is intended to reduce the occurrence of illness, help each individual lead a happier private life, and contribute to improving the productivity of the workplace.

Man is said to be a cerebral and spiritual animal; yet the vitally important area of mental health is usually neglected until a problem manifests. A full and happy life implies mental as well as physical well-being. For this reason, it is important to conduct comprehensive periodic examinations to determine the state of one's physical and mental health. With this need in mind, the Japan Productivity Center has devel-

Table 12–1. Scales

Work adjustment
  A 1   Feeling of adequacy about work
      2   Relationship with supervisor
      3   Relationship with colleagues
      4   Belongingness
      5 (R) Pressure from work
      6   Motivation to work
      7   Accuracy of work
      8   Satisfaction with evaluation
      9   Prospects for the future
Physical condition
  B 1 (R) Eyes
      2 (R) Ears
      3 (R) Respiratory system
      4 (R) Cardiovascular system
      5 (R) Mouth
      6 (R) Stomach
      7 (R) Large and small intestine
      8 (R) Musculoskeletal system
      9 (R) Skin
    10 (R) Nervous system
    11 (R) Urogenital system
    12 (R) Frequency of illness
    13 (R) Fatigue
    14 (R) Multiple complaints
    15 (R) Irregularity of daily life
Mental health
      1   Premelancholic
      2 (R) Depressive
      3   Hyperthymia
      4   Hypomanic
      5 (R) Schizothyme
      6 (R) Hebephrenia
      7 (R) Paranoia
      8   Visköses temperament
      9 (R) Seizure
    10 (R) Explosive temper
    11   Attention-seeking
    12 (R) Suggestable
    13 (R) Insecure
    14 (R) Obsessive-compulsive
    15 (R) Hypochondriacal
    16 (R) Anxiety
    17 (R) Feelings of inferiority
    18 (R) Unstable
    19 (R) Weak-willed
    20 (R) Socially irresponsible
    21 (R) Addiction
Personality profile
      1   Inquiring mind
      2   Control of emotion

(continued)

Table 12–1. (*Continued*)

3	Spontaneity
4	Goal attainment
5	Empathy
6	Introversion-extroversion
7	Adaptiveness–assertiveness
8	Persistence–flexibility
9	Endurance–immediate reactiveness
10	Reality oriented–future oriented

oped the JMI Health Examination System. JMI, or "Japan Productivity Center Mental Health Inventory," is designed to determine not only the physical and mental health of individual employees but also the overall condition of an entire organization.

The JMI Health Examination System consists of four basic categories: workplace adjustment, physical condition, mental health, and personality profile. The examination is comprised of 56 scales (Table 12–1) and 596 questions, all of which must be answered by a company's employees. The results of each examination are carefully analyzed, and a report is made on each employee. In some cases, a written report includes a recommendation that an employee seek the advice of a specialist. The contents of each report are confidential; and because the privacy of each individual is closely guarded, employees are more likely to give frank answers to personal questions. As a result, the information about the state of their health is reliable.

A comprehensive report is then submitted to the company and labor union regarding the overall health of the organization and groups within it. All data are classified by department, occupation, age, sex, and so on. The names of individuals are not included in the report. In this way, the health of the organization can be understood while individual privacy is protected. For organizations and groups consisting of fewer than ten people, no comprehensive reports are submitted. Using this process, both the company and the labor union are able to grasp the organization's state of health, and each is therefore in a better position to offer practical advice on how to improve it.

A psychiatrist or counselor interviews each employee in a department or group; and in some cases the employee is advised to use an autogenic training method or yoga to improve his or her health. Autogenic training and yoga are often recommended because they are ideal for improving mental flexibility. Although most people possess a sufficient amount of physical flexibility because they have developed it continuously since childhood, the same cannot be said for their mental flexibility. In its most extreme forms, mental inflexibility can result in neuroses and psychosomatic disorders. Stage fright, for example, stems from a lack of mental flexibility and in most cases can be eliminated through autogenic training.

Within any organization or group characterized by poor health, there are employees who are in good health and those who are unhealthy without actually being sick. The reason the organization as a whole is in poor health is because there are more unhealthy employees than there are healthy ones. It is virtually impossible to improve the health of an entire organization simply by singling out employees who are unhealthy and then trying to treat them. Rather, the organization must be dealt with as a single entity. Through group recognition, the individual members can work together to en-

Table 12-2. JMI and Consultations between Supervisors and Subordinates

		T		U	
	t	M	SD	M	SD
Work adjustment					
A 1	6.732***	49.32	10.56	42.10	9.03
2	12.083***	50.07	9.67	38.33	8.16
3	7.873***	50.46	9.41	40.65	11.00
4	6.257***	51.98	9.73	44.04	11.18
5	4.191***	49.65	9.58	44.19	11.54
6					
7	2.134*	52.50	9.28	49.99	10.32
8	5.934***	52.38	9.65	45.49	10.11
9	4.808***	52.28	8.80	46.96	9.70
Physical condition					
B 1	3.691***	52.98	8.01	48.39	11.17
2	2.344*	52.14	8.61	49.53	9.80
3	4.179***	51.68	8.88	47.27	9.17
4	3.897***	52.35	7.91	47.72	10.64
5	2.373*	51.76	8.95	49.14	9.65
6	3.532***	52.13	8.68	48.20	9.78
7	3.780***	51.74	9.28	47.00	11.10
8	3.062**	51.91	8.67	48.35	10.28
9	2.035*	51.25	9.35	48.95	9.85
10	3.709***	52.32	8.50	48.10	10.06
11					
12	3.911***	52.98	8.20	48.59	9.95
13	4.613***	53.72	8.53	47.90	11.28
14	3.853***	53.05	8.70	48.60	10.20
15	5.099***	50.17	8.92	44.72	9.30
Mental health					
C 1					
2	4.168***	52.50	8.90	46.61	12.72
3	5.969***	49.43	9.71	43.42	8.52
4	4.656***	48.68	9.49	44.98	6.30
5	4.567***	51.85	9.34	46.47	10.33
6	3.046**	51.95	8.66	48.28	10.70
7	3.026**	51.45	8.78	48.19	9.41
8					
9	3.298**	52.59	7.86	49.20	9.06
10					
11					
12					
13	3.298***	50.42	9.86	46.04	11.75
14	3.442***	50.84	9.37	46.47	11.24
15	4.950***	53.59	9.39	48.12	9.75
16	3.599***	52.33	8.57	47.71	11.49
17	2.535*	52.58	8.55	49.43	11.09
18	3.015**	50.78	9.54	46.93	11.29
19					
20	2.770**	51.30	10.15	47.70	11.42
21					

(*continued*)

Table 12-2. (*Continued*)

		T		U	
	t	M	SD	M	SD
Personality profile					
D 1	3.387***	49.06	10.12	45.21	9.78
2					
3	5.771***	50.30	9.59	44.79	8.00
4	3.912***	48.67	9.87	44.70	8.57
5					
6	6.267***	50.08	10.04	44.08	7.93
7					
8	−3.324***	49.95	9.57	53.54	9.30
9					
10					

T = Group giving frank answers; U = Group not giving frank answers; R = reverse; M = mean; SD = standard deviation.
* p < 0.05; ** p < 0.01; *** p < 0.001.
Note: Some spaces in these tables were left blank because there were no significant deviations. Under normal circumstances, all blanks are filled in.

courage disease prevention and the maintenance of good health, two ideas that have more than proved their worth during the latter half of this century.

The following is an excerpt from a report that contains data from 400 companies that have used the JMI Health Examination System. It clearly shows the relation between health and productivity.

JMI AND CONSULTATIONS BETWEEN SUPERVISORS AND SUBORDINATES

The first example compares two groups in the same factory (Table 12-2). The members in the two groups were asked if they were able to discuss their jobs frankly with their supervisors. A total of 499 said "yes" (average age 33.2 years), and 88 answered "no" (average age 30.8 years). When the groups' JMI Health Examination System results were compared, it was found that only 14 of the 56 scales were not significantly different; the remaining scales showed significant differences.

Significant differences in A (workplace adjustment)
   A7: $p < 0.05$
   A1,A2,A3,A4,A5,A8,A9: $p < 0.001$
Significant differences in B (physical condition)
   B2,B5,B9: $p < 0.05$
   B8: $p < 0.01$
   B1,B3,B4,B6,B7,B10,B12,B13,B14,B15: $p < 0.001$
Significant differences in C (mental health)
   C17: $p < 0.05$
   C6,C7,C9,C13,C18,C26: $p < 0.01$
   C2,C3,C4,C5,C14,C15,C16: $p < 0.001$
Significant differences in D (personality profile)
   D1,D3,D4,D6,D8: $p < 0.001$

Table 12–3. JMI and Sales Per Branch

		V		W	
	t	M	SD	M	SD
Work adjustment					
A 1	5.016***	53.94	10.25	50.38	10.04
2	6.025***	52.83	9.41	48.56	10.55
3	6.433***	53.43	8.76	48.74	11.36
4	10.410***	53.26	9.70	45.73	10.71
5	3.817***	50.84	10.00	48.15	10.09
6	5.960***	53.77	10.76	49.45	10.05
7					
8	5.219***	52.08	10.05	48.49	9.65
9	6.828***	53.32	9.43	48.54	10.34
Physical condition					
B 1					
2					
3	2.205*	51.28	9.83	49.75	9.94
4					
5	2.172*	53.51	8.68	52.16	8.99
6					
7					
8					
9					
10					
11					
12					
13	2.523*	54.20	8.88	52.57	9.43
14					
15					
Mental health					
C 1					
2	3.401***	53.99	7.80	51.81	9.94
3	5.388***	54.60	9.80	50.93	9.66
4					
5	2.288*	52.37	9.23	50.78	10.34
6	4.151***	53.92	7.29	51.45	9.20
7	5.239***	54.05	7.03	50.57	10.80
8					
9	2.423*	52.97	7.97	51.53	8.80
10					
11	3.241**	51.84	10.16	49.50	10.35
12					
13	2.454*	52.85	9.35	51.22	9.56
14					
15	2.428*	53.26	8.95	51.64	9.88
16	2.200*	52.81	8.97	51.34	9.89
17					
18					
19					
20					
21					

(continued)

Table 12–3. (*Continued*)

		V		W	
	t	M	SD	M	SD
Personality profile					
D 1	5.727***	53.57	10.74	49.38	10.23
2	3.184**	52.82	10.31	50.52	10.30
3	5.207***	52.80	10.32	49.12	9.92
4	5.433***	51.69	9.81	47.91	10.00
5	5.141***	52.66	10.23	48.93	10.43
6	5.079***	54.65	10.90	50.96	9.99
7	2.037*	51.38	9.99	49.98	9.68
8					
9					
10					

The JMI results show that if a subordinate is able to frankly discuss any aspect of his job with his supervisor, he has good results for factors A, B, C, and D. If a supervisor makes himself available to subordinates and listens to them with an open mind, the subordinates' overall health improves and the productivity of the workplace is high.

JMI AND SALES PER BRANCH

The second example looks at two branches of the same department store, V branch and W branch (Table 12–3). This example examines the relation between sales and factors A, B, C, and D.

Branch	No. of workers	Sales/person/year	V/W (%)
V	509	$235,000	107
W	339	$220,000	100

The marketing environments in which these two branches function are essentially the same; however, V branch's environment is more competitive. Supervisor in V branch often discuss business with their subordinates, and their sales results are high. Let us compare these two branches using their JMI results.

Significant differences in A (workplace adjustment)
A1,A2,A3,A4,A5,A6,A8,A9: $p < 0.001$
(A7 was the only scale without a significant difference.)
Significant differences in B (physical condition)
B3,B5,B13: $p < 0.05$
Significant differences in C (mental health)
C5,C9,C13,C15,C16: $p < 0.05$
C11: $p < 0.01$
C2,C3,C6,C7: $p < 0.001$

Table 12–4. JMI and Traffic Accidents

	t	Group 1		Group 4	
		M	SD	M	SD
Work adjustment					
A 1					
2					
3					
4					
5	4.115***	48.96	10.62	40.40	10.89
6					
7	3.637***	50.66	9.66	44.36	9.05
8					
9					
Physical condition					
B 1					
2					
3					
4					
5					
6					
7					
8					
9					
10					
11					
12					
13	2.996**	52.54	9.64	46.51	10.55
14					
15	2.749*	51.35	9.79	45.96	10.27
Mental health					
C 1					
2					
3					
4					
5					
6	2.415*	52.00	8.36	44.93	15.44
7					
8					
9					
10	2.227*	51.37	9.75	46.17	12.27
11	−2.686*	51.74	9.81	57.49	11.23
12	33.633***	49.68	9.76	42.87	9.81
13	2.303*	51.08	9.78	45.62	12.46
14	2.387*	51.58	9.36	45.44	13.54
15					
16	2.958**	51.00	9.64	43.92	12.58
17					
18	2.718*	51.33	9.63	45.29	11.67
19	2.951**	50.74	10.14	43.86	12.24
20	2.621*	51.16	10.01	44.91	12.53
21					

(*continued*)

Table 12–4. (*Continued*)

	t	Group 1		Group 4	
		M	SD	M	SD
Personality profile					
D 1					
2	3.039**	51.70	10.20	45.98	9.84
3					
4					
5					
6					
7					
8					
9	3.452***	50.14	10.97	56.00	8.83
10					

Significant differences in D (personality profile)
D7: $p < 0.05$
D2: $p < 0.01$
D1,D3,D4,D5,D8: $p < 0.001$

Although significant differences were found with factor A, few differences were found for factor B apart from the workers' tendency to catch colds, have sore throats, or be fatigued. For factor C, significant differences were found in depression, cheerfulness, sense of isolation, and assertiveness. The results for factor D showed significant differences in the degrees of initiative, energy, and the number of introverts and extroverts.

JMI AND TRAFFIC ACCIDENTS

The next example looks at the relation between mental health and the number of traffic accidents (Table 12–4). The groups sampled consisted of salesmen, and all of the traffic accidents were work-related.

Group 1
0 accidents
1,234 salesmen (average age 37.3 years)
Group 2
1 accident
267 salesmen (average age 36.0 years)
Group 3
2 accidents
66 salesmen (average age 34.5 years)
Group 4
3 accidents
28 salesmen (average age 34.1 years)

Table 12–5. JMI and Personnel Appraisals

		S		B	
	t	M	SD	M	SD
Work adjustment					
A 1					
2					
3	2.935**	57.65	4.39	50.16	11.00
4					
5					
6					
7					
8	2.526*	57.27	7.78	49.39	12.00
9	2.096*	57.88	7.13	51.92	10.91
Physical condition					
B 1	2.292*	58.18	3.18	53.13	9.75
2					
3					
4					
5					
6	2.855**	58.53	4.24	51.75	10.16
7	2.598*	58.56	4.99	52.76	8.99
8	2.539*	57.00	3.67	50.48	11.38
9					
10	2.562*	58.02	3.90	52.04	10.11
11	3.448**	57.64	2.65	52.07	7.02
12	2.348*	56.51	3.63	51.47	9.28
13	2.318*	59.56	5.65	53.33	9.55
14	2.316*	58.59	4.92	52.27	11.50
15					
Mental health					
C 1					
2					
3	4.123**	59.83	7.04	49.28	9.31
4	2.477*	55.31	9.50	47.98	9.39
5	2.231*	56.26	7.34	49.75	11.18
6	3.465**	57.65	2.49	52.36	6.64
7					
8					
9	2.266*	56.63	3.14	52.63	7.56
10					
11					
12					
13					
14					
15					
16					
17					
18					
19					
20					
21					

(*continued*)

Table 12–5. (*Continued*)

		S		B	
	t	M	SD	M	SD
Personality profile					
D 1					
2	2.571*	58.70	8.22	51.81	8.93
3	3.424**	58.24	8.75	49.15	8.15
4					
5					
6	2.256*	54.44	10.61	47.27	9.59
7					
8					
9					
10					

S = Group with highest overall evaluation; B = Group with average overall evaluation.

The JMI results for group 1 and group 4 were then compared.

Significant differences in A (workplace adjustment)
   (A5,A7: $p < 0.001$
Significant differences in B (physical condition)
   B15: $p < 0.05$
   B13: $p < 0.01$
Significant differences in C (mental health)
   C6,C10,C11,C13,C14,C18,C20: $p < 0.05$
   C16,C19: $p < 0.01$
   C12: $p < 0.001$
Significant differences in D (personality profile)
   D2: $p < 0.01$
   D9: $p < 0.001$

The members of group 4 felt overburdened by their workloads, and they complained about not being able to do their work accurately. The heavy workload made the pattern of their daily lives irregular, and their fatigue accumulated until they felt tired most of the time. Most of the workers in this group were timid by nature, lacked confidence, were susceptible to outside influences, and were liable to develop anxieties over trivial matters. The results for factor D showed them to be impulsive and often incapable of controlling their emotions.

JMI AND PERSONNEL APPRAISALS

The following example looks at two groups of engineers in the same company (Table 12–5). Group S ($m = 19$, average age 39.0 years) received the highest overall evaluation, and group B ($m = 22$, average age 40.8 years) was evaluated as average. Their JMI results are as follows.

Significant differences in A (workplace adjustment)
   A8,A9: $p < 0.05$

Table 12–6. JMI and Medical Expenses

		X		Y	
	t	M	SD	M	SD
Work adjustment					
A 1	6.078***	55.64	8.68	51.31	9.74
2					
3					
4					
5					
6	5.024***	53.89	9.90	50.03	10.03
7					
8					
9	4.356***	51.22	9.46	48.07	9.31
Physical condition					
B 1					
2					
3					
4					
5					
6					
7					
8					
9					
10					
11					
12					
13					
14					
15					
Mental health					
C 1					
2					
3	2.135*	52.46	10.43	50.81	9.63
4					
5					
6	2.828**	53.80	7.12	52.12	8.22
7					
8					
9					
10	3.513***	52.68	8.94	50.20	9.36
11					
12					
13					
14					
15					
16					
17	2.263*	53.27	8.83	51.69	9.27
18					
19					
20					
21	4.517***	51.39	8.51	47.94	11.06

(*continued*)

176

Table 12–6. (*Continued*)

		X		Y	
	t	M	SD	M	SD
Personality profile					
D 1	6.395***	54.92	9.79	50.02	10.08
2	2.427*	51.83	10.83	49.87	10.14
3					
4	2.333*	51.50	9.09	49.81	9.68
5					
6					
7	3.918**	54.24	10.99	51.03	10.28
8					
9					
10	3.746***	53.17	11.30	50.13	9.75

X = High medical cost office; Y = low medical cost office.

A3: $p < 0.01$
Significant differences in B (physical condition)
B1,B7,B8,B10,B12,B13,B14: $p < 0.05$
B6,B11: $p < 0.01$
Significant differences in C (mental health)
C4,C5,C9: $p < 0.05$
C3,C6: $p < 0.01$
Significant differences in D (personality profile)
D2,D6: $p < 0.05$
D3: $p < 0.01$

For factor D, there was a significant difference between the groups in terms of their relationships with coworkers. Differences were also observed in job satisfaction and expectations. There was a substantial difference in the overall physical condition of the two groups of engineers. The mental health evaluations showed significant differences in the cheerfulness, liveliness, and sense of isolation among members of the two groups. Similarly, the results of the personality profiles revealed significant differences in the number of extroverts in the two groups, as well as their initiative, energy, and ability to control their emotions.

JMI AND MEDICAL EXPENSES

This example shows the relation between the JMI results of two offices in the same company and their total medical expenses for 1 year after the JMI Health Examination

Table 12–7. Medical Expenses of Two Offices in One Company

Office	No. of workers	Av. age	Medical expenses	1985/1986 ratio	Diagnostic rate (%)
X	348	37.3	$ 9.29	104	61.0
Y	326	39.0	$13.23	119	63.8

Table 12–8. JMI Results versus Physicians' Diagnoses

Subjects	Percent of people	No. of healthy people	Depression	Total No.
Healthy people (no medication and not seeing a physician)	100	80	0	80
Depression diagnosed by a physician	96.7	2	58	60
Total	98	82	58	140

System was conducted (Table 12–6). Calculations were based on data collected from April 1985 to March 1986 (Table 12–7).

Significant differences in A (workplace adjustment)
A1,A6,A9: $p < 0.001$
Significant differences in B (physical condition)
No significant differences were found.
Significant differences in C (mental health)
C3,C17: $p < 0.05$
C6: $p < 0.01$
C10,C21: $p < 0.001$
Significant differences in D (personality profile)
D2,D4: $p < 0.05$
D7: $p\ 0.01$
D1,D10: $p < 0.001$

These results show that although there were no significant differences for factor B, medical expenses were high and the employees had several professional consultations. In the area of workplace adjustment, the respondents said that their jobs were uninteresting, and therefore they lacked ambition and the motivation to work. The results for factor C showed that, overall, the workers were depressed and felt isolated, and many of them had inferiority complexes combined with explosive tempers. This picture goes a long way toward explaining why alcohol consumption was so high. The results for factor D showed that the respondents were unable to control their emotions and lacked initiative.

JMI AND THE CONSISTENCY OF RATE OF DOCTORS' DIAGNOSES

Table 12–8 shows the consistency rate of JMI results and physicians' diagnoses.

13
Psychosocial Factors in the Workplace

Gunn Johansson and Gunnar Aronsson

This chapter addresses psychological and social factors in the workplace that may foster or inhibit the development of disease. It is written from a Scandinavian perspective. Scandinavia has had strong labor movements and a high level of unionization. The unions have not limited their activities to wage negotiations but have formed action programs and policies on a variety of issues of importance to their members, such as welfare policy, education, and labor market policy. A characteristic feature of the Swedish labor market has been the ideology of mutual understanding and cooperation between employers' organizations and trade unions. Occupational health and safety is one area of collaboration between the two parties; agreements on new technology is another.

Until the mid-1960s industry was generally regarded as a resource for political reform and for increased private and public consumption. Any possible human or social costs associated with prevailing means of increasing productivity were compensated for by an increased standard of living and greater leisure time. In Scandinavian research, the idea that scientific management and human relations were antagonistic sets of ideas started to emerge around 1960. Similar discussions started in the labor movement as a consequence of (a) increasing difficulties for older and less educated individuals to keep up with structural change, (b) increasing awareness of physical and chemical risk factors for health, absenteeism, and recruitment, and (c) increasing signs of dissatisfaction with monotonous work and other labor conditions (30).

Technological change and working conditions were major topics during the 1966 Congress of the Swedish Trade Union Confederation. As a result, the unions exerted political pressure to raise funds for research on the work environment, and they eventually developed their own policies concerning work science. Management responded early to these signs. Programs for work reform at the shop floor level were introduced, some of which have become internationally known, such as group assembly at Volvo and Saab-Scandia.

In 1972 a Work Environment Fund was founded to provide resources for research into working life issues, and in 1977/1978 a new legal framework was introduced for the regulation of industrial relations and working conditions. Recently, preparations have been initiated to revise this legislation on the basis of experiences gathered during the 1980s (61).

- The *Act of Codetermination* gives trade unions the right to influence decisions at all levels in the company, and all questions related to work and work environment are open for collective bargaining.
- The *Work Environment Act* specifies that working methods, equipment, and material should be adapted to humans from a physiological and a psychological point of view. Work must also be organized to promote self-determination and vocational responsibility.

Local health and safety promotion on the job is organized by safety committees including employee and employer representatives. Through an agreement between employers and unions, training of both safety delegates and foremen occurs during paid working hours and is financed by the employer. It is estimated that about 650,000 people have completed the basic occupational safety and health course, and an advanced training program reaches another 30,000 to 40,000 people per year.

This local organization of health and safety promotion has led to articulated formulations of problems (including those of a psychosocial character); it has also influenced scientific research and offers a channel for intervention. These unique circumstances have influenced Swedish research on work, stress, and health. They also explain why some types of research in work sites can be carried out with less resistance in Scandinavia than in some other countries. There is more trust and understanding between the parties in the labor market and, generally, between them and researchers.

RESEARCH ON WORK, STRESS, AND HEALTH

Our analysis of work and stress is based on current consensus about stress as a transactional, dynamic process mediated by the central nervous system (5,9,12). Characterizations of the stress process have emphasized the interaction between stressors, transmission processes, and recipients. Thus behavioral, biological, and emotional stress reactions develop as a result of the mismatch between internal demands and resources and external demands and resources (4).

Although the role of stress in health and disease has been studied in various sectors of human life, the work setting seems well suited for the purpose. First, large groups of adults are systematically exposed to fairly similar conditions during a large part of their waking hours. Second, when adverse conditions are identified, they can often be modified and the consequences evaluated in terms of health and well-being.

The research reported in this chapter deals with four dimensions that have emerged as particularly important for stress and worker health (52).

1. Quantitative overload, i.e., too much to do, time pressure, repetitive work flow in combination with one-sided job demands and high demands on attention.
2. Qualitative underload, i.e., too narrow and one-sided job content, lack of stimulus variation, no demands on creativity or problem-solving, or low opportunities for social interaction.
3. Lack of control, especially in relation to work pace and working methods.
4. Lack of social support at home and from fellow workers.

Our approach can be illustrated by the model shown in Figure 13–1, which has appeared in different versions but was first developed at the Institute for Social Re-

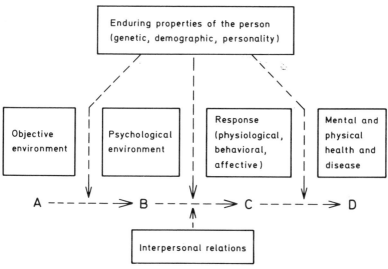

Figure 13–1. Theoretical framework for research on the effects of work role on health. From French and Kahn (24, 43).

search at the University of Michigan (24,43). It outlines some of the most important factors involved in a process leading from psychosocial conditions in the environment to health/disease. Research in this area has often been restricted to pairs of these factors. Epidemiological approaches to occupational health concentrate on relations between objective environment and health/disease (Fig. 13–1, A–D); exerimental stress research on objective conditions and immediately measurable responses (A–C); sociological quality of working life research on the psychological experience of objective environments (A–B); and certain types of clinical stress research on the interaction between enduring properties of the person and psychobiological responses to stressors.

The studies to be reported here combine three or more of the elements outlined in Figure 13–1. Field studies have usually used interviews of a few "key individuals," questionnaires filled in by a large group of individuals, on-the-job measurements of biological and behavioral reactions obtained from limited but theoretically pertinent subgroups, and health examinations (cf. 20,23). Certain elements that form part of psychosocial work conditions, e.g., machine-paced versus self-paced work, have been studied under controlled conditions in the laboratory. In those cases, a limited number of subjects have been studied intensely in terms of subjective and biological reactions as well as individual characteristics.

An important feature of our research program is the monitoring of physiological functions during work. One of the assumptions underlying the use of physiological and biochemical techniques in human stress and coping research is that the environmental load to which a person is exposed can be determined by measuring cardiovascular function through blood pressure and heart rate, adrenal medullary activity through urinary excretion of epinephrine (adrenaline) and norepinephrine (noradrenaline), and pituitary-adrenal activity reflected in the excretion of cortisol. Urinary estimates reliably reflect the level of circulating hormones (2). They are particularly convenient in field settings where urine samples may be obtained without interference with daily routines of the individual (19,23).

The role of specific environmental factors in the selective activation of the two hormone systems has been the object of intense interest among researchers in this area. Evidence has revealed a complex pattern of endocrine stress responses in which the individual's possibilities for active involvement and control are of crucial importance (64). Thus Lundberg and Frankenhaeuser (19,53) emphasized effort and distress as two factors of major importance. They claimed that an adrenaline increase is associated with effort as well as with distress, whereas cortisol increases primarily in response to distress. Distress occurs, for instance, in unpleasant situations with limited individual control. According to their experiments, the cortisol response may even be suppressed in situations of effort if at the same time the individual is allowed to exert control. Arthur (8) reached a similar conclusion on the basis of a literature review of research concerning adrenocortical hormones. He suggested that adrenocortical hormones peak during anticipation of a stressful event, not during confrontation with it.

Because of the complex interaction between objective conditions, subjective appraisal of the situation, and biological response, biological indicators alone are insufficient for evaluating the emotional quality of the reaction. The qualitative aspect can be tapped only through the individual's self-report. For this purpose the participants in our studies give quantitative self-ratings of mood and arousal using a method based on psychophysical scaling techniques (38).

Adrenaline and noradrenaline usually facilitate both mental and physical adjustment to acute environmental demands. However, a growing body of evidence indicates that frequent or long-lasting physiological activation has a potentially damaging impact (64), especially on the cardiovascular system (34).

Initially, our interest was directed toward basic features of different production technologies, such as mechanization and automation, especially with regard to stimulus overload or underload (20,21). We first focused on psychosocial factors representative of conditions in a wide range of highly mechanized, mass-producing industries (27). Work on the assembly line, for instance, is characterized by the machine system's rigorous control over the worker. The job is understimulating in the sense that it offers no options for varying pace or content and few opportunities for social interaction. Body posture and movement are narrowly restricted. At the same time these tasks contain elements of overload such as a forced work pace and demands for sustained attention.

REPETITIVE INDUSTRIAL WORK

The first example of our research concerns work in a highly mechanized sawmill (40). A nationwide study of the ergonomics of Swedish sawmills had already provided detailed data on physical and psychosocial components of the work environment, reactions to these environments, and health status of the employees. In practically all the larger sawmills it was possible to identify what might be called a high-risk group, whose tasks were characterized by repetitiveness and short (about 10-second) work cycles. The work demanded that these workers keep continuously attentive and alert, as they were to make complex judgments about the raw material at a high speed. Production was arranged in a way that placed these workers in a "bottleneck" in the flow of material and production. Therefore they also carried a great deal of responsibility for the productivity as well as for their own and their workmates' income (they were all on group piece rate). Most of these characteristics are typical of other, similar assembly-line type of tasks. The high-risk group in the selected sawmill was compared to a control group in the same plant. The members of the control group were engaged in maintenance and repair work. Major differences in job content between the groups are shown in Table 13–1. In contrast to the high-risk group, the control group could move about more freely, regulate their own pace of work, and interact with mates.

Other important differences between the two groups, presented in Table 13–2, concerned health status. Thus the high-risk group displayed a higher frequency of sleep disorders, headaches, gastrointestinal disorders, cardiovascular disease, and nervous tension.

We measured urinary catecholamine output at 2-hour intervals during an 8-hour shift and also (to obtain baseline measures) during a work-free day at home. At the same points in time the workers made self-ratings of mood and alertness using a graphic scale with endpoints defined. Factors that might influence the secretion of catecholamines, e.g., the consumption of nicotine and alcohol-containing beverages and physical exercise, were kept under control.

Figure 13–2 shows the excretion of the two catecholamines during work, expressed as a percentage of the corresponding baseline measurements collected during work-free time. The adrenaline group averages ranged between 12.6 and 75.3 pmol/minute for baseline and between 24.4 and 84.1 pmol/minute for work conditions. The corresponding measures for noradrenaline were 56.7 to 237.6 pmol/minute and 78.0 to 283.7 pmol/minute, respectively.) The control group reached a peak level in the morning, followed by a slow decline toward the end of the shift. The high-risk group started off at a level twice as high as the corresponding baseline level; after a temporary decline, the excretion increased continuously to its maximum at the end of the day. The pronounced increase in the adrenaline level toward the end of the day was interpreted as attempts to counteract the buildup of fatigue. The fatigue had to be compensated for in terms of effort, and as a result the high-risk group left the workplace in a state of high physiological activation. This finding is in agreement with

Table 13–1. Psychosocial Factors in the Work Environment of Two Groups of Sawmill Workers

High-risk group
    Cycle time shorter than 10 seconds
    Machine-paced work
    Continuous demands for attention
    Physical constraint
Control group
    Cycle time longer than 1 minute
    Self-paced work
    Possibility to move around
    Possibility to leave for 10 minutes
    Freedom to interact with mates

Source: Johansson et al. (40).
All jobs were rated by the same expert.

Table 13-2. Relative Frequency of Symptoms Among Two
Groups of Sawmill Workers

Symptom	High-risk group (%)	Control group (%)
Joint disorders	50	22
Peripheral circulation	21	11
Headaches	36	0
Intestinal disorders	7	0
Low-back disorders	43	11
Nervous tension	36	0

Source: Johansson et al. (40).
Data are based on a combination of self-reports and clinical tests.

statements by these workers during interviews. They claimed that it usually took them an hour or two after work to get sufficiently relaxed for interaction with their family and for other activities.

When evaluating these data it is worth mentioning that the two groups were comparable with regard to physical conditions, such as exposure to noise and dust. The two groups were also comparable in significant aspects other than work conditions: They were of equal age and background. They all lived in a rural area where most of them spent their leisure time in similar ways, e.g., fishing, hunting, and boating. Housing conditions were similar for all of them. It is also worth noting that the high-risk group had been selected for their demanding jobs because of their personal qualifications. They held jobs that were of great economic importance for their employer. It is reasonable to assume that they represent a positive selection at the time of appointment to the job, with regard not only to skill but to health, absenteeism, and so on.

In an attempt to identify specific factors that induced the psychological and neuroendocrine stress responses, the data were broken down into new subgroups ac-

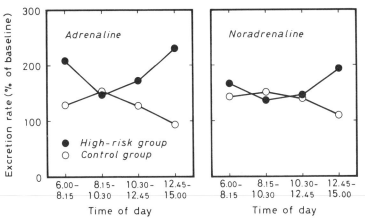

Figure 13–2. Average excretion of adrenaline and noradrenaline during an 8-hour shift in two groups of sawmill workers. Measurements have been transformed into percentages of corresponding baseline measurements obtained during nonwork conditions. From Johansson et al. (40).

cording to the level of repetitiveness, physical constraint, and control of work pace as indicated by expert ratings. The resulting subgroups were small, but the results formed a meaningful pattern (Fig. 13–3). Objectively assessed repetitiveness, i.e., little variation between work cycles, was positively associated with levels of catecholamine output and levels of irritation. Similarly, machine pacing was associated with larger catecholamine output and more irritation than self-paced work. Finally, there was a positive relation between, on the one hand, objectively assessed physical constraint and, on the other, high pituitary-adrenal medullary activity and irritation.

The tendency for work on the assembly line to affect catecholamine output was also reported in a study of individuals working alternately on and off the assembly

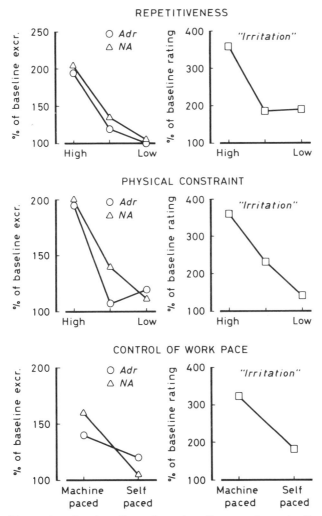

Figure 13–3. Mean values for adrenaline and noradrenaline excretion and self-ratings of irritation in a group of sawmill workers under conditions differing with regard to repetitiveness, physical constraint, and control of work pace. Values obtained during work have been expressed as percentages of baselines obtained under nonwork conditions. From Johansson et al. (40).

line (63). In this case no self-reports or health indicators were available, but on-the-job measurements formed a clear pattern: Averaged over a 4-day period, urinary adrenaline measures were significantly higher during assembly line work than in other tasks. These results were confirmed when a subsample of the workers were studied again after 6 months, and a recent study by Lundberg and co-workers (54) lent further support to the notion that assembly-line work is associated with a considerable increase of antonomic arousal as measured by catecholamine output, blood pressure, and heart rate.

Timio and his coworkers (63) performed the same procedure in a second group for comparison of piece-rate work and fixed salary. They found that these workers excreted significantly larger amounts of catecholamines during periods of piece-rate payment than during periods of fixed salary. An early semiexperimental study by Levi (51) showed a fourfold increase of adrenaline excretion under piece-rate conditions compared to salary conditions.

Thus psychobiological research has shown that the poor work satisfaction, high absenteeism, and high frequency of health complaints associated with fragmented, repetitive industrial work is paralleled by arousal of endocrine stress reactions during performance of the job. A natural conclusion is that this type of work should become the object of health promotion through job redesign.

It may be argued that assembly work, organized according to tayloristic principles, will soon be abandoned as a result of new technology being introduced. It is true also that organizational experiments are being performed to find alternatives to the traditional organization of assembly work. Although systematic and independent evaluation is scarce—especially with regard to health—practically oriented analyses have reported promising results in terms of job satisfaction and productivity (18). However, the experiments have been local and restricted to Western industrialized countries. In many developing countries and in some East European countries, industrial production will continue to apply traditional forms of work organization for a considerable time to come. Furthermore, statistics recently published by the Swedish Metal Workers Union (62) reveal that only a minority of their members have been affected by organizational experiments. Finally, the introduction of computers in administrative and clerical work in economically developed countries has transferred the principles of work organization from the shop floor to the office.

OFFICE AUTOMATION

One of the most common applications of computer technology in the office is the switch from paper files to centralized, computer-based information systems. This development has created fragmented and repetitive tasks in the form of data-entry work. Instead of distributing this necessary but monotonous task among large groups of employees, it has often been assigned to special groups of clerical workers. In an initial phase of the process, the task of these clerical workers may be to enter old, accumulated data into the computer base and later, when the system has been established, to continuously update it.

In a study of an insurance company (37), we compared two groups of female employees. One-half of them were directly affected by the computer system. They spent more than half their work-day in intense interaction with the computer system by means of a visual display terminal (VDT). They used their terminals either to feed data from documents into the computer system or to serve customers by personal contact or over the telephone. The rest of the participants constituted a control group of secretaries and typists who spent their workday typing, answering the telephone, and so on. The control group had no contact with the computer system.

The two groups were matched for age and were equivalent in terms of family conditions, education, and time of employment. A research design similar to the one used in the sawmill was applied. In addition to interview and questionnaire data that had already been collected for a larger group, we collected biochemical and physiological measurements and self-reports. These data were collected during and after workdays as well as during and after a work-free day, which was spent by the women in their homes.

Figure 13–4 shows the adrenaline excretion for the two groups during and after work. As before, work measures have been expressed as a percentage of baseline measures. (Average daytime measures of adrenaline excretion on the job were 38.2 pmol/minute for the VDT group and 25.1 pmol/minute for the control group. Corresponding measures of noradrenaline excretion were 157.1 and 149.9 pmol/minute, respectively.) During work, the VDT operators excreted significantly higher levels of adrenaline than the control group. It is interesting to note that this difference remained and even increased somewhat during the evening after work. This result is in agreement with self-reports by these women (Fig. 13–5), indicating that those who spent their day in intense VDT work felt more tired after work than did the control group. That is, they took longer to unwind after a day's work.

Figure 13–6 presents blood-pressure measurements obtained on five occasions during a day's work. The upper pair of curves represent the systolic pressure and the lower pair the diastolic pressure for both groups. There is a consistent tendency toward higher blood-pressure measurements among the VDT operators than in the control

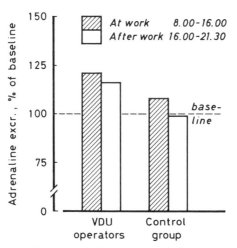

Figure 13–4. Average excretion of adrenaline during and after work for two groups of insurance clerks. All values are given as percentages of baseline measures obtained on a separate work-free day spent at home. From Johansson and Aronsson (37).

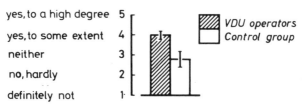

Figure 13–5. Perceived fatigue after a day's work, reported by two groups of insurance clerks. From Johansson and Aronsson (37).

group. The differences cannot be explained by reference to a difference in habitual levels. Average baseline measures of blood pressure taken at the corporate health unit were equal for the two groups. It can therefore be assumed that the difference in blood pressure between the groups was at least partly due to differences in work conditions.

At the time of the investigation there was only one hyperactive person in the group. She belonged to the VDT group and was excluded from these statistical analyses. At the time of this study, the average exposure time to the intense VDT work was 4 years. The higher blood pressure level for VDT operators was paralleled by significantly higher levels of triglycerides. A 7-year follow-up study did not provide evidence that the blood pressure difference during work had persisted. However, intense VDT work was still associated with higher hormone output during work (7).

Similar conditions were investigated in a French study of VDT work (17). In a simulated but realistic data-entry task, performance and physiological reactions were monitored for 2 hours. The patterns of response showed a performance decline and an increasing amount of electroencephalographic (EEG) theta activity during the first hour. A rebound was then noted, first in the EEG record, where theta and alpha activity diminished and beta increased. The authors interpret the results as showing how a repetitive task induces low arousal and a decline of performance until a compensatory

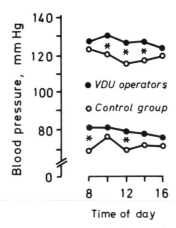

Time of day

Figure 13–6. Mean blood pressure measurements during an 8-hour work day for two groups of insurance clerks. The upper pair of curves represent systolic pressures, the lower pair diastolic pressures. Asterisks signify statistically significant differences between groups. From Johansson and Aronsson (37).

effort at the cerebral level intervenes and results in increased arousal and improved performance.

A more recent study (16) showed that during a 2-hour period of data-entry work the imbalance between arousal and task demands appeared in machine-paced as well as self-paced work. These two studies were limited to the work sessions. Our own study of data-entry clerks suggested, however, that the compensatory effort takes place at the expense of psychoneuroendocrine mobilization and a buildup of fatigue that extends into work-free hours.

Research has confirmed the impression that extensive, monotonous VDT work, and data-entry work in particular, leads to fatigue, poor work satisfaction, uneven performance, somatic complaints (e.g., eye strain, headache, and upper back and neck tension), and, in some cases, more absenteeism (16,59,68). This accumulation of aversive outcomes results from a combination of monotonous work devoid of intellectual stimulation, dependence on technical equipment, forced work pace, physical constraint, and high demands for attention, i.e., high work load in combination with strict limitation of individual control.

There is growing recognition that the impact of computer-mediated work on stress and health is strongly dependent on the character of the tasks performed (6,7,58,65) and that any general statements about computer technology, stress, and health tend to be misleading (35). Apart from the data-entry tasks, we still know little about the mental load and stress reactions associated with various computerized tasks, such as data acquisition, interactive communication, programming, and computer-aided design. The need for a taxonomy of VDT work has been emphasized (50) and is necessary as part of future occupational health strategies.

SUPERVISORY MONITORING OF COMPLEX TECHNICAL PROCESSES

The consequences of new technology in production industries have been different from those observed in the office. An interesting example are the supervisory tasks in process industries. Nuclear power plants belong in this category, and similar conditions exist in chemical plants, refineries, dairies, and the paper and pulp industry, where production is based on the continuous flow of liquids, gas, or energy. Although centralized remote control of such processes has been applied for a long time, the introduction of computers has accentuated certain elements in the operator's task that tends to increase the mental demands on the operator (36).

These conditions were investigated in a field study of two groups of control room operators (39) in which monotony was the major object of study. One of these groups performed process control work dominated by passive supervisory control. They monitored stable, continuous processes such as oxygen production and power generation. In a monotonous work situation their task was to remain passive but alert until disturbances in the production process called for their action. They had only limited possibility to predict the character of the next disturbance and the time of its occurrence. It was a situation of stimulus underload that provided little personal control.

The second group was involved in active production planning and control. They used telephones, radio, and computer communication to coordinate activities in several parts of a steel mill. These operators worked under time pressure and at a high level of stimulus input. Their situation involved elements of stimulus overload, but they had good opportunities for personal control over their own work as well as that of others. It must be emphasized that both groups carried a large responsibility for efficient and safe production.

The results showed that both groups markedly increased their urinary output of adrenaline during daytime work compared to baselines, a finding in agreement with results from laboratory research showing that understimulation as well as overstimulation give rise to an adrenaline increase (22,41). Their excretion levels were comparable to those obtained for the sawmill workers described above, and the two operator groups did not differ significantly in terms of catecholamine output.

Instead, differences were found in their experience of the work situation. Subjective workload was higher in active production planning and control, as was the perceived time pressures. Passive supervision was associated with feelings of monotony but also with more pronounced feelings of anxiety when facing process failures. The passive group also reported a vague feeling of uneasiness during the early morning hours of night shifts. Both groups were satisfied with the possibilities for learning and occupational development at work. They also reported satisfaction from the fact that they managed a difficult and complex job, but this feeling was significantly less pronounced in the passive process control group.

Our interpretation of these results is that a situation of passive supervisory control with continuous demands for attention and action readiness can give rise to effort, strain, and physiological arousal comparable to those of a job containing complex information processing and decision making under time pressure. The difference lies in the emotional quality of the experience. Whereas the effort of actively planning a coordination task tends to be associated with positive feelings, the effort experienced in a passive, uneventful situation is associated with feelings of monotony, uneasiness, uncertainty, and lack of control.

A more recent study of control room operators (57) has focused on the level of automation and on social and organizational aspects of supervisory monitoring. The results show that the combined exposure to high-level automation and social isolation represents a particularly adverse situation. Operators working under these conditions were dependent on the technical systems, they felt less confident in the performance of their work, and they reported significantly more health complaints such as headaches, extreme fatigue, and back and shoulder pain.

The shift from passive monitoring to active information processing and problem solving, which is required by the operator during a process failure, is difficult to analyze in a field setting. Therefore we attempted to study this phenomenon in the laboratory (41). Performance and stress reactions were investigated in a suddenly and unexpectedly occurring task that required selective perception and rapid information processing. Two groups performed the test, one of them after 2 hours of passive monitoring and the other after 2 hours of active involvement in the same monitoring task.

Analyses of the data showed that passive monitoring was followed by more performance errors and much more variable and unpredictable performance than active monitoring. This finding is in agreement with other experimental studies (13,66) showing that behavior efficiency is better after active involvement than after passive monitoring.

JOB DEMANDS AND RESOURCES FOR CONTROL

The examples given have emphasized the importance of the four psychosocial aspects of work mentioned in the introduction: quantitative overload, qualitative underload, lack of control, and lack of social support. In different ways they tend to support the job strain model suggested by Karasek (44) and developed by him in collaboration with others (45,46,48).

Application of this model (Fig. 13–7) requires that jobs be described in terms of two dimensions: job demands and decision latitude (control, autonomy). It predicts (Fig. 13–7) that moving along the diagonal from high control/low demand jobs ("low strain") toward low control/high demand jobs ("high strain"), one finds increasing signs of dissatisfaction and ill health. This finding has been repeatedly confirmed in analyses of representative samples of worker populations in the United States and Scandinavia (3,42,45,47,49).

The job strain model also predicts that high job demands combined with a high level of autonomy ("active jobs") (Fig. 13–7) increase the probability for growth and feelings of mastery and for active participation in social networks on and off the job (44,46).

In addition to its scientific value this model may prove useful from strategic and pedagogical perspectives. It suggests that unwanted consequences of job stress may be avoided not only through the elimination of psychosocial stressors but through the introduction of resources for control that facilitate coping by individuals and groups. An interesting example of how health outcomes may be modified by the balance between job demands and resources for control was found in a study of local transport personnel (32). A randomly selected group of 1,442 full-time bus, train, and tram drivers and guard personnel participated in this questionnaire study. In accordance with the job strain model, it was assumed that individuals working under high job demands and having few resources for control would be more vulnerable with regard to health and well-being than a group facing moderate job demands and numerous resources for control.

The job of a city bus driver is stressful, a fact that has been proved in many parts of the world (14,32,55,56). Urban public transport is characterized by the rigors of a timetable, and drivers work under time pressure determined by conditions such as traffic congestion or requests for assistance/information by passengers over which they

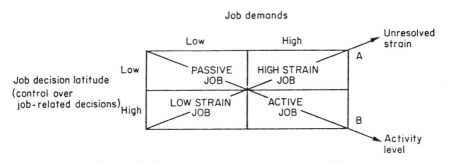

Figure 13–7. Job strain model. From Karasek (45).

have no control. In our study three stressors were included in a measure of *job demands:* frequency of (a) stressful efforts to keep the timetable; (b) conflicts between ambitions to keep the timetable and other goals, e.g., safe driving and service to the passengers; and (c) passenger behavior, e.g., complaints about conditions beyond the driver's control and conflicts, disagreements, or even threats and assaults.

Four resources were identified that would assist the bus driver in dealing with these demands: technical resources (radio and alarm systems), organizational resources (trade union support in efforts to improve work conditions), social resources (support of superiors and fellow workers), and personal resources (personal authority in the occupational role, perceived ability to handle difficult passenger contacts).

The combination of high workload and few resources for control was systematically associated with mental and physical exhaustion, back and joint pains, gastrointestinal disturbances, sleep disturbances, slight mental stress, and absence due to illness. Figure 13–8 shows one example of these associations: the absence from work due to illness more than 1 month in the past 12 months. Generally speaking, all these indicators of ill health became more frequent at higher levels of job demands, but the tendency was clearly modified by the number of resources available to the driver on the job.

It must be added that studies in several countries have identified city bus drivers as a risk group with regard to sick-leave, morbidity, and mortality (32,55,67). This trend can be illustrated with data from an epidemiological study carried out in Denmark (56) in which bus drivers in the Copenhagen area were compared to individuals in other age-matched occupational groups in terms of cardiovascular disease and mortality. The

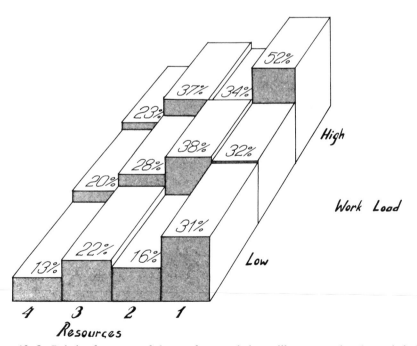

Figure 13–8. Relative frequency of absence from work due to illness more than 1 month during the past 12 months as reported by city bus drivers. From Gardell et al. (32).

total mortality rate in this all-male group was identical among bus drivers and the reference group. However, mortality due to ischemic heart disease was significantly higher among bus drivers. The prevalence of self-reported angina pectoris was also higher among bus drivers than in the reference group at all age levels between 30 and 69 years.

FUTURE RESEARCH

Considerable scientific knowledge has been accumulated concerning the role of psychosocial factors in job stress. In combination with results obtained in human and animal research exploring pathogenic mechanisms, it forms a sound basis for worksite intervention. Such intervention should first concern such factors as work schedules, machine-pacing, and repetitive, fragmented, and specialized simple tasks which have repeatedly been shown to contribute to somatic disturbances and perceived strain.

One priority in future research should be careful, systematic, long-term evaluation of such interventions in terms of health as well as productivity. So far, evaluations have usually concerned productivity and job satisfaction or health-related behavior such as absenteeism or accident rates with little reference to economic results. Methods are being developed for economic evaluation of the balance between costs and benefits in this area, and it still remains to be proved that costs associated with job redesign would be wasted money. However, this kind of evaluation is a demanding task that requires a multidisciplinary approach and intimate collaboration between researchers, employees, and corporate officials who carry responsibility for long-term planning, productivity, and human resource development.

Because traditional models of efficiency and organization of work have provided good economic returns, there has been considerable resistance among those responsible for effective production when attempts have been made to increase the autonomy and complexity of job roles. However, the radical transformation of production methods, work routines, and job demands brought about by computer technology may demand a reconsideration in this respect, even without reference to any humanistic or health and safety values. It is our impression that production managers and engineers in process industries, for instance, have now taken an interest in the human aspect of the production processes. Their motive seems to be that margins for efficiency increases tend to diminish in the technical sphere, and that new forms of work organization may soon be one of the few remaining means of increasing efficiency.

The skepticism regarding alternative forms of work organization has led to a tendency, more pronounced in the United States than in Scandinavia, to address demands for change to the individual rather than to the organizational level, thus "turning social and technical problems in the work environment into a private problem" (31). Several worksite health-promotion programs aiming at a change of health-related behaviors and life styles have been successful, at least in a short-term perspective (10). However, research results such as those reviewed here clearly indicate that the individual approach must be supplemented by organizational and technical change. In the Scandinavian countries this approach is formalized and based on existing work environment legislation (28,33).

One other research need must be mentioned in this context. Whereas the combined effects of various chemical and physical factors in the work environment have been reported (e.g., 26), the combination of physical/chemical and psychosocial factors has received little attention. The issue has been discussed (11,25), but empirical evidence is lacking. Exploration of these interactions can be justified on theoretical grounds. There are, for instance, large numbers of physical/chemical as well as psychosocial factors in work environments that are frequently combined, the effects of which are mediated through the central nervous system (e.g., monotonous work and toxic solvents, machine pacing and noise). Again, collaboration among many experts, each with his or her own area of expertise, is necessary for successful research.

Some of the most urgent research needs in the area of work, health, and productivity seem to have this complex and multidisciplinary character (15). Therefore the formulation of research priorities may not be sufficient for the advancement of knowledge in the area. To address the most complex issues, we may need to design more complex scientific designs and approaches than those most commonly used.

Our final remarks concern worker involvement in the improvement of work conditions. Although efforts to find more democratic forms of work organization are not usually regarded as part of occupational health and safety programs, the research cited above suggests that in the long run they may contribute to the improvement of health, as well as to productivity.

There is an unfortunate lack of systematic scientific evaluation of the interesting job redesign and autonomy experiments that have been introduced, for instance, in car assembly plants. The scant documentation available claims that productivity has been maintained while these experiments have been carried out (1). A few experiments have been scientifically documented, and they seem to show a consistent pattern. One such study concerns geriatric care (60): Home care assistants took part in an attempt to decentralize the planning of work and responsibility for maintaining the prescribed level of service rather than relying on a supervisor in a traditional hierarchical organization.

Here, as was the case in similar experiments in assembly industries (29), increased autonomy had a pronounced activating and motivating effect on the workers. They gained considerably in self-confidence, job satisfaction, and perception of their job as a meaningful activity. They also tended to be more willing to take on responsibility for efficient production—and for their own work environment. These results are not surprising to those who have become increasingly aware of the workplace as an important place for social learning. Research stimulated by the job strain model has shown how helplessness and passivity can be learned on the job and spill over into the sphere of leisure. Unfortunately, these studies have only indirectly addressed health and productivity issues.

In terms of a research agenda on the psychosocial work conditions we suggest the following.

1. Better evaluation of work reform programs in terms of both health and productivity.
2. Search for a balance between intervention at the individual and systems levels.
3. Identification of resources for control and coping with job demands, and search for an appropriate balance between job demands and resources for control.
4. Investigation of interactions between psychosocial and other environmental factors, e.g., interaction between monotony and toxic solvents, noise and machine-pacing.

A final observation concerns the increased participation of women in the labor market. With more than 80% of Swedish women gainfully employed, it is embarrassing that most of our knowledge about psychosocial factors, health, and productivity, as well as theoretical models used in research and consultation, are still based on studies of primarily male samples.

ACKNOWLEDGMENTS

The research reported was supported by grants from the Swedish Work Environment Fund, The National Board for Technical Development, and the Swedish Council for Research in the Humanities and Social Sciences.

REFERENCES

1. Agurén, S., Bredbacka, C., Hansson, R., Ihregren, K., & Karlsson, K. G. (1985). *Volvo Kalmar revisited: ten years of experience; human resources, technology, financial results.* Stockholm: Efficiency and Participation Development Council SAF, LO, PTK.

2. Åkerstedt, T., Gillberg, M., Hjemdahl, P., Sigurdson, K., Gustavsson, I., Daleskog, M., & Pollare, T. (1983). Comparison of urinary and plasma catecholamine responses to mental stress. *Acta Physiologica Scandinavica, 117,* 19–26.

3. Alfredsson, L., Karasek, R. A., & Theorell, T. (1982). Myocardial infarction risk and psychosocial work environment: an analysis of the male Swedish working force. *Social Science and Medicine, 16,* 463–7.

4. Appley, M. H., & Trumbull, R. (eds.). (1986). *Dynamics of stress: physiological, psychological, and social perspectives.* New York: Plenum.

5. Appley, M. H., & Trumbull, R. (1986). Development of the stress concept. In M. H. Appley & R. Trumbull (eds.). *Dynamics of stress: physiological, psychological, and social perspectives* (pp. 3–18). New York: Plenum Press.

6. Aronsson, G. (1989). Changed qualification demands in computer mediated work. *Applied Psychology: An International Review, 38,* 57–71.

7. Aronsson, G., & Johansson, G. (1987). Work content, stress and health in computer-mediated work: a seven year follow-up study. In B. Knave & P-G. Widebäck (eds.). *Work with display units 86: selected papers from the International Scientific Conference on Work with Display Units* (pp. 732–8). Amsterdam: Elsevier.

8. Arthur, A. Z. (1986). Stress as a state of anticipatory vigilance. *Perceptual and Motor Skills, 64,* 75–85.

9. Baum, A., Singer, J. E., & Baum, D. S. (1981). Stress and the environment. *Journal of Social Issues, 37,* 4–35.

10. Cataldo, M. F., & Coates, T. J. (eds.). (1986). *Health and industry: a behavioral medicine perspective.* New York: Wiley.

11. Cottington, E. M., & House, J. S. (1987). Occupational stress and health among factory workers: a multivariate relationship. In A. Baum & J. E. Singer (eds.). *Handbook of psychology and health,* (Vol. 5, pp. 41–62). Hillsdale, NJ: Lawrence Erlbaum Associates.

12. Cox, T. (1978). *Stress.* London: Macmillan.

13. Ephrath, A. R., & Young, L. R. (1981). Monitoring vs. man-in-the-loop detection of aircraft control failures. In J. Rasmussen & W. B. Rouse (eds.). *Human detection and diagnosis of system failures* (pp. 143–54). New York: Plenum Press/NATO Scientific Affairs Division.

14. Evans, G. W., Palsane, M. N., & Carrere, S. (1987). Type A and occupational stress: a cross-cultural study of blue-collar workers. *Journal of Personality and Social Psychology, 52,* 1002–7.

15. Evans, G. W., Carrere, S., & Johansson, G. (1990). A multivariate perspective on environmental stress. *Archives of Complex Environmental Studies, 1,* 1–5.

16. Floru, R., & Cail, F. (1987). Data entry task on VDU: underload or overload? In B. Knave & P.-G. Widebäck (eds.). *Work with display units 86: selected papers from the International Scientific Conference on Work with Display Units* (pp. 756–67). Amsterdam: Elsevier.

17. Floru, R., Cail, F., & Elias, R. (1985). Psychophysiological changes during a VDU repetitive task. *Ergonomics, 28,* 1455–68.

18. Forslin, J. (1990). *Det klippta bandet. En VOLVO-industri byter kultur [The broken line: cultural change in a VOLVO industry].* Stockholm: FArådet Norstedts. [In Swedish.]

19. Frankenhaeuser, M. (1986). A psychobiological framework for research on human stress and coping. In M. H. Appley & R. Trumbull (eds.). *Dynamics of stress: physiological, psychological and social perspectives* (pp. 101–16). New York: Plenum Press.

20. Frankenhaeuser, M., & Gardell, B. (1976). Underload and overload in working life: a multidisciplinary approach. *Journal of Human Stress, 2,* 35–46.

21. Frankenhaeuser, M., & Johansson, G. (1981). On the psychophysiological consequences of understimulation and overstimulation. In L. Levi (ed.). *Society, stress and disease. Vol. IV: Working life* (pp. 82–89). Oxford: Oxford University Press.

22. Frankenhaeuser, M., Nordheden, B., Myrsten, A-L., & Post, B. (1971). Psychophysiological reactions to understimulation and overstimulation. *Acta Psychologica, 35,* 298–308.

23. Frankenhaeuser, M., Lundberg, U., Fredriksson, M., Melin, B., Tuomisto, M., Myrsten, A.-L., Hedman, M., Bergman-Losman, B., & Wallin, L. (1989). Stress on and off the job as related to sex and occupational status in white-collar workers. *Journal of Organizational Behavior, 10,* 321–46.

24. French, J. R. P., Jr., & Kahn, R. L. (1962). A programmatic approach to studying the industrial environment and mental health. *Journal of Social Issues, 18,* 1–47.

25. Gamberale, F. & Kjellberg, A. (1990). Behavioural and psychophysiological effects of the physical work environment. *Scandinavian Journal of Work Environment and Health, 16,* suppl. 1.

26. Gamberale, F., Annwall, B. A., & Hultengren, M. (1978). Exposure to xylene and ethylbenzene. III. Effects on central nervous functions. *Scandinavian Journal of Work Environment & Health, 4,* 204–11.

27. Gardell, B. (1981). Psychosocial aspects of industrial production methods. In L. Levi (ed.). *Society, stress and disease. Vol. IV: Working life* (pp. 65–75). Oxford: Oxford University Press.

28. Gardell, B. (1981). Strategies for reform programmes on work organization and work environment. In B. Gardell & G. Johansson (eds.). *Working life: a social science contribution to work reform* (pp. 3–13). Chichester: Wiley.

29. Gardell, B. (1982). Worker participation and autonomy: a multilevel approach to democracy at the workplace. *International Journal of Health Services, 12,* 527–58.

30. Gardell, B. (1987). Efficiency and health hazards in mechanized work. In J. C. Quick, R. S. Bhagat, J. E. Dalton, & J. D. Quick (eds.). *Work stress: health care systems in the work place* (pp. 50–71). New York: Praeger.

31. Gardell, B. (1987). *Organization of work and human nature: an overview of research on the human need to master technology.* Stockholm: Swedish Work Environment Fund.

32. Gardell, B., Aronsson, G., & Barklöf, K. (1981). *The working environment for the local public transport personnel.* Stockholm: Swedish Work Environment Fund.

33. Gardell, B., & Gustavsen, B. (1980). Work environment research and social change: current developments in Scandinavia. *Journal of Occupational Behaviour, 1,* 3–17.

34. Henry, J. P., & Stephens, P. M. (1977). *Stress, health, and the social environment: a sociobiologic approach to medicine.* New York: Springer-Verlag.

35. Johansson, G. (1987). Growth and challenge vs. wear and tear of humans in computer mediated work. In B. Knave & P-G. Widebäck (eds.). *Work with display units 86: selected papers from the International Scientific Conference on Work with Display Units* (pp. 725–31). Amsterdam: Elsevier.

36. Johansson, G. (1989). Stress, autonomy and the maintenance of skill in supervisory control of automated systems. *Applied Psychology: An International Review, 38,* 45–56.

37. Johansson, G., & Aronsson, G. (1984). Stress reactions in computerized administrative work. *Journal of Occupational Behaviour, 5,* 159–81.

38. Johansson, G., & Barklöf, K. (1980). *Factor structure of self-reported mood and arousal among blue-collar workers.* Reports from the Department of Psychology, University of Stockholm, no. 562.

39. Johansson, G., & Sandén, P.-O. (1989). *Mental load and job satisfaction of control room operators.* Reports from the Department of Psychology, University of Stockholm, no. 698.

40. Johansson, G., Aronsson, G., & Lindström, B. O. (1978). Social psychological and neuroendocrine stress reactions in highly mechanized work. *Ergonomics, 21,* 583–99.

41. Johansson, G., Cavalini, P., & Pettersson, P. (1986). *Psychobiological reactions to unpredicted performance stress in a monotonous situation.* Reports from the Department of Psychology, University of Stockholm, no. 646.

42. Johnson, J. V. & Hall, E. (1988). Job strain, work place social support, and cardiovascular disease: a cross-sectional study of a random sample of the Swedish working population. *American Journal of Public Health, 78,* 1336–42.

43. Kahn, R. L. (1981). Work and health: some psychosocial effects of advanced technology. In B. Gardell & G. Johansson (eds.). *Working life: a social science contribution to work reform* (pp. 17–37). Chichester: Wiley.

44. Karasek, R. A. (1976). *The impact of the work environment on life outside the job* (doctoral dissertation). Massachusetts Institute of Technology. Distributed by the Institutet of Social Research, University of Stockholm.

45. Karasek, R. A. (1981). Job socialization and job strain: the implications of two related psy-

chosocial mechanisms for job design. In B. Gardell & G. Johansson (eds.). *Working life: a social science contribution to work reform* (pp. 75–94). Chichester: Wiley.

46. Karasek, R. & Theorell, T. (1990). *Healthy work: stress, productivity, and the reconstruction of working life*. New York: Basic Books.

47. Karasek, R. A., Gardell, B., & Lindell, J. (1987). Work and non-work correlates of illness and behavior in male and female Swedish white-collar workers. *Journal of Occupational Behaviour, 8,* 187–207.

48. Karasek, R. A., Russel, R., & Theorell, T. (1982). Physiology of stress and regeneration in job related cardiovascular illness. *Journal of Human Stress, 3,* 29–42.

49. Kauppinen-Toropainen, K., Kandolin, I., & Mutanen, P. (1983). Job dissatisfaction and work-related exhaustion in male and female work. *Journal of Occupational Behaviour, 4,* 193–207.

50. Landy, F. J. (1987). Human computer interactions in the workplace: psychosocial aspects of VDT use. In M. Frese, E. Ulich, & W. Dzida (eds.). *Psychological issues of human–computer interaction.* Amsterdam: North Holland.

51. Levi, L. (1972). Conditions of work and sympatho-adrenomedullary activity: experimental manipulation in a real-life setting. Acta Medica Scandinavica, Supplement 528.

52. Levi, L., Frankenhaeuser, M., & Gardell, B. (1986). The characteristics of the workplace and the nature of its social demands. In S. G. Wolf & A. J. Finestone (eds.). *Occupational stress: health and performance at work* (pp. 54–67. Littleton, MA: PSG Publishing

53. Lundberg, U., & Frankenhaeuser, M. (1980). Pituitary-adrenal and sympathetic adrenal correlates of distress and effort. *Journal of Psychosomatic Research, 24,* 125–30.

54. Lundberg, U., Granqvist, M., Hansson, T., Magnusson, M., & Wallin, L. (1989). Psychological and physiological stress responses during repetitive work at an assembly line. *Work and Stress, 3,* 143–53.

55. Mulders, H. P. G., Meijman, T. F., O'Hanlon, J. F., & Mulder, G. (1982). Differential psychophysiological reactivity of city bus drivers. *Ergonomics, 25,* 1003–11.

56. Netterström, B., & Laursen, P. (1981). Incidence and prevalence of ischaemic heart disease among urban busdrivers in Copenhagen. *Scandinavian Journal of Social Medicine, 9,* 75–79.

57. Sandén, P-O., & Johansson, G. (1990). *Job content and technology in process control: con-* *sequences for mental load and job involvement.* Reports from the Department of Psychology, Stockholm University, No. 725.

58. Smith, M. J., Cohen, B. G. F., Stammerjohn, L. W., & Happ, A. (1981). An investigation of health complaints and job stress in video display operations. *Human Factors, 23,* 389–400.

59. Stellman, J. M., Klitzman, S., Gordon, G., & Snow, B. R. (1987). Comparison of well-being among non-machine interactive clerical workers and full-time and part-time VDT users and typists. *Journal of Occupational Behavior, 26,* 95–114.

60. Svensson, L. (1986). *Grupper och kollektiv [Groups and collectives].* Stockholm: Swedish Center for Working Life [in Swedish].

61. Swedish Government Reports (1990). *Arbete och hälsa [Work and Health].* Report from the Swedish Work Environment Committee. [In Swedish.]

62. Swedish Metal Workers Union. (1989). *Solidarisk arbetspolitik för det goda arbetet [A work policy of solidarity for the good work].* Report to the 1989 Congress of the Swedish Metal Workers Union.

63. Timio, M., Gentili, S., & Pede, S. (1979). Free adrenaline and noradrenaline excretion related to occupational stress. *British Heart Journal, 42,* 471–4.

64. Ursin, H., & Murison, R. (eds.). (1983). *Biological and psychological basis of psychosomatic disease.* Oxford: Pergamon Press.

65. WHO (1989). Work with display terminals: psychosocial aspects and health. Report on a World Health Organization meeting. *Journal of Occupational Medicine, 31,* 957–68.

66. Wickens, C. D., & Kessel, C. (1981). Failure detection in dynamic systems. In J. Rasmussen & W. B. Rouse (eds.). *Human detection and diagnosis of system failures* (pp. 143–54). New York: Plenum Press/NATO Scientific Affairs Division.

67. Winkleby, M., Ragland, D. R., Fisher, J. M., & Syme, S. L. (1988). Excess risk of sickness and disease in bus drivers: A review and synthesis of epidemiological studies. *International Journal of Epidemiology, 17,* 255–62.

68. Wright, I. (1987). Identification and prevention of work-related mental and psychosomatic disorders among two categories of VDU users. In B. Knave & P. -G. Widebäck (eds.). *Work with display units 86: selected papers from the International Scientific Conference on Work with Display Units* (pp. 595–604). Amsterdam: Elsevier.

14
Work Values and Work Performance: Critical Commentary from a Comparative Perspective

Raymond G. Hunt

Freud described the healthy individual as one who could work (and love) effectively. Sullivan called work one of the "fundamentally important aspects of all living" (38, p. 326); and Erich Fromm called work an "inescapable necessity for man," an imperative, however, that could also be "his liberator from nature, his creator as a social and independent being" (13, p. 177).

Studs Terkel, meanwhile, introduced his book *Working* on another note, saying that "being about work, [it] is, by its very nature, about violence—to the spirit as well as to the body. It is about ulcers as well as accidents, about shouting matches as well as fistfights, about nervous breakdowns as well as kicking the dog around. It is above all (or beneath all), about daily humiliations" (40, p. xi).

Terkel acknowledged, of course, "the happy few who find a savor in their daily job," but he wondered if "these satisfactions . . . [don't] tell us more about the person than the task." Terkel's concern then, and Fromm's too, is with the meaning of work to society and its individual members, with the interconnections of tasks and human attributes and the outcomes of those interconnections of tasks and human attributes and the outcomes of those interconnections. The questions put by both men are about how people come to terms with the demands of work and with what results. They are questions, in short, about the values people seek to maximize and the environments in which they do it.

This chapter is concerned with the comparative analysis of values. Motivating the project is the basic question of how work behavior (and its "products," i.e., satisfaction and production) is linked with characteristics of the individual and how these personal characteristics vary, if they do, as a function of national, cultural, or other (environmental) conditions. It also explores ways in which information bearing on these points can be used to guide practical policy in the American workplace, if in fact it can be used this way.

The discussion includes reflections on the nature of values, work values in particular, and their relations to culture on one hand and performance and human well-being on the other. These reflections prompt us to consider certain methodological problems associated with the conceptualization of value-behavior linkages, some others having to do with the language and strategy of comparative cross-cultural research, and still others involved in the drawing of practical managerial lessons from cross-cultural examples. Reasons to question the utility of "culture" as an explanation for variations in work performance and productivity are explored herein, and it is suggested that values generally have little directly to do with productivity. This conclusion leads to the recommendation that closer attention be paid to the environmental contingencies of behavior and to systematic study of linkages between these factors and both productivity and human well-being.

ON THE NATURE OF VALUES

In common usage, the concept of "value" typically is thought of as referring to the goals to which behavior is oriented. Locke, for instance, in a widely influential treatment, distinguished between needs, which are requirements of existence, and values, which are "that which one acts to gain and/or keep" (23, p. 1304). Values, Locke suggested are "subjective," in that they are things that, so to speak, one has in mind. Needs, on the other hand, are "objective," existing separately from anything a person wants or even thinks about. Locke integrated the two constructs (needs and values) by proposing that values serve "to direct [man's] actions and choices so as to satisfy his needs" (23, p. 1306). Values, then, as Smith (37) had earlier suggested, are decision standards according to which one selects alternative courses of action, presumably on the basis of the attractiveness of their expected outcomes. Elizur (11), in the Lockeian manner, expressly described values as goals and choice criteria—things a person believes it is important to get or to avoid. At any rate, it is commonly assumed that individuals acquire values and norms via participation in a social system.

Indications are many that value orientations vary over social systems (e.g., nations) and their subsystems (e.g., social classes). Value measures also vary interindividually: Ronen and Kraut (33), for instance, found differences among individuals to be about 2.5 times as great as those between countries, which suggests that values and value systems may be linked to microsocial as well as macrosocial and, probably, nonsocial as well as social life conditions (1). The possibility exists, then, that culture—the macrolevel collective properties of societies—may have much to do with generalities of conduct—the broad "aims" and "tone" of populations of people (10)—but may have rather less to do with its specifics. Figure 14–1 shows work values combining with other factors to generate psychological and other reactions among workers as well as work performance itself. Performance becomes "productivity" when it is evaluated, by the worker or another party, as, for example, when the dollar value of work output is factored against the cost of its labor inputs.

The significance of values has generally been couched in terms of a bearing on individual (and collective) motivation to work (2, especially pp. 1647 ff). Customary models of performance in organizations (9) treat motivation (and by implication work values) as a primary (if not the only) determinant of work output, including job satisfaction. Thus work values plainly seem to qualify as factor inputs to productivity and may be responsible for a significant portion of the variance in it, not only as between individuals but also among workers and managers (21,39) and nations (24). Moreover, given as much as 25% shared variance between work and life satisfaction,

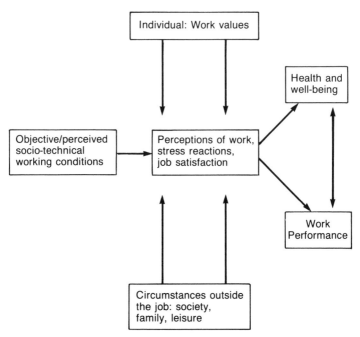

Figure 14–1. Model of relations between various factors and work outcomes. After Gardell (14).

the importance of work values to perceived quality of life and personal well-being is clear enough (32). Thus work values have arguable practical as well as theoretical interest.

A wide variety of specific definitions and measurements of work values exists; and a number of attempts at empirical specification of the domain and structure of work values have been undertaken. In a large study, Hofstede (18), for example, employed factor analytical methods to identify four dimensions of work values he called Power Distance (authority relations), Uncertainty Avoidance, Individualism, and Masculinity. Similarly, Bond (5) used factor analysis of results from his Cultural Values Survey (which is not specific to work values) to generate four factors that overlapped extensively with those of Hofstede. Pryor (30), meanwhile, found that three factors explained most of the variance in responses to his Work Aspect Preference Scale, factors somewhat but, allowing for the usual terminological differences, not greatly different from those of Hofstede or of Bond. Similarly, the Meaning of Work (MOW) International Research Team (26), in an eight-nation survey of nearly 9,000 individuals, conceived the "meaning" of work in terms of three structured dimensions. One of these dimensions, "work centrality," has to do with "general belief about the value of working in one's life" (26, p. 17). A second dimension, "societal norms about working," refers to "work ethic" questions of entitlement and obligation ("rights and duties") as bases of work orientation. Finally, what are customarily called "work values" the MOW researchers considered under the heading "work goals": "valued working outcomes/preferences." Via factor analysis, they identified four work value dimensions: Expressive (e.g., interesting work), Economic (e.g., pay), Comfort (e.g., hours), and Learning/Improvement Opportunity (e.g., promotion).

The conception of work values we have used was formulated by Elizur at Bar Ilan University, Tel Aviv. Elizur has been especially interested in developing an empirically based definition of work values. Accordingly, he has used facet analyses and smallest space techniques to "formally define the universe of observations and to test hypotheses about the relationship between the definitional framework and the structure of the empirical observations" (11, p. 380). This work led to a two-faceted definition of work values. The first facet (A), Elizur called Modality of Outcome. It includes three elements; i.e., work outcomes may be material (e.g., wages or working conditions), social (e.g., interpersonal relations and their affective accompaniments), or psychological (e.g., interest, achievement, independence). These elements Elizur called "instrumental," "affective," and "cognitive," respectively.

A second facet of work value is the Relation (of outcome) to Task Performance. This facet has two elements: (a) "rewards," which are performance-contingent outcomes such as status, recognition, or pay; and (b) "resources," which are noncontingent benefits resulting from simple membership in the system, such as hospitalization insurance, work conditions, and various workplace services (e.g., day care). Using a multiitem questionnaire, the specific items of which are construed simply as a sample of all conceivable items, Elizur used smallest space analyses to "validate" his bifaceted definitional framework for work values.

We have been using this model and its associated instrumentation in cross-national

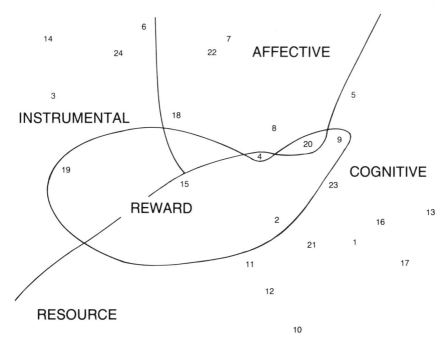

Figure 14–2. Structure of work values: U.S. sample. $n = 154$; two-dimensional SSAI (smallest space analysis index); coefficient of alienation = 0.21.

comparative studies with some interesting outcomes. One of these studies (by Estvan Beck of the Karl Marx University of Economics in Budapest, Elizur, and me) was a comparison of work values in seven countries: United States, China (PRC), Korea, Taiwan, Holland, Hungary, and Israel. Using a 24-item questionnaire (in English), items were classified a priori according to facets such that for the Modality of Outcome facet, pay, hours of work, security, benefits, and work conditions were defined as "instrumental values"; relationship with the supervisor and coworkers, recognition, esteem, and opportunity to interact with people were defined as "affective"; and responsibility, achievement, influence, interest, feedback, meaningful work, use of abilities, independence, company status, and contribution to society were considered "cognitive" work values. For the Relation to Task Performance facet, meanwhile, pay, recognition, feedback, advancement, and status were classified as "rewards" and the remaining items as "resources."

Given a matrix of pairwise similarity coefficients between items, Smallest Space Analysis (SSA) maps the items into a space of prespecified dimensionality, each item represented by a point. The proximity of points in the space is then a function of their similarity, and one may examine the configuration of points to determine if the space can be partitioned into regions corresponding to the facets and their elements. The results of such an examination, with partition lines drawn among the 24 work values

Table 14–1. Rank Order of Work Values of Samples from Seven Countries

Work values	Holland	USA	Israel	Korea	Taiwan	China	Hungary
Cognitive values							
Advancement	6	3	2	8	4	9	24
Feedback	16	9	11	22	14	11	8
Status	24	23	13	24	22	17	23
Achievement	2	2	1	1	1	1	2
Job interest	1	1	3	3	2	8	7
Meaningful work	13	13	9	13	16	14	4
Personal growth	4	4	7	4	6	5	13
Use of ability	8	6	14	5	11	2	6
Responsibility	11	8	8	11	5	6	15
Contribution to society	23	24	24	27	24	4	20
Independence	5	7	5	19	10	7	16
Company	22	17	20	17	21	18	21
Work influence	7	14	17	16	18	15	18
Organizational influence	17	19	19	20	20	13	22
Affective values							
Recognition	12	12	15	10	8	16	3
Coworkers	3	18	12	6	13	12	14
Esteem	15	5	6	18	3	3	9
Interaction	10	21	23	23	23	23	19
Supervisor	9	11	4	7	9	10	1
Instrumental values							
Pay	18	15	10	14	15	20	5
Benefits	19	16	16	12	12	19	17
Security	14	10	18	2	7	22	10
Convenient hours	21	22	21	15	19	21	12
Work conditions	20	20	22	9	17	24	11

measured, is illustrated for the U.S. sample by Figure 14–2. The structures for the other six nationality samples varied but were basically similar.

Given this structural similarity, we proceeded to a comparative analysis of the relative locations of the specific items within regions in regard to their proximity to nearby regions. Some interesting national (cultural?) differences appeared. For instance, the item "supervisor" tends to be located in the "cognitive" region for the China, Korea, and Hungary samples. In the other samples, including Taiwan, it is found in the "affective" region. Several other such variations were observed, suggesting a measure of cross-national (cross-cultural?) variability in work value structures. Hence not all nominal work values can be expected to have the same meaning in different contexts. This point was emphasized, too, by the MOW team (26) in its (mainly European) international comparisons of work value structures and national profiles of the "meaning of work." We shall refer to it again shortly.

Elizur, Beck, and I also evaluated the relative importance of the 24 work values measured, with the results displayed in Table 14–1. Substantial variability is evident. In the Chinese example, for instance, "instrumental" values tend generally to be low in importance, whereas they are considerably higher in the Korean (another Confucian society) and Hungarian (another socialist political economy) samples. Thus in a context of structural similarity, cross-national variability can be observed in both the

Table 14–2. Importance of 24 Work Values by USA and PRC Samples

Value item (abbreviated)	USA			PRC			Sign
	Mean	SD	Rank	Mean	SD	Rank	
Achievement	1.45	0.58	1	1.33	0.65	1	ns
Advancement	1.64	0.91	4	2.05	1.03	9	*
Benefits	2.00	0.81	15	2.66	0.99	20	*
Company	2.20	0.90	18	2.56	1.09	17	*
Society	2.93	1.14	24	1.74	0.78	3	*
Work hours	2.51	1.01	23	3.07	1.13	23	*
Coworkers	2.16	0.83	17	2.39	1.03	13	ns
Esteem	1.62	0.68	3	1.75	0.79	4	ns
Feedback	1.90	0.84	12	2.20	0.86	11	*
Independence	1.89	0.86	11	1.95	0.90	7	ns
Organizational influence	2.33	0.93	21	2.40	0.92	14	ns
Work influence	1.99	0.78	14	2.44	0.89	15	*
Interest	1.48	0.71	2	1.97	0.89	8	*
Security	2.07	1.03	16	3.09	1.13	24	*
Status	2.32	0.88	20	2.53	0.87	16	ns
Meaningful work	1.88	0.74	9	2.24	0.90	12	*
Growth	1.67	0.77	6	1.84	0.82	5	ns
Social	2.34	0.96	22	2.74	0.89	21	*
Pay	1.97	0.77	13	2.63	0.89	19	*
Recognition	1.85	0.72	8	2.57	0.94	18	*
Responsibility	1.83	0.77	7	1.95	0.88	6	ns
Supervisor	1.88	0.80	10	2.13	0.98	10	*
Ability use	1.66	0.61	5	1.59	0.78	2	ns
Work conditions	2.28	0.89	19	2.89	1.02	22	*

Note: 1 = very important to 6 = very unimportant; ns = not significant.
*indicates two-tailed *t*-test $p \leq 0.05$ or greater.

relative meaning and the importance of specific values, probably reflecting the varied circumstances of individuals in the several countries represented.

In another (actually earlier) study using the same 24-item work values questionnaire, Meindl, Lee, and I, together with Elizur compared groups of Chinese (PRC) and U.S. junior-level managers' work values (25). Between-group differences were found for 15 of the 24 values, along with indications that the American group sought to obtain more and a greater variety of work outcomes than did other groups (Table 14–2). The Chinese, by contrast, placed a heavily concentrated emphasis on "contributing to society," suggesting a more ideologically based orientation to work consistent with the deemphasis on instrumental values found by Elizur, Beck, and me (8). Despite the variability, however, a strongly covergent pattern of importance ratings was found between the two samples (Fig. 14–3), and "achievement" was the single most important value for both groups (although a difference of meaning is distinctly possible).

The Meindl/Hunt/Elizur/Lee study also included measures of achievement motivation, individualism-collectivism, and several demographic variables. Correlations of these variables with the 24 work values are shown in Table 14–3. It was not surprising that the Chinese showed stronger "collectivist" orientations and more emphasis on "friendships" in work settings.

Meanwhile, factor analytical treatments of the 24 work values in the two samples yielded some provocative outcomes. The first factor in the U.S. sample, for example,

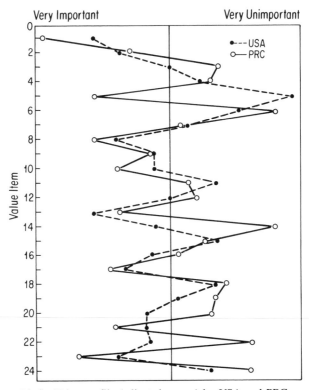

Figure 14–3. Value profile (adjusted means) by USA and PRC samples.

Table 14–3. Correlations Between the Value Items and Selected Variables[a]

		Independent variables								
Value item	Mach[b]		Work collectivism		Age		Education		Job level	
Achievement	38*	(22*)	26*	(27*)	−12	(−03)	06	(11)	19*	(13)
Advancement	22*	(18*)	−07	(26*)	−08	(−24*)	36*	(08)	11	(−09)
Benefits	02	(−19*)	−02	(12)	−04	(−19*)	−08	(−20*)	−14	(01)
Company	03	(14*)	02	(12)	−12	(−05)	27*	(04)	06	(0)
Society	0	(23*)	10	(14*)	−03	(−14*)	−05	(09)	11	(−10)
Work hours	−24*	(−28*)	−15	(07)	−04	(−13*)	−02	(0)	−19	(−02)
Coworkers	−25*	(−09)	09	(05)	13	(−18*)	02	(−17*)	12	(−12)
Esteem	0	(05)	07	(09)	−01	(−20*)	17*	(−05)	−20	(0)
Feedback	06	(08)	05	(−01)	−01	(02)	07	(03)	04	(−17*)
Independence	−08	(29*)	−11	(−19*)	02	(07)	01	(19*)	−14	(13*)
Organizational influence	06	(27*)	−08	(13*)	−14	(09)	02	(16*)	−01	(28*)
Work influence	05	(25*)	0	(05)	04	(11)	19*	(22*)	02	(15*)
Interest	15	(27*)	−06	(01)	−20*	(17*)	04	(25*)	03	(−11)
Security	−20	(−24*)	−02	(18*)	03	(21)	−18*	(−28*)	0	(04)
Status	07	(−08)	−08	(01)	06	(−09)	08	(−14*)	−05	(0)
Meaningful	19*	(15*)	−06	(03)	−15	(−03)	05	(14*)	−13	(−03)
Growth	15	(28*)	−11	(02)	25*	(−05)	13	(11)	−13	(−08)
Social	10	(−01)	09	(27*)	−13	(−13*)	0	(−09)	04	(04)
Pay	−03	(04)	−05	(05)	−13	(−04)	0	(−21*)	04	(05)
Recognition	11	(08)	−02	(20*)	−07	(−21*)	10	(03)	−08	(0)
Responsibility	−01	(27*)	22*	(21*)	07	(−21*)	22*	(07)	−09	(−08)
Supervisor	01	(−16*)	02	(11)	−16	(20*)	−07	(−16*)	18*	(−07)
Ability use	15	(24*)	06	(03)	06	(−05)	06	(08)	11	(− 0)
Work conditions	−15	(−27*)	−09	(10)	−02	(−09)	−08	(−27*)	03	(−11)

Note: All variables were recoded so that positive correlations indicate direct relations and negative correlations indicate inverse relations. Decimals have been omitted.

[a] The U.S. sample is shown in parentheses.
[b] Achievement motivation.
* Indicates $p < 0.05$ or greater.

was a clear "extrinsic" factor (i.e., benefits, security, pay, work conditions). This factor was thus dominated by "instrumental" values; but it also included a "cognitive" value (status), implying an instrumental significance of that value. [In the Chinese sample, status grouped in a factor with two other "cognitive" items (work and organization influence); in the U.S. group these two items factored with two different "cognitive" items (independence and responsibility).] No "instrumental" (or "extrinsic") factor emerged in the Chinese group, which is consistent with the Elizur/Hunt/Beck findings.

Obviously, these results (and others like them by investigators such as Hofstede, Bond, and the MOW group) demonstrated interesting empirical similarities and differences across national groups that are typically presumed to reflect properties of their cultures. Such an assertion, however, risks banality: It amounts to a statement of the obvious, something surely true by definition. What we therefore need to do is move beyond demonstrational differences (or similarities) and become more specific about the perhaps variable ways in which work values (or any values for that matter) are associated with specific interacting conditions of life and work. Whether "culture" is a useful construct for this purpose is at least debatable.

METHODOLOGICAL ISSUES IN COMPARATIVE STUDIES

In its search for cross-cultural/cross-national universals, comparative research confronts serious methodological difficulties, not the least of which is the problem of language and translation. This problem actually is embedded in a larger one of arguable singularities of culture and the feasibility of nomothetic social science (7). Schermerhorn (34) examined the language-translation issue in an interesting way, i.e., by taking as problematical the practice of using a shared language, usually English, when conducting research among bilinguals. This approach, of course, is what we have done, by and large, in our comparative studies of work values. Schermerhorn, however, compared the distributions of responses by samples of subjects answering questions in a second language (English) with others responding to nominally the same questions in their first language (Chinese). He found some noteworthy differences, the substance of which need not concern us here.

Schermerhorn's findings, although intriguing, were not in themselves compelling. Therefore we have been following up on his work using our work values measures in a quasiexperimental study of subjects' responses to English-language and Chinese-language versions of the same questionnaire. The (still incomplete) study employs multiple administrations of the questionnaire to the same respondents under conditions where some complete first a native-language version and later a second-language version; others do the reverse; and still others complete a native- or a second-language version twice.

Preliminary results of this research (17) suggested that conclusions on the translation problem may depend on the method used to investigate it. On the one hand, we have found simple item correlations to be low and variable across instrument administrations; but at the same time, profiles of value rankings have been consistently congruent.

The issue in this research, is not simply a practical one of the quality of translation but a more basic one of essential validity and the relativity of meanings (as in arguments about cultural biases in IQ tests). It implicates not only large and obvious intergroup variation but intragroup differences as well. The issue itself has been framed in terms of the anthropological–linguistic constructs of *etic* and *emic*. Emics are phenomena particular to a given society. Etics are universal, or at least multicultural (4). The contrast of etic and emic echoes the general methodological distinction, usually applied at the level of individual psychology, between nomothetic and idiographic sciences (42).

The validity question raised by Schermerhorn can be conceived as a potential confusion of emics and etics. A questionnaire (e.g., our work values questionnaire) originally written in a specific language (e.g., English), because of the intimate linkage of language and culture, can be expected to express a specific emic. Translation of the questionnaire to another language, e.g., Chinese, entails two fundamental assumptions. The first is that the first-language *emic* has been effectively represented in the new orthography. This assumption is one that is "tested" by one or another "back translation" strategy (7) in which a questionnaire is translated into a second language and then independently retranslated into the original language for comparison. The second assumption is more basic: that the first-language emic is, in fact, an etic, a universal—or at least an emic shared by other groups. Berry (4) has spoken of this "ethnocentric" presumption as involving an "imposed etic." [Triandis et al. (41), called them "pseudoetics".] Testing the etic status of a construct is a complex task (7). We cannot go into it here, but the essential methodological point was well put by Berry: "Our major problem is how to describe behavior in terms which are meaningful to members of a particular culture (an emic approach) while at the same time to compare validly behavior in that culture with behavior in another or all other cultures (the etic aim)" (4, p. 12).

Granting that we have not settled this problem—in terms, that is, of the comparability of cross-language measurements of work values—we would nevertheless like to think that the facet analytical technique of identifying value *structures,* for example, is a suitable way of testing for and identifying what Berry (4) called a "derived etic," a defensible generalization about, in our case, the structure of work values, as an emergent from phenomena observed in a variety of contexts. [For other evidence on this incidental point see Griffeth et al. (15).]

A still more basic validity question remains, however. Simply put: What exactly do measures of work values measure? Structural analyses of questionnaire results alone cannot answer this question. However, we have seen that a conventional answer to the question is that, at one level, they measure dispositional attributes of individuals and at another level normative attributes of societies (i.e., culture). We have also noted, however, the conjectural quality of these equations and earlier mentioned an alternative attributional interpretation of "values."

Following a related line of thought, Nord et al. turned the causal equation upside down, observing that "espoused work values in society may often be a result of work activity rather than a cause of it" (28, p. 67). Such an observation suggests some possibilities for us to consider. One already mentioned is that measurements of "work values" may be simply descriptions (self-reports?) of aspects of work activity. Another, not incompatible with the first, is that they are ways by which individuals make retrospective sense of their experiences, at work and elsewhere, or parts of personal and collective mythologies whereby they explain to themselves and others the manifold ambiguities of their work and lives. Hence, as Nord et al. suggested, instead of viewing work values as "ideals to achieve" we may be ahead of the game to think of them as personal and social constructions, bearing complex interactive relations with various features of social and intellectual life.

For scholars as well as everybody else, these constructions may serve to simplify the complexities and uncertainties of living, but the phenomena they signify are not simple. Consider the notion of a Protestant work ethic and its alleged instrumental significance for economic growth and development. Drawing heavily on the historical analyses of D. T. Rodgers, Nord et al. (28) claimed, for instance, that these values never were shared by the American working class during the period of U.S. industrialization. It (the work ethic) was—and continued to be—a belief system of the middle class for whom it served, among other things, to conceal the "coercive forces that made people work" (see also 16). As an ideology, the work ethic myth (and various managerial tenets associated with it) admittedly may have had substantial appeal to workers as well as others. For the former, "who chafed at labor, the appeal to the moral centrality of work was too useful to resist. Pitched in the abstract, it turned necessity into pride and servitude into honor; it offered a lever upon the moral sentiments of those whose power mattered" [quoted in Nord et al. (28, p. 28)]. In general, the work ethic served as an ideological means of reconciling the irreconcilable— "the harsh realities and the belief in voluntary free labor" (28, p. 46). Empirically, however, a connection between the Protestant work ethic and economic performance, individual or collective, remains an assertion, not a fact. [See also the MOW Team report (26), Chapter 6.]

In the same vein, *The Economist*[1] has suggested that Japanese workers have been induced to "sacrifice their all for GNP growth" by having "drummed into them the idea that they are a small, poor, vulnerable island race." Whether such sentiments per se account for Japan's economic success is doubtful. As *The Economist* pointed out, the Japanese have evidently been willing to accept a variety of inefficiencies, expensive food and housing, and other inconveniences as an apparent "price for protecting jobs" and sustaining social stability. The Chinese populace, however, was similarly convinced of China's destiny and challenge and the need for great human effort and sacrifice during the Great Leap Forward of 1958–1960; yet that campaign was hardly notable for its economic accomplishments (12).

We should note, as did Nord et al., that mythologies of the "left" have been no less mythological than that of the work ethic, certainly not those nostalgically oriented to preindustrial conditions of work. Work, then, by all appearances was no more intrinsically fulfilling (and therefore motivating) than it is now. (Compare the testimony of people moving from the countryside into eighteenth century American factories, found in sources such as Anthony Wallace's 1978 book *Rockdale,* and the replication of those experiences in contemporary China.)

What of demonstrable correlations between work values and behavior or, more particularly, productivity? Bond (5), for example, reported strong correlations between values (measured via his Cultural Values Scale) and gross national product (GNP) per capita for 22 nations and for their 20-year economic growth patterns. He speculated that the mechanism linking values with economic performance may be found in an interactive model wherein values, in concert with arrays of institutional and other conditions, "release" an entrepreneurial "spirit" and associated action (viz., deployment of resources). Thus "in each society whose structural conditions predispose to growth, the entrepreneur is the supplementary catalyst" (5). Because "structural conditions" may vary from time to time, the entrepreneurial values and "spirits" that "fit" them are different. Hence what makes for economic productivity today may not be what made for it yesterday and may not do it tomorrow.

Conditions change of course. Unfortunately, we continue to remain unsure of what "causes" work performance, the relation to it of "values," or what these "values" are. Nor are we sure to what extent our causal models, tied as they are to motivational assumptions, are more than psychological word games, professional story-telling, or retrospective sense-making.[2] Which brings us to the question of what it is we can (or dare) say on the subject of productivity improvement.

POLICY ISSUES

Normally, cross-cultural (etic–emic) criticism of research concentrates on the sins of Western investigators who thoughtlessly impose their Euro-American emics (which, of course, they believe are etics) on other groups. The practice, however, has another side that manifests in contemporary curiosity about the "secret" of Japanese industrial achievement and, in particular, the mysteries of the Japanese management methods which are presumably responsible for that country's high productivity. Attention in the West has naturally fastened on a variety of visible Japanese techniques, e.g., quality control circles and just-in-time production methods, as well as the apparent willingness of Japanese people to work hard, long, and carefully.[3] The search, then, is for a Japanese emic that is convertible to a kind of borrowed etic for use in the West. Just how "Japanese" are Americans prepared to become, however?

Quality circles, for example, now are widespread in U.S. factories, often with disappointing results and rarely with much recognition of their dissimilarity to the Japanese model. What has happened is that a variable array of more or less superficial features of the Japanese quality control circle have been seized on as an etic, without regard to the root context of the Japanese variety (i.e., its emic character). Meanwhile, the quality circle in the United States is inevitably integrated into emic properties of American life. Hence the label is the same but the phenomena differ: The etic here is merely verbal, truly pseudo.

Consider just one portion of the emic difference. Hofstede (18) has demonstrated large differences between the United States and Japan on his individualism index (IDV); and he discussed at length the numerous intercultural variations associated with this contrast. In the low IDV case (Japan), for example, is what Hofstede referred to as a "we consciousness" and a personal identity based in the social system. In the high IDV case (United States), on the other hand, is an "I consciousness" and a personal identity based in the individual. In a work setting, high IDV (United States) suggests such things as emotional independence from the company, desires for freedom and challenge from the job, preferences for individual decisions, and a calculative commitment to the company. By contrast, low IDV (Japan) connotes emotional dependence on the company, emphasis on training and use of skills, reliance on group rather than individual decisions, and a moral commitment to the company. Obviously, then, quality circles subsist in sharply different "emic contexts" in Japan and the United States. The quality circle in Japan in fact expresses a Japanese work emic. In itself the quality circle, as a technique, is at most of secondary significance to performance. It is the work emic that counts. As Boulding argued long ago, productivity "is a product of the whole culture, of all its institutions and ideas, and it is meaningless to separate out a single part of the culture and say [it] produces the product" (6, p. 164). In what sense, then, can the Japanese emic be considered an attractive solution to American industrial performance problems?

This question is not answered here except to say that it seems unlikely that solutions to *American* productivity and work performance problems are going to be found in *Japanese* emics anymore than the Japanese "miracle" is attributable per se to Deming's (American) technique of statistical quality control. The problem at this point is that we have no reliable productivity etics. Answers to American problems therefore must be found within an American framework, in an essentially American emic. Indeed, attempts to do otherwise risk making matters worse, not better.

CLOSING ARGUMENTS

Obviously mine is not an argument that proscribes instruction from non-American sources and comparative emics. What it means is that managerial and other work performance facilitation strategies must be harmonious with broader interactive fundamentals of American beliefs, institutions, and other durable circumstances. Of course it may mean that some things cannot be done in America, at least not as well or as easily as they can be done somewhere else in the world.[4] Such is life.

That American individualism, for instance, poses certain operational problems in a corporate setting can hardly be doubted. Those values, however, are emic realities within which work systems are framed in the United States. Bellah et al. (3), in a review of individualism and commitment in American life, showed how much the ways we think about success, freedom, and justice are linked with our institutions and the particular ways in which individuals relate to them.

An article by B. F. Skinner sounded a similar theme, but from a different perspective and with different implications. Skinner began by noting that, in the West especially, many people are bored, even depressed, are not enjoying their lives, do not like what they do, and do not do what they like. "In a word, they are unhappy" (36, p. 568). Skinner blamed this "malaise" on cultural practices that have promoted the "pleasing effects" of the consequences of behavior at the expense of "strengthening effects."

At work, for example, specialization, routinization, and bureaucratization tend to separate workers from the *consequences* of their work. For many people (maybe most) the conditions of work are therefore not reinforcing (put differently, do not consort well with customary work values such as individual achievement and so forth). The result presumably is alienation from work and a redirection of interest to extra-work sources of satisfaction. To retain and control a workforce under these conditions, Skinner suggested, managements inevitably take recourse to coercive methods and problematical generalized secondary reinforcers—money, in particular.[5] In effect, companies say to workers: "Come to work, play by the rules, and we'll please you by giving you money to buy the things that really please you."

The idea, as Skinner said, is "work or suffer the consequences"; and the eventual result, of course, is an absence of worker commitment, absenteeism, and resentment (even sabotage). Furthermore, most of the popular remedies, such as participative management, Skinner pointed out, have not worked, largely he maintained, because they miss the point—the point, of course, being the contingencies of reinforcement for working.

Measures of work values, whatever their form, may give an indication of what it is that is apt to "reinforce" work performance. In an individual case, such measures can provide a glimpse of a person's understanding of what it is that is apt to reinforce his or her work behavior. Aggregated, these measures can be used to describe a pattern of expectation for populations of people or communities. Actual workplace performance is no simple function of these values (or of macrocultures). Recall for a moment Skinner's distinction between the "pleasing" and "strengthening" effects of reinforcement and our finding about the particular work value "status." In a U.S. sample, we found this value to be linked with others (e.g., pay, working conditions) of an "instrumental" nature. In a Chinese sample, however, it factored differently. Thus status apparently has a different meaning in the two samples, and, by implication, probably a different behavioral function. One may infer, then, that high status jobs are attractive to U.S. workers because, like Herzberg's "hygiene factors," they are associated with "pleasing" things such as high pay. However, awards of status may, in general, be of little moment as a means of strengthening work performance.

Assuming, however, that one does wish to strengthen work performance, it follows from this example that simple surveys of workers' values may be undependable guides to how to do it. Expressed work values may describe only what workers find (or have found) "pleasing" about their jobs (or workplaces) or think they should find "pleasing" about them, not what it is that would "strengthen" their work performance. Workers, obviously, may consider a job or workplace "pleasing" for any number of reasons unrelated to its performance contingencies (e.g., good pay, good friends, good conditions), a circumstance that may account for the disappointment that has often attended organizational performance improvement programs tied to workers' attitudes. It is worth remembering in this connection that, at one and the same time, Japan has one of the world's most productive workforces and one of the most *dis*satisfied.

In order to understand performance or to change it (improve it?), environmental contingencies (including, to be sure, prevalent belief systems) eventually must be examined directly. Japanese or American workers do not behave the way they do at work merely *because* of their values, although knowing something about those values may tell us something helpful about possible ways of affecting their performance. Workers behave as they do chiefly because of properties of their workplaces—the incentives, work methods, and control systems there. Understanding this point is key to productivity improvement (22,26). Describing a shift at Saab-Scandia in Sweden, for example, from autonomous work groups—widely touted for their human relations and motivational benefits in production environments—to automated-robotized engine assembly using solitary worker-attendants, Simonsen (35) reported increased monotony and regrets at losses of the social benefits of autonomous work groups, accompanied, however, by *increased* engine quality, which clearly is a productivity improvement.

If values are descriptions of preferences, they may, as has been said, be advisory about what may reinforce worker behavior. It seems likely, though, that examinations of relations between measured work values (preferences) and workplace experience can explain only variations in job satisfaction, and experience abundantly shows that it does not help at all to understand or predict work performance (19). To do that (and to comprehend broader collective performance contingencies), it is necessary to know the complex interacting technical, operational, organizational, and interpersonal workplace conditions that control it.

HEALTH, WELL-BEING, AND WORK VALUES

What, then, one may ask, does any of this discussion have to do with health? Conceptually, at least, the connection is plain enough. Speaking broadly, there are two essential and potentially interacting outcomes of work: goods or services ("production") and "welfare" (individual and collective benefits and costs). Welfare outcomes include such obvious rewards for working as pay, but they also include direct and indirect physical and psychosocial consequences of work participation. The "spillover" from work experience (e.g., job satisfaction) to persons' general psychic well-being (i.e., satisfaction with life), already noted, may be substantial. How substantial this spillover is probably depends on how important the job is to an individual (31) (what the MOW

Team speaks of as work centrality, which, for example, is high among Japanese and Yugoslavs but much lower for Britons and Germans). Thus to generalize the case, one may expect *individual* work values to moderate relations between work and its *personal* outcomes and for particular *distributions* of these values within social aggregates to be associated with population *prevalence rates* for those outcomes. A similar argument can be made, as suggested earlier, for productivity; and one could expect interactions among the various measurements.

Consider again Figure 14–1, which is adapted from Gardell's (14) outline model of behavioral investigations (in Scandinavia) of monotony and stress and their consequences for worker health and life activity.[6] Note the posited role of personality (read: work values) influencing both perceptions of work conditions and the translation of these perceptions into health-related phenomena and social participation. Note too the assumption in the model of a mediation by the worker's personal characteristics of the relation between working conditions and health and well-being. Obviously there is much room here for individual and collective effects from work values.

Gardell observed that Scandinavian studies show that worker "perceptions of monotony, coercion, mental strain and social isolation are considerably more common and more intense among workers engaged in tasks that have been impoverished with respect to self-determination, variation, qualifications and social contact, compared with workers in freer, more responsible jobs" (14, p. 12). Certainly values come into play when answering questions about the importance of self-determination, social contact, responsibility, and the like. Indeed, Gardell sensibly observed that "what is monotonous to one person may be deeply satisfying to another" (14, p. 12), depending, one presumes, on personal characteristics such as values and perhaps off-setting effects of other valued workplace features. Some workers, for instance, enjoy routine assembly-line work because of the opportunities its low demand for attention provides for social interaction with other workers; and they resist "job enrichment" programs. Clearly it is a matter of values.

To the extent, then, that workplace factors are linked with human health and well-being, it is reasonable to suppose that work values function as important moderators of these relations, in much the way Rice, McFarlin, Near, and I have suggested that "work importance" is likely to moderate relations between psychosocial work and general life outcomes.[7] Plausible as it seems and reasonable as it plainly is to raise questions of the associations between human values and organizational productivity on the one hand and human well-being on the other, the strange fact is that these questions have not been asked in any systematic way. Consequently, the state of the art is not far advanced.

More attention has been given to the matter in Scandinavia than anywhere else perhaps. Much of it, however, as in Sweden, is oriented toward making it "easier to put up with the job" (which was the title to Simonsen's 1987 article mentioned above). Oscarsson and Dockerty (29), for example, as they summarized the program of the Swedish Work Environment Fund, although emphasizing the utilization of new technology, in fact oriented chiefly toward controlling its human impacts. "Technological development," they asserted, "by itself guarantees neither economic growth nor long-term competitiveness, nor the social welfare of individuals, companies, regions and nations" (29, p. 11). This point may well be true, but it is also a normative statement of values. Many questions remain to be settled about the factors that mediate the outcomes of work. At the risk of banality, much careful research is needed in this area.

NOTES

1. See *The Economist, 307,* (7554), 33–35 (June 11, 1988).
2. It is true, of course, that our stories can become "words to live by" and thus become conceptual constraints on decisions and actions—even self-fulfilling prophesies. They are therefore factors to consider in analyses of behavior—but not necessarily as preeminent determinants and certainly not as discovered truth.
3. According to the MOW Team's data (26), Japanese workers exhibit the highest "work centrality" and longest work week (48.9 hours) of the eight nations surveyed. According to Nonaka (27), the principal problem with Japanese labor-intensive "compressive management" practices is exhaustion.
4. Bond (5), for instance, proposed that "those values that are related to growth in one historical period may be different from those which potentiate growth in another." Thus "individualism" may have made for success in one era and "collectivism" in another.
5. Nord et al. (28) also discussed the operational structures and the workplace factors that seemingly compelled managements to employ coercive methods in order to obtain work.
6. Gardell's model is substantially similar to the well known ISR model (20, p. 584).
7. Note that Rice et al. failed to demonstrate this moderator effect using measures of job and life *satisfaction* because, they argued, "importance" was already reflected in the satisfaction measures and so could not serve as a "third variable" affecting relations between those measures. Importance weightings can nevertheless be important, they concluded, but only when used correctly.

REFERENCES

1. Altman, I., & Chemers, M. M. (1980). Cultural aspects of environment-behavior relations. In H. C. Triandis & R. W. Brislin (eds.). *Handbook of cross-cultural psychology* (Vol. 5, pp. 73–120). Boston: Allyn & Bacon.
2. Barrett, G. V., & Bass, B. M. (1976). Cross-cultural issues in industrial and organizational psychology. In M. D. Dunnette (ed.). *Handbook of industrial and organizational psychology* (pp. 1639–86). Chicago: Rand McNally.
3. Bellah, R. N., Madsen, R., Sullivan, W. M., Swidler, A., & Tipton, S. M. (1985). *Habits of the heart: individualism and commitment in American life.* Berkeley, CA: University of California Press.
4. Berry, J. W. (1980). Introduction to methodology. In H. C. Triandis & J. W. Berry (eds.). *Handbook of cross-cultural psychology* (Vol. 2, pp. 1–28). Boston: Allyn & Bacon.
5. Bond, M. H. (1987). Invitation to a wedding: Chinese values and economic growth. Presented at the Conference of International Union of Psychological Sciences, Hong Kong.
6. Boulding, K. E. (1953). *The organizational revolution.* Chicago: Quadrangle.
7. Brislin, R. W. (1980). Translation and content analysis of oral written material. In H. C. Triandis & J. W. Berry (eds.). *Handbook of cross-cultural psychology* (Vol. 2, pp. 389–444). Boston: Allyn & Bacon.
8. Chang, S. (1985). American and Chinese managers in U.S. companies in Taiwan: a comparison. *California Management Review, 27,* 144–56.
9. Cummings, L. L., & Schwab, D. P. (1973). *Performance in organizations: determinants and Appraisal.* Glenview, IL: Scott, Foresman.
10. DeVos, G. A., & Hippler, A. E. (1969). Cultural psychology: comparative studies of human behavior. In G. Lindzey & E. Aronson (eds.). *Handbook of social psychology* (2nd ed., Vol. 4, pp. 323–417). Reading, MA: Addison-Wesley.
11. Elizur, D. (1984). Facets of work values: a structural analysis of work outcomes. *Journal of Applied Psychology, 69,* 379–89.
12. Fairbank, J. K. (1987). *The great Chinese revolution: 1800–1985.* New York: Harper & Row.
13. Fromm, E. (1955). *The sane society.* New York: Rinehart.
14. Gardell, B. (1987). *Work organization and human nature.* Stockholm: Arbets-Miljofonden.
15. Griffeth, R. W., Horn, P. W., DeNisi, A. S., & Kirchner, W. K. (1985). A comparison of different methods of clustering countries on the basis of employee attitudes. *Human Relations, 38,* 813–40.
16. Gursslin, O. R., Hunt, R. G., & Roach, J. L. (1960). Social class and the mental health movement. *Social Problems, 7,* 210–17.
17. Hunt, R. G., Meindl, J. R., Pillai, R., Wilderom, C., & Yu, K. C. (1989). The problem of translation in cross-cultural research: an ex-

ploratory study of work values in the PRC. Presented at the First European Congress of Psychology, Amsterdam.

18. Hofstede, G. (1984). *Culture's consequences: international differences in work-related values* (abridged edition). Beverly Hills, CA: Sage.

19. Iaffaldano, M. T., & Muchinsky, P. M. (1985). Job satisfaction and job performance: a meta analysis. *Psychological Bulletin, 97,* 251–73.

20. Katz, D., & Kahn, R. (1978). *The social psychology of organizations* (2nd ed.) New York: Wiley.

21. Katzell, R. A., & Yankelovich, D. (1975). *Work, productivity and job satisfaction.* New York: Psychological Corporation.

22. Kelly, J. E. (1982). *Scientific management, job redesign and work performance.* New York: Academic Press.

23. Locke, E. A. (1976). The nature and causes of job satisfaction. In M. D. Dunnette (ed.). *Handbook of industrial and organizational psychology* (pp. 1297–1350). Chicago: Rand McNally.

24. McClelland, D. C., & Winter, D. G. (1969). *Motivating economic achievement.* New York: Free Press.

25. Meindl, J. R., Hunt, R. G., Elizur, D., & Lee, W. (1986). Work values and achievement orientations: comparing the U.S.A. and China. In *Proceedings HRMOB Annual National Conference,* (Vol. 1, pp. 28–32).

26. MOW International Research Team. (1987). *The meaning of work.* London: Academic Press.

27. Nonaka, I. (1988). Toward middle-up-down, management: accelerating information creation. *Sloan Management Review, 29,* 9–18.

28. Nord, W. R., Brief, A. P., Atieh, J. M., & Doherty, E. M. (in press). Work values and the conduct of organizational behavior. In B. Staw & E. Cummings (eds.). *Research in organizational behavior* (Vol. 10). Greenwich, CT: J.A.I. Press.

29. Oscarsson, B., & Dockerty, P. (1987). *New technology, working life and management in Sweden.* Stockholm: Swedish Work Environment Fund.

30. Pryor, R. G. C. (1987). Differences among dif-

ferences: in search of general work preference dimensions. *Journal of Applied Psychology, 72,* 426–33.

31. Rice, R. W., McFarlin, D. B., Hunt, R. G., & Near, J. P. (1985). Job importance as a moderator of the relationship between job satisfaction and life satisfaction. *Basic and Applied Social Psychology, 6,* 297–316.

32. Rice, R. W., McFarlin, D. B., Hunt, R. G., & Near, J. P. (1985). Organizational work and the perceived quality of life: toward a conceptual model. *Academy of Management Review, 10,* 296–310.

33. Ronen, S., & Kraut, A. (1977). Similarities among countries based on employee work values and attitudes. *Columbia Journal of World Business, 12,* 89–96.

34. Schermerhorn, J. R. (1987). Language effects in cross-cultural management research: an empirical study and a word of caution. Presented at the Academy of Management, New Orleans.

35. Simonsen, T. (1987). Easier to put up with the job. *Working Environment 1987 in Sweden* (annual, pp. 48–51). Stockholm: Swedish Work Environment Association.

36. Skinner, B. F. (1986). What is wrong with daily life in the Western world? *American Psychologist, 41,* 568–74.

37. Smith, M. B. (1969). *Social psychology and human values.* Chicago: Aldine.

38. Sullivan, H. S. (1953). *The interpersonal theory of psychiatry.* New York: Norton.

39. Tannenbaum, A. (1980). Organizational psychology. In H. C. Triandis & R. W. Brislin (eds.). *Handbook of cross-cultural psychology* (Vol. 5, pp. 281–334). Boston: Allyn & Bacon.

40. Terkel, S. (1974). *Working.* New York: Pantheon.

41. Triandis, H. C., Malpass, R. S., & Davidson, A. (1972). Cross-cultural psychology. In B. Siegel (ed.). *Biennial Review of Anthropology* (pp. 1–84). Stanford, CA: Stanford University Press.

42. Zavalloni, M. (1980). Values. In H. C. Triandis & R. W. Brislin (eds.). *Handbook of cross-cultural psychology* (Vol. 5, pp. 73–120). Boston: Allyn & Bacon.

V
MANAGING FOR HEALTH AND PRODUCTIVITY

There are a number of reasons management must be concerned about the health of its staff members. One of the most obvious is that unhealthy workers are unlikely to be as productive as their healthy counterparts in terms of individual efforts or joint efforts with other members of the work organization. Furthermore, ill employees sometimes are unable to come to work.

Another major consideration is the cost of illness to the work organization. Walsh (Chapter 15) points out the problems of adequately estimating illness costs inherent in considering only insured costs or limiting one's attention to illnesses that derive directly from the work experience. Brenner (Chapter 16) moves to the societal level of analysis and considers other costs. This approach, however, makes it more difficult for the organizational manager to deal with health and productivity problems, as the indirect costs tend to exceed direct costs when viewed from this level. In analyzing the costs of illness in the workplace, Walsh notes the importance of adhering to the employer's perspective, as the cost to companies in terms of reduced productivity seems to be greater for direct illness; companies are not usually responsible or interested in indirect costs.

The direct approach to reducing the cost of illness has its drawbacks. For example, it is difficult to justify health-promotion programs in economic terms, as most employers tend to do. As Fielding points out in Chapter 17, these programs are likely to have an impact on the costly utilization of health care services only over extended periods as risks for serious health problems are gradually reduced.

One of the main ways managers envision that improved health status influences productivity is through its effect on absenteeism. Reduced absenteeism alone may demonstrate the value of health promotion and disease prevention activities. Some have argued that the effect of health status on absenteeism is mediated through its effect on softer productivity variables such as job satisfaction.

In any case, the way to determine the impact of programs intended to improve the health of workers is through adequate program evaluation. Unfortunately, rigorous evaluation has been the exception, rather than the rule, for assessing the value of worksite health-promotion efforts. There are many reasons, including the willingness of management in earlier efforts to be content with the good will and increased morale engendered by such efforts. The costs of good evaluation also have not seemed justified in the short-term perspective of many businesses, and there are methodological problems to be overcome. However, Fielding points out the obvious anomaly in business not investing in sufficient program evaluation given the general recognition by management of the importance to success of tracking the results of other investments. He underscores the need for more evaluation efforts and highlights some future evaluation priorities, not the least of which is the need for enhanced quantification of the interrelations of health and productivity at work.

15
Costs of Illness in the Workplace

Diana Chapman Walsh

Estimating the economic costs of illness in the workplace is a monumental undertaking that has yet to be tackled in an adequately comprehensive way. This chapter locates such a project in the established literature, discusses a few of the more nettlesome complexities it entails, identifies sources and types of partial estimates already at hand, and sketches in broad outline what is known about a few of the costs of illness at work, pinpointing the most serious gaps in knowledge of this field. Most importantly, perhaps, it begins to grapple with questions of definitions that are essential for establishing ground rules for future debate on this subject. A serious attempt to specify much more rigorously than in the past what those costs are and who is underwriting them could influence both public policy and private sector decisions. Better data on the driving forces behind costs could influence how much is invested in programs to modify preventable illness by altering the work environment, promoting the worker's health, or adopting some combination of strategies informed by a clearer picture of the sources of preventable illness costs.

Definitional ambiguities are evident in the term "costs of illness in the workplace." Putting the accent on *costs* in the workplace directs attention to those expenses incurred by employers or business firms and raises questions about variations within and across companies in the coverage their benefit plans provide different groups of employees, dependents, and retirees. Attending only to insured costs introduces serious distortions. Alternatively (or in addition), the focus could be limited to *illness* in the workplace, implying only "occupational illnesses" that arise in some way out of the work experience. However, it leaves unanswered questions of etiology: whether, for example, an employee's heart attack was triggered by stresses on the job, not irritants at home, bad genes, even bad luck, or some murky mix of causes. From the outset the discussion requires confronting arbitrary distinctions that are difficult to sustain. Table 15–1 summarizes the conceptual framework that was used to organize this review.

COST OF ILLNESS METHODOLOGY: OVERVIEW

The effort to quantify a disease's impact forces hair-splitting choices. A virtue of the enterprise is to make underlying assumptions explicit in the hope that decisions will be better informed (35). Rapid inflation in health care costs in recent decades and the

217

Table 15-1. Conceptual Framework for Estimating the Costs of Illness in the Workplace

Direct costs	Indirect costs	Psychosocial costs
The Firm		
Goods and services covered through the employee benefit plan (e.g., emergency services, drugs, appliances and medical supplies, home care services, dental care)	Wage replacement programs (insured or paid out of current assets) including short-term and long-term disability, workers' compensation	Impact of preventable illness or death on morale and organizational effectiveness, loss of "institutional memory".
Costs of financing and administering the employee benefit plan	Death benefits, life insurance and pension costs related to premature mortality	
Costs of company-funded preventive and palliative health services (e.g., occupational health, employee assistance, health-promotion programs)	Costs of turnover and diminished productivity, quality of product, and competitiveness	
The Worker		
Deductibles and copayments for covered services (above) and out-of-pocket expenses for goods and services covered partially or not at all (e.g., modifications to the home, special diets, clothing, transportation)	Unreimbursed earnings foregone owing to morbidity (work-loss days for temporary short-term illness; lost earnings for chronic debility) or mortality	Deteriorations in self-esteem, quality of life; disfigurement; loss of function; pain, grief, isolation; unwanted job changes; diminished career opportunities; impact on family, coworkers, and friends
Society		
Government subsidies (tax deductionss and welfare payments) for illnesses experienced by current and former workers and their dependents.	Loss of productivity; impact on the gross national product and on competitiveness in world markets	Effect of illness and disability on work ethic, national confidence, and pride
Costs of administering state and federal agencies regulating prevention and the delivery of services to workers (including parts of OSHA, NIOSH, ERISA, EPA, and others)	Costs of administering state and federal agencies regulating income replacement programs, workers' compensation and disability boards, and others	

proliferation of new technologies have stimulated growing interest in the cost of ill health and a leap in the number of studies examining the economic burden of various diseases. These estimates complement evaluation research in cost-effectiveness and cost-benefit analyses comparing alternative strategies to advance the public health. Data generated from such research can support policy analyses of competing bids for investment of society's scarce resources in technologies and activities purporting to enhance health and extend life.

The conceptual origins of cost-of-illness studies go back two or three centuries (9); modern techniques were later refined and applied in a series of reports that began to appear during the late 1950s (8,23,32,52). Rice's landmark 1966 study (38) and a follow-up by Cooper and Rice (5) developed a comprehensive framework as well as accounting procedures that obviated double counting and invited comparison of the relative economic costs, nationwide, of 16 major disease categories.

Rice and her colleagues have continued to update the estimates of illness costs on a national scale (39). Meanwhile, more than 200 cost-of-illness studies were published between 1959 and 1979, most limited to a particular population or geographic area and to one or a few categories of illness. Variations from one to another in the assumptions, methods, and data used have created large inconsistencies that have been impossible to reconcile (18). Nevertheless, there is now general agreement on a basic vocabulary and accounting approach, which were codified in a set of guidelines for use by the U.S. Public Health Service by a 1978 task force convened and chaired by Rice (19).

The two reigning methodologies for estimating the indirect costs of illness are the "human capital" (or "output accounting") approach and the "willingness-to-pay" method. Each contributes a different perspective and addresses different basic questions; it has been suggested that the ideal valuation of illness costs would employ both approaches (21).

The human capital model is more widely used and portrays an individual as someone capable of producing a stream of output over the years, valued at the level of average earnings for someone of his or her group (where "group" is typically defined by age and sex but occasionally, in more refined analyses, by other variables as well, including education, residence, industry, and occupation (40). Illness or injury can intrude on this earning capacity and result in indirect costs.

Direct costs are expenditures for prevention, detection, treatment, and rehabilitation services for the illness or impairment in question. Indirect costs are from "productivity foregone" as a result of it: contributions to the economy that victims of the disease would in theory have made had they not been disabled or died. Because both types of cost reduce the goods and services available for other social purposes— because they are applied to treat the illness in question (direct costs) or are not produced at all (indirect costs)—the two types can be combined in a summary statement of the total economic cost of a particular disease or injury.

Few studies pay more than lip service to a third broad category of costs. These "psychosocial" costs of illness refer to decrements in the quality of life for victims and their families, friends, coworkers, caregivers, and others. Granting the importance of these intangible costs, most analysts, with a few exceptions (33), sidestep them as difficult to quantify and monetarize in a convincing way.

Another methodological distinction within the human capital framework is whether estimates take a "prevalence" or an "incidence" approach. Incidence-based studies are rarer and more difficult because they project the likely course and duration of a disease from the time of onset in order to extrapolate potential costs, including information on treatment costs and effects. Conducting such a study involves an elaborate culling of the literature for fragments of data of uneven quality collected for widely ranging purposes (14,37).

Prevalence-based estimates, by contrast, assign the costs of the illness to the year of death, irrespective of its time of onset, and compute the present value of future earnings lost. National-level prevalence-based studies can work from established data sets. The bulk of direct costs are captured in the U.S. National Health Accounts published by the National Center for Health Statistics and the Health Care Financing Administration. Despite gaps and inaccuracies in these data (43), they do provide a strong foundation for studies of this kind (18). Raw data required for computing most of the indirect costs are available from the National Health Interview Survey, the Bureau of Labor Statistics, and the United States Census (39). Using these national data usually encourages the construction of measures at a high level of aggregation, as for example breaking down average wages by age and sex alone and looking at broad age groups (under versus over age 65). Finer-grained classifications (e.g., working status, occupation, education, and age) yield cost estimates that would be more accurate for specific groups of workers and would be useful for estimating costs of illness related to occupation (18). A difficulty is that occupation is not routinely available on current records that are used to compute wage rates, one of many complications that begins to arise as one moves from the aggregate national level to "costs of illness at work."

FIRST APPROXIMATION

One way to say something about the overall costs of illness at the workplace is to begin with existing national cost-of-illness estimates and qualify them to apply specifically to workers on the job. This approach requires narrowing the population to noninstitutionalized working-age adults who have been in the workforce for at least some segment of the year(s) being studied. Unfortunately, most of the national data are reported in such a way as to preclude this reaggregation. Table 15–2 provides summary data from the 1980 national study (30). Both the $146.2 billion in direct costs for those under age 65 and the $162 billion in mortality costs include costs for infants and children: their health care when they are sick and their foregone earnings if they die. Health care costs for infants and children are often included in employee benefit plans and, because of this financing artifact, are in an important sense direct costs (at the workplace) of illnesses (experienced elsewhere). Lost wages of children who die before

Table 15–2. Economic Cost of Illness, United States, 1980

Parameter	Costs (billions of dollars)			
	All	Men	Women	Under 65 years
Direct cost	211.1	87.6	123.5	146.2
Indirect cost				
Morbidity[a]	67.8	48.3	19.5	64.1
Mortality[b]	175.9	123.5	52.2	161.8
Total costs	454.8	259.6	195.3	372.2

Source: Rice et al. (39).

[a]Work-loss days dervied from the National Health Interview Survey; number of persons unable to work from the Bureau of Labor Statistics, number in institutions from the U.S. Bureau of the Census.
[b]Present value of lifetime earnings discounted at 4%.

entering the workforce, however, should not be considered a cost of illness at work. The $68 billion in morbidity costs include employed adults, women usually keeping house, and people unable to work or institutionalized. Logically, only the first group incurs workplace-related costs, but we lack sufficient detail to adjust the figure appropriately.

Salkever (40) did take as his unit of analysis noninstitutionalized working-age adults but estimated only morbidity costs and omitted women. Nevertheless, the estimates he derived, summarized in Table 15–3, allow a beginning approximation of indirect costs of illness at work. The 1980 total of $51.9 billion (in 1975 dollars) comprises $28.1 billion of earnings lost by men unable to work at all, $11 billion for days lost by active workers, and $12.7 billion for "debility costs," defined as "earnings reductions, for people who work, caused by long-term health problems." Assuming that morbidity costs for men are roughly 2.5 times those for women (39), the total costs for both sexes would be approximately $72.6 billion.

The difference between this estimate and that in Table 15–2 ($73 billion versus $68 billion in morbidity costs) reflects Salkever's more thorough accounting of "debility" costs and an inconsistency in the estimates of people unable to work by the U.S. Bureau of Labor [used by Rice et al. (46)] and the (higher) number derived from the National Health Interview Survey [and used in Salkever's analysis (48)]. Even if we could reconcile this difference, the crucial issue the Salkever data highlight is which of these illness expenses are properly workplace costs. To approach that question we need to grapple with alternative perspectives and the complex question of who bears the costs.

The national illness-cost estimates can finesse many problems and take a social perspective where all costs count, no matter who actually pays. Introducing the question "whose costs?" muddies the waters but is a necessary part of struggling with the notion of workplace costs. Table 15–1 summarized sources of direct, indirect, and psychosocial costs for the three principal payers: the employer (or the firm), the employee (or the worker), and residual uncovered costs borne by "society" at large in the form of tax subsidies and welfare payments of various kinds. For our purposes attention is confined to direct and indirect costs *to business firms*. In so doing, I am arguing that "costs of illness in the workplace" are costs to business firms, not illness costs incurred by workers owing to their work or outlays by society to pay for the health impact of work. This point is not to minimize the importance of personal and social costs associated with working or to discourage efforts to quantify those costs. It is to assert that if, as a matter of policy, we want business firms to absorb costs

Table 15–3. Morbidity Costs, Noninstitutionalized Working-Age Men (Ages 17–64), 1980

Estimated annual frequencies (No.)	
Persons unable to work	2.7 billion
Work-loss days	272 billion
Working persons with long-term health problems	5.4 billion
Estimatd annual morbidity costs, 1975 dollars	
Earnings losses for persons unable to work	$28.1 billion
Productivity losses from work-loss days	$11.0 billion
Debility costs	$12.7 billion
Total morbidity costs	$51.9 billion

Source: Salkever (40).

currently being borne by workers or by society we need regulations designed to internalize those costs.

COMPLEXITIES, CONFOUNDERS, AND PITFALLS

If the costs of a given illness were a fixed number, the challenge would be to allocate them accurately across the three payer groups and then repeat the process for all other illnesses relevant to work. For risk factors, there would be the additional step of estimating the probability of contracting the disease, at different exposure levels (37). However, because incentives flowing from various payment schemes probably alter the absolute numbers (e.g., when the firm offers a dental plan, workers and their families visit dentists more), variations in the distribution of costs, across firms, and through time confound the absolute numbers in unpredictable ways. The most important complexity, then, and one that is seldom discussed is the impact of transfer payments on the utilization of health services.

Second, when the perspective shifts to that of the firm, conceptual distinctions between direct and indirect costs begin to blur. The health system's "indirect costs" are really direct costs to the firm: The firm exists to produce a product, and employees' illnesses result in lost, delayed, or degraded output, with direct bearing on the bottom line. The "direct costs," or outlays for illness care, are consequential for American industry chiefly because of the peculiar health care financing system that grew up after World War II.

That same system brings dependents' health care into a complete accounting of workplace costs and, on a growing scale, that of retirees. Had we in the United States a national health service (such as the one in Britain), costs for employees' personal care for nonoccupational illness or injury and costs for all the care required by dependents and retirees would be external to the workplace and could be omitted from this discussion. Illness costs at the workplace would comprise indirect costs plus the costs of caring for illness or injury arising from work (45). In fact, more than one-half of persons covered under employer plans are insured as dependents, and a full 17% of all *workers* in 1979 were covered as spouses' dependents rather than as primary beneficiaries through their own places of work (4). In addition, at least 19 states mandate one or more kinds of continued coverage (after job termination, divorce, death of the covered spouse, during layoffs or strikes, and so on, depending on the specifics of the state statute or regulations) (6), and these laws are likely to proliferate as the problem of gaps in insurance takes on growing salience for policy. Therefore the third major challenge is to specify the relevant population and to limit the focus manageably.

Fourth, although we know that more than 60% of the civilian U.S. population has health insurance through an employer group plan, such plans vary widely in the scope of services offered. A few studies have been done to identify factors influencing whether employees have coverage. Variables such as firm size and industry type as well as the employee's seniority, wage, full-time work status, and union membership are significant (29). Employees of small firms and firms with high concentrations of minimum-wage jobs are significantly less likely to have access to an employer group health plan. Also, where employees are offered plans, further variations arise from the choices they make concerning which (if any) combination to elect. The possibilities have multiplied with the diversification of managed health care and the growing popularity of flexible benefits, or "cafeteria plans."

Fifth, any confusion this maze of benefits creates is magnified by the fragmentation of existing records on employee health. In the case of large employers, employment-based health insurance is often funded and is sometimes administered by the firm on its own, but most companies have multiple administrative contracts. Claims data are generated and manipulated by commercial insurers and "the Blues" [more than 800 private insurance companies were writing policies in the United States in 1983 (16)], health maintenance and preferred provider organizations, third- and fourth-party administrators, benefit consultants, and data management firms; some of the latter specialize in claims analysis or case management, others in the collection, consolidation, and interpretation of primary data, e.g., through "health risk appraisal" instruments. Entrepreneurialism and keen competition in this rapidly evolving market render potentially rich databases inaccessible to policy research.

Sixth, the fragmentation of records is accompanied by splintered responsibility inside most business firms. Stewardship for aspects of health is typically spread among several functional units (e.g., human resources and benefits, the medical unit, employee assistance, and finance). Also, most large firms are highly decentralized and have great difficulty piecing together a coherent and complete profile of the health needs of all their employees, who are distributed in multiple plant sites and with a remarkably long list of jobs. As just one example, we and others have made concerted but often frustrated efforts to integrate medical care claims data (obtained from insurance carriers) with absenteeism tapes (maintained at local plants) in order to build detailed case files that would track an employee's illness career from the first day off work, through layers of the health care system, until the first day back (49). The number of successful matches in which the records are complete is always disappointing for reasons that are never clear, except that available data sources are inflexible and unwieldly. Developed for specific purposes—medical care claims records to pay providers expeditiously, absenteeism reporting for the paymaster, occupational illness and injury records for regulatory compliance, workers' compensation files for risk management—these disparate data streams combine awkwardly and produce at best distant approximations of the information necessary to conduct health services research.

Outside research too has reinforced a patchwork view of worker health. Studies tend to emphasize specific interventions (the impact on attendance or job performance of occupational alcoholism programs, the effect on utilization of different levels of copayment, the relative efficacy of hypertension interventions of graded intensities), or they examine specific risk factors (smoking, substance abuse, low-back pain, or known or suspected toxins). Interactive and synergistic effects among these domains of health are generally overlooked, but they are certainly confounding factors that we have no way to control adequately. What we can do is examine illustrative data that some companies possess and draw a few tentative conclusions about what we know now and still need to learn about the costs of illness at work.

"DIRECT" (HEALTH CARE) COSTS TO EMPLOYERS

Direct costs to the firm (Table 15–1) include three major categories: (a) health care goods and services used by employees and their dependents and covered through the employee benefit plan; (b) the overhead costs of funding and administering the plan (seldom more than 10 to 15% of the annual premium); and (c) budgeted company outlays for preventive and palliative services, including the operating costs of occupational health and safety, employee assistance, and health-promotion units or programs.

Health Care Financed Through Private Insurance

More than 80% of the civilian noninstitutionalized population in the United States (192 million Americans) had some private health insurance at the end of 1983; most of these persons (more than 80%) are insured in whole or in part through an employer's group health plan (16). Table 15–4 shows the relative importance of public and private third-party payment over the two decades ending in 1985, when private insurance paid $113.5 billion in medical care costs—about 31% of the nation's total spending for such care (47).

Federal third-party payments (Medicare and Medicaid) account for about the same proportion of total personal health care costs as does private insurance. Yet the two government programs cover only about 18% of the population, compared to the 73% whose care is financed through private insurance. Also, the costs of Medicare and Medicaid have been climbing faster than costs to other payers: Outlays by the two government programs grew 17% between 1970 and 1982, compared to 14% growth in expenditures from private insurance. The public sector has been the largest purchaser of health services since 1974 (4).

Nevertheless, private sector payors have become increasingly concerned about trends in their costs. Many have invested in data systems they hope will help pinpoint "hot spots that are sources of trouble." Most large corporations now have basic accounting data regarding where their health care dollars are being spent: Utilization reports provide data for active employees, dependents, and retirees; on inpatient admissions, charges, and days; outpatient visits and charges; and derivative statistics (e.g., admissions, days, and visits per thousand covered lives; per capita costs, and trends over time) compared to national and regional norms. These data are generally classified in various ways: (a) by plant site and other relevant company variables, such as job level, union eligibility, and employment status (exempt/nonexempt/hourly pay class; employee/dependent/retiree); (b) by a few demographic variables, usually just

Table 15–4. Personal Health Care Expenditures, by Payment Source, United States, 1965–1982[a]

Year	All payments ($)	Direct patient payments		Private insurance		Other private[b]		Public programs[c]	
		$	%	$	%	$	%	$	%
1965	35.9	18.5	51.6	8.7	24.2	0.8	2.2	7.9	22.0
1970	65.4	26.5	40.5	15.3	23.4	1.1	1.7	22.4	34.3
1975	117.1	38.1	32.5	31.2	26.7	1.6	1.3	46.3	39.5
1980	219.7	63.0	28.7	67.5	30.7	2.7	1.2	86.5	39.4
1985	371.4	105.6	28.4	113.5	30.6	4.9	1.3	147.5	39.7

Source: Waldo et al. (47).
[a]All figures are in billions of dollars.
[b]Spending by philanthropic organizations, industrial in-plant health services, and privately financed construction.
[c]Federal spending ($112.6 billion in 1985 including $19 billion for Medicare and part of $39.8 billion for Medicaid) and state and local spending ($34.8 billion in 1985).

age and sex; (c) by health service variables including, for inpatient care, major service and primary diagnosis, surgical procedure, and the like; for outpatient care, location, specialty, and sometimes type of episode. Special studies are often done of areas where some costs might be saved through more aggressive management: cesarean section, surgery that could be done on an outpatient basis, "high-cost" cases (e.g., costing over $10,000).

Table 15–5 summarizes illustrative data from a nonrepresentative sample of a few large employers who had reports such as this one conveniently at hand and were willing to share them. It demonstrates the idiosyncrasies of company accounting systems and how many variables would have to be held constant to make meaningful comparisons among firms. The ranges appearing here—from $1,200 to $2,600 per employee per year for "medical costs," and $1,700 to $4,400 per employee per year for those labeled "health" care costs, and, in terms of percent of payroll, from 3.6% to 7.6% for medical and 6.2% to 10.8% for health—reflect differences in assumptions and sources of data, underlying characteristics of populations and worksites, and the coverage and incentives built into diverse benefit plans. These disparities discourage meaningful comparisons across firms and even across different locations operated by a single firm.

A "wild card" in aggregate and per capita company costs is the issue of retirees. Of Americans over 65 years of age, at least 6.3 million (about one-fourth) have some kind of employer-provided health insurance coverage (7). Growth in early retirement together with the aging of the population will accelerate the number of retirees in years to come. As it is, in some older smokestack industries the number of retirees now exceeds the number of active employees. Projections of the unfunded liability associated with already-promised medical coverage for current retirees range from $100 billion to nearly $3 trillion (7). Many companies and the U.S. Congress have been reassessing policies and practices on this question of financing health care for retirees. The situation is volatile, and available statistics are highly unstable; but a full accounting of the costs of illness at the worksite would have to grapple with them.

Direct Costs by Specific Condition

The cost-of-illness studies and most company utilization reports array the distribution of costs by major diagnostic group. Again, inconsistencies in accounting procedures and assumptions, as well as variability in underlying characteristics of companies, plants, workforces and jobs make it foolish to generalize. For illustration, four case studies from tapes supplied by a single large national insurance carrier are shown in Table 15–6. A hierarchy, by major diagnostic category, is shown for inpatient claims of employees only (outpatient claims and dependents have been excluded from this analysis). Nine diagnostic groups make the top five list for one of the four firms; only circulatory diseases and neoplasms make the top five on every list. The number of claims roughly corresponds to the number of admissions; ranking varies by number versus dollar amounts because of variations in length of stay and intensity. Variations from company to company presumably reflect demographics of the workforce and perhaps geographical patterns in medical practice, among other factors.

The main conclusion to be drawn from the data in Table 15–6 is that they reflect the patterns of illness in general working-age populations and say nothing specifically

Table 15–5. Distribution of Company Costs for Health-Related Insurance: Companies A to H

Parameter	A	B	C	D^k	E	F	G^s	H
Costs ($ millions)^a								
Medical	83.8	65.0	9.8	62.3	24.1	777.0	—	66.0^t
HMO	30.4	20.2	1.6	33.5	10.2	15.5	—	4.9
Other^b	33.1^h	85.6	—	23.2^l	0.4	60.7^p	—	7.6^u
Total medical	147.3	85.6	11.4	128.0	27.8	853.2	—	78.5
Dental	18.1	8.2	1.2	13.6	4.4	115.0	—	9.3
Sick pay/STD/S&A^a	4.8^i	36.9	0.6	12.8	10.6^o	195.5^q	—	19.3^v
Workers' comp.^{d}	11.2	32.7	0.9	15.8	1.5	—^{r}	—	5.8^w
Life^e	6.4	—	2.2	9.3	1.1	42.2	—	2.6
LTD^f	—	—	0.3	—	0.3	8.9	—	—^{x}
Total	187.9	163.4	16.6	179.5	45.7	1,214.8	—	115.5
Per employee/costs/year^g								
Medical	2,442	—	1,183	1,927	1,987	2,615	2,434	2,033^y
Dental	300	—	124	259	314	353	343	288
Sick pay/STD	79	—	62	163	758	599	465	126^z
Life	107	—	228	233	79	129	183	80
Workers' comp.	186	—	93	295^m	107	—	—	54^{aa}
LTD	—	—	—	—	21	27	—	—
Total	3,114	—	1,690	2,877	3,266	3,724	4,425	2,581
Percent of payroll								
Medical	7.5	3.6	4.3	7.1	5.9	7.6	—	8.7
Dental	0.9	0.35	0.5	—	0.9	1.0	—	1.0
Sick pay/STD	0.2	1.5	0.2	—	2.3	1.7	—	0.45
Life	0.3	—	0.8	0.7	0.2	0.4	—	0.3
Workers' comp.	0.6	1.4^j	0.3	1.1	0.3	—	—	0.7
LTD	—	0.01	0.1	0.6	0.1	0.8	—	—
Total	9.2	6.9	6.2	8.5^n	9.7	10.8	—	11.15

^{a}All costs are for 1986 except those for company A, which are for 1987. None include retirees; all include dependents. Inconsistencies in assumptions and accounting rules make comparisons virtually meaningless, as the footnotes below testify.
^{b}"Other" includes PPO contracts and special provisions (e.g., vision and prescription drup coverage) in some of the companies' benefit packages (see other footnotes for more detail).
^{c}STD = short-term disability; S&A = sickness and accident insurance. This category is sui generis from one company to the next, depending on contractual relationships with employees and company policies and procedures. The generic category is either income replacement for days missed from work owing to illness or company costs of replacing disabled workers.
^{d}Workers' comp. = workers' compensation programs, which are administered by individuaal states, making it difficult for some large multistate corporations to provide aggregate data on costs in this category.
^{e}Some companies look on life insurance costs as part of their health-related expenditures on the logic that preventive interventions might reduce premature mortality and life insurance claims paid. Many view life insurance in a class with pensions—essentially separate from medical outlays.
^{f}LTD = long-term disability. There is considerable variability in the terms under which different companies cover long-term disability.
^{g}Denominators may be inconsistent from company to company because not all eligible employees opt for coverage in the medical plan and the per employee costs may or may not reflect that fact. Also, the demographics of the workforce and the numbers and ages of dependents are not reflected consistently in these denominators.
^{h}Includes PPOs, major medical, and "other medical."
^{i}This item is called "weekly income" in company A's accounting scheme.
^{j}aThe denominator for the percentage is larger than for the others because all employees (full- and part-time) are covered for Workers' Compensation but not for medical care.
^{k}Full-time *salaried* employees only.
^{l}Includes flexible benefit account outlays.

226

Table 15–5. (*Continued*)

---

*m*Total *all* benefits (including pension, flexible benefit account, and statutory benefits such as FICA, federal and state unemployment, tuition): $7,503.45/employee/year.
*n*Other payroll loading factors: vacation 0.2%; pension 4.8%; company matched savings 0.5%; FICA 6.5%; federal unemployment 0.2%; state unemployment 0.4%; tuition 0.2%; total 22.5%.
*o*Sick pay only.
*p*Includes $10.7 million for a vision care benefit.
*q*Includes $128.7 million in benefit payments beginning on the eighth calendar day of illness and $67.8 million in departmental payments for absences of less than one calendar week.
*r*Not available at the corporate level because it varies by state jurisdiction.
*s*Political and labor considerations precluded company G from providing any absolute numbers.
*t*There is uncertainty in the accuracy of this figure owing to the claims lag and the dollar value of uncashed claims payments.
*u*Not included here are costs of "health and safety programs ($7.6 million or 0.9% of compensation).
*v*Includes both short-term disability ($3.5 million) and accidental death and dismemberment insurance ($600,000) payments as well as sick pay ($15.2 million).
*w*A significant difference ($4.3 million) between the actual workers' compensation losses reported by the safety department and the dollar value reported by the finance department could not be explained at this time.
*x*Employees pay any portion of the life insurance premium they choose above the company contribution of one times the employees' annual base salary.
*y*Includes medical costs only. HMO aveage capitation (per employee) rate was $2,311 (average family and single rates).
*z*Includes STD and accidental death and dismemberment ($4.1 million). Sick pay is not included; it would raise the percent of payroll to 2.1%.
*aa*Per capita estimates from the workers' compensation department were used. Finance department data show a per capita figure of $468, which is *clearly* too high. See note *w*.

about the work-relatedness of disease. The national cost of illness studies show the greatest losses owing to diseases of the circulatory system ($85 billion), followed by injury and poisoning ($83 billion), and then neoplasms ($51 billion), diseases of the respiratory system ($33 billion), and mental disorders ($31 billion) (39). Other than injuries and poisonings (in which younger groups figure importantly), this profile resembles the one in Table 15–6.

In contrast, a hierarchy of preeminent *occupational* diseases and injuries appears in Table 15–7. Developed in 1983 by the National Institute for Occupational Safety and Health (NIOSH), the suggested list of ten leading work-related diseases and injuries reflects criteria that took account of the incidence, prevalence, and severity of conditions, as well as a judgment about their "amenability to prevention" (31).

Occupational Illness and Injuries. Available statistics on occupational injuries and illnesses are notoriously sparse, and estimates of the direct costs of treating them simply do not exist. Highly politicized in struggles over whether proposed standards are excessive or insufficiently protective (30), the cost debate in occupational health often reduces to a clash of competing world views: on the one hand, concerning social justice and the pricelessness of life and limb and on the other about the vulnerability of profit margins and the imperative of conserving American jobs.

Data on the incidence of workplace illnesses and injuries are reported annually by the Bureau of Labor Statistics (BLS), based on records required by the Occupational Safety and Health Act of 1970. The 1985 survey, which sampled 280,000 establishments, reported 5.5 million injuries and illnesses: 7.9 per 100 full-time workers. Of 3,750 work-related deaths recorded, one-third were highway fatalities (on company business). Injuries occurred at a rate of 7.7 per 100 (28). Total economic costs, direct and indirect, are placed at more than $20 billion a year (11, p. 386). Elsewhere, NIOSH estimated that some 10 million workers are injured on the job each year— about 3 million seriously and "at least" 10,000 fatally; other organizations have cited other numbers, and the discrepancies are striking even at this general level (36).

Table 15–6. Inpatient Claims, By Top Five Diagnoses, Employees Only (Dependent Claims Excluded), 1985: Four Illustrative Companies[a]

| Primary diagnostic category | No. of claims | | | | | | | | Dollars of paid claims ($ thousands) | | | | | | | |
	A No.	A Rank	B No.	B Rank	C No.	C Rank	D No.	D Rank	A $	A Rank	B $	B Rank	C $	C Rank	D $	D Rank
Circulatory disease	31	1	280	1	103	1	94	4	226.7	1	1,232	1	332.7	1	557.3	1
Digestive system disorders	-*-		244	2	90	3	129	3	-*-		563.5	2	227.0	4	431.6	2
Neoplasms	19	2	179	5	34	5	66	5	152.2	2	33.9	5	240.4	2	334.5	3
Mental illnesses	9	4	-*-		42	4	-*-		60.1	5	-*-		238.0	3	-*-	
Genitourinary system	-*-		223	4	93	2	137	2	-*-		342.1	4	156.0	5	311.7	4
Respiratory disease	14	3	-*-		-*-		-*-		70.2	4	-*-		-*-		-*-	
Nervous system disorders	4	5	-*-		-*-		-*-		104.2	3	-*-		-*-		-*-	
Injuries/poisonings	-*-		328	3	-*-		-*-		-*-		405.0	3	-*-		-*-	
Pregnancy	-*-		-*-		-*-		174	1	-*-		-*-		-*-		310.5	5
Total (above)	77		1,254		362		600		613.6		2,877.0		1,194.2		1,945.6	
Total (all diagnoses)	173		2,250		882		1,150		830.4		4,130.7		1,833.4		3,058.9	

Source: Analysis of data tapes made available by a large insurance carrier. Thanks are owed to Robert St. John for the analytical work.

*Not in top five.

[a]Company A is a national engineering firm with about 10,000 employees; total payments for 2,166 claims employees only (inpatient and outpatient): $1.9 million. Company B has 18,220 employees and a rich benefit plan; total payments for 4,655 employee claims: $6.8 million. Company C is a heavy construction firm located on a small metropolitan area; the data here represent a 20% sample of its 11,000 claimants (excluding dependents) for whom $17 million was paid in claims. Company D is a California computer services firm whose 6,477 employee claimants incurred $7.2 million in inpatient and outpatient claims.

Table 15–7. Suggested List of Ten Leading Work-Related Diseases and Injuries[a]

Occupational lung diseases: asbestosis, byssinosis, silicosis, coal workers' pneumoconiosis, lung cancer, occupational asthma
Musculoskeletal injuries: disorders of the back, trunk, upper extremity, neck, lower extremity; traumatically induced Raynaud's phenomenon
Occupational cancers (other than lung): leukemia; mesothelioma; cancers of the bladder, nose, liver
Severe occupational traumatic injuries: amputations, fractures, eye loss, lacerations, traumatic deaths
Occupational cardiovascular diseases: hypertension, coronary artery disease, acute myocardial infarction
Disorders of reproduction: infertility, spontaneous abortion, teratogenesis
Neurotoxic disorders: peripheral neuropathy, toxic encephalitis, psychosis, extreme personality changes (exposure-related)
Noise-induced loss of hearing
Dermatological conditions: dermatoses, burns (scaldings), chemical burns, contusions (abrasions)
Psychological disorders: neuroses, personality disorders, alcoholism, drug dependency

---

Source: National Institute for Occupational Safety and Health; Reprinted by the Association of Schools of Public Health (2).
[a]The conditions listed under each category are to be viewed as selected examples, not comprehensive definitions of the category.

Incidence rates for occupational illness are more suspect still. The orthodox numbers are 100,000 deaths and 390,000 new cases a year, but these figures are crude. Only 125,000 new cases were reported in the 1985 BLS report, which certainly understated chronic and long-term latent illnesses. They are difficult to identify or to ascribe to exposures on the job; meanwhile, more than two-thirds of the new cases reported by BLS were skin diseases or repetitive-trauma conditions, well recognized for associations with work (28). Musculoskeletal injuries are a high-visibility problem on the job; afflicting some 19 million workers, they are the leading cause of disability, lost earnings, and workers' compensation payments. Lower-back problems alone amass an estimated $14 billion a year in direct and indirect costs (2). This number illustrates the problem with occupational illness cost estimates. As costly as they are, low-back problems do not account for 70% of the total costs of occupational illness and injuries, leaving a residual of only $6 billion for all the rest. In one study, back injuries accounted for 33% of all workers' compensation dollars (1), but workers' compensation rates are strongly biased against occupational disease.

We know that millions of workers are currently exposed on the job to factors that may elevate their risk of cardiovascular disease, the leading cause of death and disability in the United States (22,42). Millions more work with agents that are known or suspected carcinogens. How many workers have had significant exposures at some time during their careers is not known, but for asbestos alone that number is something over 27 million (34). Although occasional special studies attempt to quantify costs for a sample of employees exposed to a particular hazard, only fragmented data exist at this time.

Information is available on medical care secured through workers' compensation, reflecting the direct cost component of this two-pronged program, but here too inconsistencies preclude definitive statements. Total hospital and medical expenditures financed through workers' compensation at the federal, state, and local levels were placed at $6.4 billion in 1983, a figure that Table 15–8 shows has risen more slowly than general medical inflation (19). Another interpretation suggests rapid growth in workers' compensation costs, which jumped from 1% to 2% of payroll during the

Table 15–8. Trends in Workers' Compensation Costs and Benefits

Calendar year	Estimated workers covered (millions)	Total benefits ($ millions)	Benefits/ worker	Medical and hospitalization ($ millions)	Percent of total	Compensation payments ($)	Percent change from previous year
1940	25	256	$10.24	95	37	161	
1949	35	566	16.17	185	32	381	121.1[a]
1950	37	615	16.62	200	32	415	
1959	44	1,210	27.50	410	34	800	96.7[a]
1960	45	1,295	28.78	435	34	860	
1969	59	2,634	44.64	920	35	1,714	103.3[a]
1970	59	3,031	51.37	1,050	35	1,981	15.0
1973	66	5,103	77.32	1,480	29	3,623	68.3[b]
1974	68	5,781	85.01	1,760	30	4,021	13.2
1975	67	6,598	98.48	2,030	31	4,568	12.4
1976	70	7,597	108.53	2,380	31	5,217	15.1
1977	72	8,623	119.76	2,680	31	5,943	13.5
1978	75	9,734	129.79	2,960	30	6,775	12.9
1979	79	11,872	150.28	3,470	29	8,402	22.0
1980	79	12,027	152.24	3,520	29	8,507	1.3
1981	80	13,562	169.53	3,930	29	9,632	12.8
1982	78	16,263	208.50	5,860	40	11,403	19.9
1983	79	17,589	222.65	5,690	32	11,899	8.1
1984	83	19,529	235.29	6,370	33	13,159	11.0

Source: Social Security Bulletin, 1980;43(10):5 and 1981;44(9):9–13;1986;49(2):5–11;1986;49(12):19–24; and U.S. Department of Commerce, Bureau of the Census, *Statistical Abstract of the United States 1985.* Washington, DC, GPO Table 632.

[a]Ten-year change.
[b]Three-year change.

1970s (11). However interpreted, these data also grossly underreport chronic conditions emanating from work exposures. Without better record-keeping and a firmer epidemiological base, putting dollar figures on occupational ill health is like painting bulls'-eyes around arrows already shot into a blank target.

Behavioral Risk Factors for Chronic Illnesses. The cost of behavioral risk factors has been estimated more closely than has that of environmental hazards. Table 15–9 updates Fielding's collection of "very conservative" estimates of the costs of "preventable problems." Direct costs typically comprise less than one-third of the total, but they of course include all social costs, not just those at work. The workplace implications of alcohol abuse and smoking have received the closest attention, and we briefly review here the estimates of their costs, both direct and indirect.

Comprehensive estimates of the economic costs of alcohol abuse were developed first. Berry and Boland (3) did the original work, which was subsequently updated and refined at the Research Triangle Institute (RTI) by teams led by Cruze in 1980 (6) and Harwood in 1984 (15). The RTI studies built inductively from specific events, in preference to the population-specific approach Berry's group had used. The two methods differ in the types of bias they introduce. Underestimation is the danger of the illness- or event-specific strategy: It is difficult to identify the full range of alcohol-related events. Inferring costs from a presumed population at risk tends to err the other way: Confounding is everywhere, making it difficult to avoid overstating the marginal costs incurred by problem-drinking groups.

Table 15–10 summarizes the estimated economic costs of alcohol and alcohol abuse in 1983, a total of $117 billion in direct and indirect costs. The "core" costs are closely associated with alcohol itself: direct costs of prevention and treatment and indirect costs of productivity foregone. "Other related costs" attach to secondary effects of alcohol abuse: motor vehicle accidents, fires, and crimes, as well as the social expenditures for managing these problems.

Assigning an appropriate share of these costs to the workplace has not been done. What one finds instead are fairly loose statements about costs to industry, to particular companies, or among groups of "high-cost employees" as well as claims about costs averted through successful interventions (10). The workplace-related costs can be separated conceptually into the four-way matrix in Table 15–11, but meaningful dollar values cannot be estimated for the four cells. What does emerge from this breakdown is

Table 15–9. Estimated Costs of Health Risks and Illnesses

Risk	Year	Costs	Direct as % of total costs	Standardized to 1982 dollars[a]
		Costs (billions of dollars)		
Alcohol abuse	1983	24.3	20	112.71
Smoking	1984	23.3	30	25.35
Cancer	1975	6.41	28	39.04
Coronary heart disease	1975	2.49	18	23.14
Motor vehicle injuries	1975	4.77	33	24.28
Stroke	1975	27.05	28	97.39

Source: Harwood et al. (15), Rice et al. (39), Hartunian et al. (14).
[a]Using implicit price deflators from Statistical Abstract of the U.S., 1987, Table 699, p. 417.

Table 15–10. Economic Costs to Society of Alcohol
Abuse and Alcoholism, United States, 1983

Types of cost	Cost ($ millions)
Core costs	
Direct	
Treatment[a]	13,457
Health support services	1,549
Indirect	
Mortality[b]	18,151
Reduced productivity	65,582
Lost employment	5,323
Other related costs	
Direct	
Motor vehicle crashes	2,697
Crime	2,631
Social welfare administration	49
Other	3,673
Indirect	
Victims of crime	194
Incarceration	2,979
Motor vehicle crashes	590
Total	116,875

Source: Harwood et al. (15).

[a]For alcohol abuse and alcoholism, liver cirrhosis, other illnesses, motor
vehicle crashes, and other injuries.
[b]At 6% discount rate.

that an overemphasis on the manifest costs may abet a tendency to deny the importance of alcohol problems, encouraging false economies. Often it is argued that more spending to prevent or treat manifest problems would yield savings in latent costs. For example, it is frequently asserted that abuse of alcohol is a decisive, but overlooked, factor behind many hospital admissions, perhaps as many as one-third of all hospitalizations of men (13). Moreover, it has been shown that when alcoholics stop drinking, they use fewer medical services (20). More work is needed, however, to pinpoint these associations and describe their cost implications in the context of work. This need is even more pronounced in the case of other substance abuse and mental disorders, which together with alcohol problems certainly account for a large, if unknown, share of direct and indirect costs in the workplace when the latent costs are included.

Smoking is the other behavioral risk factor analyzed extensively, but here too we know much less about costs than about health effects. Kristein (25,26,27) has developed the most thorough analysis of how much smoking costs businesses (Table 15–12). His accounting scheme deviates from those noted in other cost-of-illness (or risk factor) research reports. Also, confounding factors seem inadequately controlled, and justifications for some of the assumptions seem weak (e.g., compared to nonsmokers, smokers use one-half again the health care, have twice the accidents, miss work two more days a year, and waste 8 minutes a day in smoking rituals). Kristein's estimates nevertheless are considerably more conservative than others in the literature (51), but the field badly needs a systematic and temperate accounting of the costs of smoking to

Table 15–11. Economic Costs of Alcoholism to Industry: Typology

Manifest costs	Latent costs
Direct costs	
Insurance premiums for covered alcoholism treatment	Insurance claims for any health care for conditions in which alcohol abuse is an important underlying but undiagnosed factor (employees and dependents)
Costs of the company medical department and the employee assistance program related to the identification and management of alcohol-related problems	
Indirect costs	
Absenteeism, productivity losses, turnover, waste, accidents where alcohol abuse is clearly implicated	Labor force management costs (e.g., absenteeism, turnover) where alcohol abuse is implicated but unacknowledged
Grievances and disciplinary actions for alleged alcohol-related offenses	Potential legal liability for "job-related" alcohol abuse under workers' compensation and tort liability systems
	Damage to labor relations, public image, company morale

employers and the benefits of smoking reduction, as was done from the individual smoker's perspective by Oster and colleagues (37).

Such a study would have to reckon with our problem of who pays, an issue Schelling (41) raised in an essay challenging the notion that smokers inflict costs on others. He argued that "the main economic burden" associated with diminished productivity falls on smokers themselves and their families and only indirectly on the wider economy. Also, he asserted, smokers' *net* direct costs are not necessarily higher. Because lung cancer kills quickly "it is not at all evident that over their lifetimes smokers incur greater medical-care costs than nonsmokers"; distinctions must be drawn between total and net costs.

These and other conceptual and methodological challenges await resolution before we will have satisfactory estimates of workplace costs of other risk factors. Examples are hypertension (said to claim almost 125,000 workers' lives every year and 29 million workdays at a cost of $2 billion in lost earnings) and elevated cholesterol (an important modifiable factor for atherosclerosis, believed to cost the national economy more than $80 billion a year in lost wages, lost productivity, and medical care costs). Job accidents too comprise an understudied but obviously important source of workplace illness costs (17), accounting for perhaps $33.4 billion in 1983, including some $3.8 billion in medical expenditures (16, p. 63).

The final component of direct costs—company expenditures for in-house or contract health services for employees—is proprietary information few firms willingly share. Anecdotal comments suggest that annual occupational health budgets in Fortune-100-sized corporations tend to cluster in the $2 million to $5 million range, and seldom grow much beyond $10 million, but these impressions may be wrong. One firm (that asked to remain anonymous) conducted an internal "cost valuation" audit of its occupational health programs nationwide. The 16 facility medical clinics responding to the pilot survey (there were four nonrespondents) covered 97,000 employees, em-

Table 15–12. Summary of Kristein's Estimates of Economic Costs to Businesses of their Employees' Smoking

"Cost centers"	Assumptions	Estimated excess cost to business per smoking employee ($)
Insurance		
Medical insurance premiums	Smokers use 50% more health care services than do nonsmokers.	75–100
Other insurance premiums	Excess fire insurance premiums are needed.	5
	Smokers are twice as likely to have accidents, elevating workers' compensation costs.	17–34
	Smokers die younger; therefore group life insurance premiums are elevated.	20–33
Absenteeism and sick pay	Smokers miss 33–45% more days of work (ca. 2 days/year at $40/day).	40–80
Productivity Losses	Smokers waste 1 minute/ working hour, or 8 minutes/day.	166
"Involuntary" smoking	Involuntary smokers incur 20% of the risk of pack-a-day smokers.	27–56
Occupational illnesses	Synergistic effects between smoking and occupational toxins increase occupational health liability and disability costs.	72
Total costs		336–601

Source: Kristein (27).

ployed 24 physicians and 90 nurses, and represented a total (1985) expenditure of $9.6 million, ranging from $156,000 to $1.2 million. Per capita expenditures for these in-house dispensaries averaged about $100 a year (range $65 to $460). Even collecting this rudimentary accounting data on a companywide basis is a step many large companies are only just beginning to contemplate.

"INDIRECT" (WORK-RELATED) COSTS TO EMPLOYERS

Indirect costs to the firm (Table 15–3) are productivity decrements or other organizational impacts when employees who are ill or injured lose some or all of their capacity to perform their jobs. The distinction between direct and indirect costs points out an irony. In some ways it seems reasonable to argue that the health system's "indirect costs" are really direct costs to the firm. If companies exist to produce a product and if illness results in lost, delayed, or lower-quality output, it has direct bearing on the bottom line. That the "direct costs" of illness are as serious a concern as they are for American industry is an artifact of the peculiar health care financing system that grew

Table 15–13. Absence Rates for Full-time Wage and Salary Workers, Nonagricultural, By Reason, May 1985

Measure	1980	1985	1980–1985 change No.	1980–1985 change %
Absent workers				
Total number of workers[a]	64,043	77,698	13,655	21.3
Total absent	3,926	3,683	−243	−6.2
Total incidence rate[b]	6.2	4.7	−1.4	−23.0
Illnesses and injuries	3.6	2.6	−1.4	−27.8
Miscellaneous reasons	2.6	2.1	−0.5	−19.2
Hours lost				
Weekly hours usually worked	2,693,930	3,276,410	582,480	21.6
Weekly hours lost	89,823	86,279	−3,544	−3.9
Total inactivity rate[c]	3.3	2.7	−0.7	−21.2
Illnesses and injuries	2.1	1.6	−0.5	−23.8
Miscellaneous reasons	1.2	1.1	−0.1	8.3
Hours lost per absent worker				
Usual weekly hours per worker	42.1	42.2	0.1	0.2
Total severity rate[d]	56.1	57.2	1.1	2.0
Illnesses and injuries	61.4	61.9	0.5	0.8
Miscellaneous reasons	48.9	51.6	2.7	5.5

Source: Klein (24).
Data are given in thousands.
[a]Includes incorporated self-employed workers.
[b]Number of workers absent as a percent of the total working.
[c]Number of hours absent as a percent of the total number of hours usually worked.
[d]Number of hours absent as a percent of the number of hours usually worked by absent workers.

up after World War II. As a result, American industry's concerns about direct (medical) costs have tended to overshadow concern about the indirect (productivity) costs. Yet the latter are much more clearly within industry's control, much more unequivocally the "responsibility" of a business firm (49).

The first type of indirect costs are those replacing wages when workers are ill.

1. Incidental absenteeism costs can be insured (through short-term disability coverage, often called a "sickness and accident" plan) or paid out of current assets. Firms make various arrangements for different classes of employees; hourly workers are more likely to be covered by insurance and salaried employees by the more permissive wage continuation arrangements. Premium costs for short-term disability insurance run about 0.5 to 2.0% of total payroll, with exceptions at both extremes (e.g., 0.006 to 3.0% of the payroll), reflecting variations in the scope of coverage. In 1983 about 64 million Americans (63% of workers) had some short-term disability coverage (16, p. 8).

2. Long-term disability programs usually are insured, typically cover only a fraction of the employee's wage (usually not more than 60%), and tend to go into effect 6 months to 2 years into a continuous absence. They may pay benefits for at least 5 years but often until age 65 or for life. Some 25 million people had private long-term disability coverage in 1983 (16, p. 8).

3. The income-maintenance portion of mandatory workers' compensation coverage also produces indirect costs. These payments replace a fraction of the wage of an

employee disabled by a work-related injury or illness. About 70% of workers' compensation outlays are for these indirect costs of cash payments for income replacement, as distinct from coverage for medical care. On average, workers' compensation runs 2.55% of payroll and ranges from 0.86 to 4.34%, depending on the state and often the experience of the firm (11, p. 369).

The second major component of indirect costs comprises death benefits to survivors of deceased employees as well as other welfare payments, such as continuing health insurance. Third, there are various indirect costs related to workforce management: recruitment, training, and other accommodations to temporary absence or turnover. They are true productivity costs but are rarely quantified carefully, at least not in the health literature. Absenteeism is the measure of indirect costs most frequently used in research on health programs at work. Absenteeism stands in as almost an omnibus proxy for "productivity." Behind this substitution lies the simple syllogism that a worker has to report for the job in order to produce anything that day. There are a few problems the syllogism overlooks, however: If mere attendance is necessary for productivity (and even that holds for only some jobs), certainly it is not sufficient. Moreover, measuring attendance turns out to be less straightforward than it may seem.

Incidental Absenteeism

Unlike nearly all other cost indicators, absenteeism rates are going down (Table 15–13). Data collected in the May 1985 Current Population Survey indicate that the average American worker lost 7.2 days of work that year, compared to 9.7 in 1980, a more than 20% decline. Possible explanations for the improvement include the 1981–1982 recession, in which many chronically poor attenders probably lost their jobs, and a variety of belt-tightening initiatives by employers were instituted to stay competitive in the economic upswing. These reductions were especially prominent in the manufacturing sector, whose employee absence rates in 1985 were lower than those in the service sector for the first time since the BLS started counting (24).

In a typical week in 1985, about 4.7% of the full-time workforce missed a scheduled day of work (owing to illness, injury, civic duties, or personal affairs); 2.6% of hours that should have been worked were lost to absences. These rates, too, represent an improvement over 1980 of about 20% (24). Extrapolating from earlier research, the overall absence rate translates to well over $37 billion in annual costs (44).

As a bridge between health and productivity, absenteeism data are weak in many ways.

1. They tend to be collected, in automated and accessible formats, only or mostly for employees earning an hourly wage. Managerial, technical, and professional workers (and companies with large concentrations of them) seem often to elude formalistic reporting of days missed from work.

2. Definitions can be elastic and loose. The BLS advocates specific rates, but their taxonomy is seldom used because appropriate denominators to construct the indices are often unavailable.

3. Concerns must be raised about the reliability and validity of reported absence rates. In our studies of problem drinking at work, employees' recall of their absenteeism correlates poorly with computerized company records (40.7% agreement, after

adjusting for known periods of hospitalization) (50). Whether more inaccuracies originate in the company's records, in respondents' recall, or clumsiness on our part is difficult to say. The headaches we have had (in other studies) trying to integrate medical claims and absenteeism files, however, inspire little confidence in company records as a panacea.

4. Philosophical nuances may influence the responses individuals give and how to interpret them. Is a day missed by a worker who has a full month of paid vacation the functional equivalent of a day missed by someone entitled to only a week? Should the absence of a parent to care for a sick child (or an adult child, caring for an elderly parent) weigh equally with the "go-to-Hell day" taken by a worker who literally has "gone fishing"? What about people who feel sick and drag themselves into work; should that not count somewhere? How much do job satisfaction and commitment figure into absence taking? Does "corporate culture" matter, and how influential are the incentives that income-replacement programs create?

Despite a sizable transdisciplinary literature addressing these and related questions (12), much room remains for doubt about the balance in "employee withdrawal behavior" between "motivation" and "ability" to attend (44). Variations in rates of missing work (and rates of return after illness) are influenced by at least the following factors and probably others: (a) Individuals differ in their ability to "rise above" pain and discomfort; (b) workers differ in motivation, commitment to the job, and the tug of counterpressures from outside responsibilities and enticements; (c) jobs differ in the demands they make and rewards they return; (d) physicians differ in the advice they give about how long to convalesce; (e) companies differ in how effectively they manage disability and absenteeism; (f) benefit plans differ in terms of the incentives they create for attending work; (g) workforces differ in their cultures and attitudes toward "the boss."

Thus even this relatively simple stand-in for the far more variegated notion of productivity taps a construct that is anything but straightforward and unidimensional. Absence is hardly a pure measure of illness effect.

WORK, HEALTH, PRODUCTIVITY, AND ILLNESS COSTS; WHERE DOES IT LEAVE US?

For years, some progressive companies have sponsored health conservation programs. More recently, health advocates have been trying to bring more companies along by cloaking such programs in an economic rationale, but the enthusiasm has papered over wide gaps in knowledge, and business managers are becoming skeptical of economic claims being made for health enhancement programs. There is the danger of some disappointed expectations and ultimately of a backlash against health protection and health-promotion programs at work unless their cost impact can be quantified more convincingly. An important step would be to estimate more fully what illness is really costing employers.

A barrier to accomplishing this task has been the tendency to approach health care costs from a social perspective because data are more easily available on that level of aggregation. It is simpler to take a social perspective and pay attention to all costs. From that perspective, the indirect costs of illness overshadow the direct costs because when the medical bills are all settled earnings losses are still being felt. Shifting to the employer's perspective tends to reverse the relation: Companies pay more for (direct) illness costs than they do for (indirect) income replacement, or so it seems.

Perhaps if companies would, or could, account more fully for their human capital costs associated with erosion in the vitality and capacity of a labor force, the indirect costs of illness (physical and mental) would loom larger than they do. Meanwhile, we face the challenge that has long stymied health advocates within business firms: Prevention of chronic illness is by definition a long-term proposition and often runs counter to short-term profit objectives of the firm.

It seems evident that in this era of international competition and cost cutting in American industry health programs are being scrutinized as never before (48). The easiest and quickest way to improve productivity is to "downsize" the labor force, as many companies are now doing. Health staffs and programs are among the first to go. The staffs' only hope (and it may be too late) is to learn to pay their own way. From a policy perspective, then, there is an urgent need for a more compelling—and more credible—picture of the costs of illness at the workplace, however preliminary, tentative, and flawed it may have to be at the start. Without such a picture, health conservation programs at work appear vulnerable indeed.

ACKNOWLEDGMENTS

Thanks are owed to Gerald Oster, Ph.D., and Lester Lave, Ph.D., for helpful critiques of the manuscript; to Edward J. Bernakci, M.D., Charles R. Buck, Sc.D., John Burns, M.D., James P. Dunn, M.D., Jeanne F. Kardos, Curtis Mikkelson, Patricia M. Nazametz, David Repko, and Brian Saylor, Ph.D., for access to data; to Robert St. John for data analysis; to Susan E. Kelleher for help with manuscript preparation; to the Pew Memorial Trust and the Kellogg National Fellowship Program for financial support.

REFERENCES

1. Antonakes, J. A. (1981). Claims costs of back pain. *Bests Review, 82*(5), 36–40.
2. Association of Schools of Public Health. (1986). *Proposed national strategies for the prevention of work-related diseases and injuries*. Published by the Association in cooperation with the National Institute for Occupational Safety and Health.
3. Berry, R., & Boland, J. P. (1977). *The economic cost of alcohol abuse*. New York: Free Press.
4. Chollet, D. J. (1984). *Employer-provided health benefits*. Washington, DC: Employee Benefit Research Institute.
5. Cooper, B. S., & Rice, D. B. (1986). The economic cost of illness revisited. *Social Security Bulletin, 39*(2), 21.
6. Cruze, A., Harwood, H., Kristiansen, P., Collins, J., & Jones, D. (1981). Economic costs of alcohol and drug abuse and mental illness—1977. Research Triangle Park, NC: Research Triangle Institute.

7. Dopkeen, J. C. (1987). Postretirement health benefits. *Health Services Research, 21*, 795–848.
8. Fein, R. (1958). *Economics of mental illness.* New York: Basic Books.
9. Fein, R. (1976). On measuring economic benefits of health programs. In R. M. Veatch & R. Branson (eds.). *Ethics and health policy* (pp. 261–87). Cambridge, MA: Balinger.
10. Fein, R. (1984). *Alcohol in America: the price we pay.* Newport Beach, CA: Care Institute.
11. Fielding, J. E. (1984). *Corporate health management*. Reading, MA: Addison-Wesley.
12. Goodman, P. S., Atkin, R. S., et al. (1984). *Absenteeism*. San Francisco, CA: Jossey-Bass.
13. Graham, G. (1982). Statement to U.S. Senate Committee on Finance, Subcommittee on Health. *Medical coverage of alcoholism treatment* (Hearing, 97th Congress, two sessions). Washington, DC: U.S. Government Printing Office.
14. Hartunian, N. S., Smart, C. N., & Thompson,

M. S. (1980). The incidence and economic costs of cancer, motor vehicle injuries, coronary heart disease, and stroke: a comparative analysis. *American Journal of Public Health, 70,* 1249–60.

15. Harwood, H. J., Kristiansen, P., & Rachal, J. V. (1985). *Social and economic costs of alcohol abuse and alcoholism* (issue report 2). Research Triangle Park, NC: Research Triangle Institute.

16. Health Insurance Association of America. (1985). *Source book of health insurance data, 1984–1985.* Washington, DC: HIAA.

17. Hingson, R. W., Lederman, R. I., & Walsh, D. C. (1985). Employee drinking patterns and accidental injury: a study of four New England states. *Journal of Studies on Alcohol, 46,* 298–303.

18. Hodgson, T. A. (1983). The state of the art of cost of illness estimates. *Advances in Health Economics and Health Services Research, 4,* 129–64.

19. Hodgson, T. A., & Meiners, M. R. (1979). Guidelines for cost of illness studies in the Public Health Service. U.S. Public Health Service, unpublished.

20. Holder, H. D. (1987). Alcoholism treatment and health care utilization. *Medical Care, 25,* 52–71.

21. Institute of Medicine. (1981). *Costs of environment-related health effects: a plan for continuing study.* Washington, DC: National Academy Press.

22. Karasek, R. A., Theorell, T., Schwartz, J. E., Schnall, P. L., Pieper, C.F., & Michele, J. L. (1988). Job characteristics in relation to the prevalence of myocardial infarction in the US Health Examination Survey (HES) and the Health and Nutrition Examination Survey (HANES). *American Journal of Public Health, 78,* 910–19.

23. Klarman, H. (1964). Syphilis control programs. In R. Dorfman (ed.). *Measuring benefits of government investments* (pp. 367–414). Washington, DC: Brookings Institute.

24. Klein, B. W. (1986). Missed work and lost hours, May 1985. *Monthly Labor Review,* November, pp. 26–30.

25. Kristein, M. M. (1977). Economic issues in prevention. *Preventive Medicine, 6,* 252–64.

26. Kristein, M. M. (1982). The economics of health promotion in the workplace. *Health Education Quarterly, 9,* 27–36.

27. Kristein, M. M. (1983). How much can business expect to profit from smoking cessation? *Preventive Medicine, 12,* 358–81.

28. Labor Month in Review. (1987). *Monthly Labor Review,* April, p. 2.

29. Mellow, W. S. (1982). Determinants of health insurance and pension coverage. *Monthly Labor Review,* May, pp. 30–32.

30. Mendeloff, J. (1980). Reducing occupational health risks: uncertain effects and unstated benefits. *Technology Review,* May, pp. 66–78.

31. Millars, J. D., & Myers, M. L. (1983). Occupational safety and health: progress toward the 1990 objectives for the nation. *Public Health Reports, 98,* 324–36.

32. Mushkin, S. (1962). Health as an investment. *Journal of Political Economy, 70*(5, part II, suppl.), 129.

33. Mushkin, S. (1979). *Biomedical research: costs and benefits.* Cambridge, MA: Ballinger.

34. Nicholson, W. J., Perkel, G., & Selikoff, J. J. (1982). Occupational exposure to asbestos: population at risk and protected mortality 1980–2000. *American Journal of Industrial Medicine, 3,* 259–311.

35. Office of Technology Assessment. (1980). *The cost-effectiveness analysis of medical technology* (publication OTA-H-126). Washington, DC: Congress of the United States.

36. Office of Technology Assessment. (1985). *Preventing illness and injury in the workplace* (publication OTA-H-256). Washington, DC: Congress of the United States.

37. Oster, G., Colditz, G. A., & Kelly, N. (1984). *The economic costs of smoking and the benefits of quitting.* Lexington, MA: Lexington Books.

38. Rice, D. P. (1966). *Estimating the cost of illness* (Health Economics Series 6, publication 947-6). Washington, DC: U.S. Government Printing Office.

39. Rice, D. P., Hodgson, T. A., & Kopstein, A. N. (1985). The economic costs of illness: a replication and update. *Health Care Financing Review, 7*(1), 61–80.

40. Salkever, D. S. (1985). Morbidity costs: national estimates and economic determinants (DHHS publication PHS 86-3393). Washington, DC: Department of Health and Human Services.

41. Schelling, T. (1986). Economics and cigarettes. *Preventive Medicine, 15,* 549–60.

42. Schnall, P. L., Pieper, C., Schwartz, J. E., Karasek, R. A., Schlussel, Y., Devereux, R. B., Ganau, A., Alderman, M., Warren, K., & Pickering, T. G. (1990). The relationship between "job strain," workplace diastolic blood pressure, and left ventricular mass index. Results of a case-control study. *Journal of the American Medical Association, 263,* 1929–35.

43. Scitovsky, A. A. (1982). Estimating the direct cost of illness. *Milbank Memorial Fund Quarterly/Health and Society, 3,* 463–91.

44. Steers, R. M., & Rhodes, S. R. (1978). Major influences on employee attendance: a process model. *Journal of Applied Psychology, 63,* 3391–3407.

45. U.S. Department of Health and Human Services. (1987). Health policy: request for grant applications. *Federal Register,* July 23, 52, 27724–31.

46. U.S. Department of Labor. (1986). *Employee benefits in medium and large firms, 1985.* Washington, DC: Bureau of Labor Statistics.

47. Waldo, D. R., Levit, K. R., & Lazenby, H.

(1986). National health expenditures, 1985. *Health Care Financing Review, 8*(1), 1–21.

48. Walsh, D. C. (1987). *Corporate physicians: between medicine and management.* New Haven, CT: Yale University Press.

49. Walsh, D. C., Connor, E., Tracey, L. V., Goldberg, G. A., & Egdahl, R. H. (1989). Posthospital convalescence and return to work. *Health Affairs,* Fall, *8,* 76–91.

50. Walsh, D. C., & Hingson, R. W., (1985). Where to refer employees for treatment of drinking problems: the limited evidence from empirical research. *Journal of Occupational Medicine,* October, *27* (10): 745–52.

51. Weis, W. L. (1981). No ifs ands or buts: why workplace smoking should be banned. *Management World,* September, pp. 38–44.

52. Weisbrod, B. (1961). *Economics of public health.* Philadelphia: University of Pennsylvania Press.

16
Health, Productivity, and the Economic Environment: Dynamic Role of Socioeconomic Status

M. Harvey Brenner

From an epidemiological perspective, one of the main issues in occupational health is the differential distribution of illnesses and mortality among occupational groups. The most fundamental discriminator of health and longevity differentials among occupations is socioeconomic status. Socioeconomic status, based on the rank ordering of occupations by skill level and income, is also the most powerful and pervasive variable in chronic, mental, infectious, trauma-related, and infant/child illnesses in industrialized (and developing) countries.

The economic and sociological literature indicates that many of the differences in socioeconomic status among individuals are a by-product of former and contemporaneous changes in the overall economic system. One purpose of this chapter is to identify some of the mechanisms whereby economic changes influence the dynamics of socioeconomic status and thus health and longevity.

The chapter begins with some prominent studies of the relation between socioeconomic status and physical and mental health. This review is followed by a discussion of the direct and indirect mechanisms whereby socioeconomic status is thought to influence health. In the next section it is argued that change in the elements of socioeconomic status within a population, and in the overall socioeconomic status of populations, is mainly a by-product of changes in the national economy: real per capita income growth based on productivity, economic instability as indicated by recessions, and policies relating to economic inequality. There are indications, however, that the first year of productivity increase may involve increased health risk associated with the stresses of adaptation to new technology, restructuring of organizations, and migration due to shifts in regional patterns of employment.

OVERALL MORTALITY AND SOCIOECONOMIC STATUS

Since the mid-1970s studies in industrialized countries of the relation between socioeconomic status and overall mortality have been uniform in showing an inverse relation (77,84,110). In the United States, for individuals in the general population

241

(1960), the basic relation was observed in studies using education, income, and occupation as measures of socioeconomic status (66). The relation has also been found among armed services personnel (100) using rank as a measure of socioeconomic status, and it has been measured in specific cities (Birmingham, Buffalo, Indianapolis) (112) and one state (Maryland) (70) using census tracts as the unit of study. Finally, even at the individual level of analysis, higher total mortality has been found associated with residence in poverty areas (51).

In Canada the inverse relation between socioeconomic status and all-cause mortality has been measured by occupational group (6) and by median household income for census tracts (85). Among western European countries, if not all countries, the United Kingdom has the longest and most consistent history of observation of the inverse relation between socioeconomic status and mortality rates beginning in the mid-nineteenth century for England and Wales (1). The basic relation is found in the decade-specific cross-sectional studies conducted by the Registrar General among men from 1911 to 1971 and among married women from 1931 to 1971 (75) and more recently in longitudinal studies of the population (46). The inverse relation in the United Kingdom appears to have become stronger (i.e., the class inequality in mortality has increased) between 1921 and 1972 for men and at least since the 1930s for women (91). These findings are consistent with observations of manual versus nonmanual occupational differences in mortality for both 1970/1972 and 1979/1983 for men and women in Great Britain. At least for men the nonmanual to manual advantage increased through the 1970s (76).

In France 12 socioprofessional categories have been used to observe the basic socioeconomic status-mortality relation. This relation has been found for men throughout the period 1956 to 1971 (72) and, following a cohort since 1954, through examination of differential mortality rates during 1966 to 1971 (68).

Among Nordic countries, Finland has provided the largest number of epidemiological studies of the socioeconomic status-mortality relation. The inverse relation was measured using five occupational groups for 1969 to 1972 (89) and 1971 to 1975 (108) in both sexes but was much stronger for men. For eastern Finland the relation was observed on the basis of income and education in a longitudinal study of men (98). Using income and educational difference measures, the basic inverse relation was found for Norway in a prospective study of Oslo men during 1972 to 1977. Even after income adjustment the educational gradients showed a clear relation, although it is especially the lowest income group that showed the highest mortality rates (56). Although for many years the relation had been observed in Sweden, the relation between occupational rank and mortality was reviewed in English only in 1986 (31).

In the Pacific region, Australian data show the inverse relation between socioeconomic status and mortality among men using a nine-occupational grouping of classes for 1968 to 1978 (81). In New Zealand the inverse relation is found among men using both the British Registrar General's classification (five occupational classes) and a classification that involves a weighting of median income and education for 1975 to 1977 (92). This relation was then extended to 1974 to 1978 using the Registrar General's classification (93). For Japan an inverse relation between social class (nine occupational categories) and mortality is seen among men, with mortality unusually low for the two highest grades and highest for miners, as is also found for England and Wales (59,60).

Similar inverse relations are observed with respect to coronary heart disease mortality in many of the above-mentioned studies. Among all of the studies in industrialized countries cited above, only in Japan was there no inverse relation found between coronary heart disease and socioeconomic status (59). In the studies cited, for overall cancer mortality there is an inverse relation to socioeconomic status for the United States, United Kingdom, Finland, France, and New Zealand. For lung cancer, again among the studies cited, there is an inverse relation found for the United States, United Kingdom, and Finland, but not for Japan. Breast cancer, by contrast, shows a higher incidence among higher socioeconomic status women (United States, United Kingdom, Finland), but a significant positive relation of socioeconomic status to survival, i.e., inverse relation to case fatality (4,33,69).

The inverse relation of socioeconomic status to mortality that is perhaps best known involves infants. This point has been documented for years in different parts of the world (2) but continues to be prominently observed in the United States (48,70,103,104,111), United Kingdom (91), and Scotland (44).

The basic inverse relation between socioeconomic status and mental disorder has been observed in more than 40 studies since at least the late 1930s. The first of the most prominent studies was done in Chicago by researchers who had mapped the city in socioeconomic terms and found that the centrally located areas, where poverty and social disorganization were most frequent, showed the highest rates of first admissions for schizophrenia (41). The landmark study in this field demonstrated the inverse relation between social class position and treatment for mental disorder based on a census in New Haven (55). This study was followed by the principal study of untreated prevalence in New York City, which found an inverse relation between socioeconomic status and degree of mental impairment (102). It is this series of studies that first raised the question of whether environmentally induced stress, related to national economic changes and most frequently found in lower socioeconomic groups, was largely responsible for the inverse relation between socioeconomic status and morbidity (73).

MECHANISMS OF THE SOCIOECONOMIC STATUS–HEALTH RELATION

Direct and indirect mechanisms underlie the relation between lower socioeconomic status and poorer health and survival. *Direct* mechanisms involve lower levels of (1) control over the human and nonhuman environment, (2) knowledge, (3) material wealth, (4) affiliation (social support and more general societal integration), and (5) mental health (i.e., self-esteem based on status, achievement, intellectual stimulation, power). Examination of this direct group of mechanisms reveals that some are intrinsic attributes of the socioeconomic status of occupations whereas others are derived.

1. *Control* is the dimension of authority that is attached to work roles. It represents administrative power over the direction of work of the individual and other employees, over exposure of workers to stressors or other health risks (e.g., physical or chemical hazards), over decisions concerning organization strategy, over hiring and terminations, and so on.

2. *Knowledge* is also a dimension of occupational role in terms of skill requirements. Specified levels of education are generally requisite to attainment of jobs ranked above particular levels. Persons with higher levels of education, in turn, tend to

be more knowledgeable of (a) health risks involving consumption, production, and infection, and (b) the means to avoid or counteract those risks.

3. *Material wealth* represents, in part, cumulative income that is differentially remunerated, via the firm and marketplace, according to the assumed value of work position and work performed. It underlies the ability of the person to demand goods and services in a market economy—from the most basic (nutrition, shelter, sanitation, communication, transportation, health care) to that which provides comfort, pleasure, relief from stress (e.g., relaxation, entertainment) and nonwork aspects of creativity and expressiveness. It is also the means of purchasing education and the services of varied specialists.

4. *Affiliation,* or the intensity and frequency of valued social relationships, is connected in a derivative manner to socioeconomic status. Thus the extent of resources such as control (i.e., administrative power), knowledge, and material wealth available to an individual makes the person relatively valuable for a social relationship in societies where status is minimally based on kinship networks.

5. *Mental health* is understood in this discussion as the overall feeling of optimism related to a *psychological sense* of control over, or confidence in, being able to negotiate the human and nonhuman environment. It is connected to the self-esteem and self-efficacy that derive from a life that is relatively fulfilling and is supported by the above identified resources of administrative power, knowledge, material wealth, and affiliation.

The second set of mechanisms in the socioeconomic status–health relation is *indirect.* Because of lower levels of *control* over the human (and nonhuman) environment, lower socioeconomic groups are more at risk to experience external shocks, especially those that involve the economy, e.g., recession and other sources of economic instability. At the same time, owing to lower levels of resources (material wealth, mental health, knowledge, and affiliation) it is less possible for lower socioeconomic groups to deflect, or otherwise mediate, such shocks. Therefore they also experience these shocks in a more severe manner.

The greater frequency of economic shocks, compounded by heightened severity (due to fewer mitigating resources), lead to more frequent and severe coping responses (i.e., stress reactions). Such responses include damage to social networks (divorce, separation, migration), emotional responses (aggression, depression, denial), and, interacting with lower knowledge levels, problems with alcohol, tobacco, drugs, and obesity.

External economic shocks thus produce a greater number and severity of *negative life changes,* which represent the summation of initial economic losses, more extended and severe economic losses due to fewer mitigating factors, and more damaging coping responses.

KEY MACROECONOMIC INFLUENCES ON CHANGE IN SOCIOECONOMIC STATUS AND HEALTH

Economic growth is the principal source of advance in socioeconomic status. It provides the basis for individual achievement, social mobility, and real income enhancement. It provides the means for financial protection of the socially, physically, and mentally disabled and disadvantaged. It is the source of "human capital" investment in future economic achievement and social mobility via education, health care, skill development, and retraining.

Economic growth provides the means for its own self-regeneration through investments in scientific and technological development. The yield of research and development, when applied to the industrial base, is increased productivity.

Economic growth is the basis of long-term improvement in a population's health. Materially, it is the foundation of improved nutrition, sanitation, transportation, communication, and health care access. Psychologically, it is requisite to the sense of control over aspects of the human and nonhuman environment by large segments of the population. Finally, investment in the health sciences, made possible by economic growth, is the source of disease prevention and increased health care effectiveness.

On the negative side, because economic growth depends on productivity, which is in turn based on technological change, there may be some short-term health costs involved in adaptation to these changes and to the obsolescence of older skills and patterns of living. Additional costs of economic growth have been related to increases in purchasing power under specified conditions. When purchasing power increased at a rate that greatly exceeded society's knowledge of health risks involved in specific types of consumption, epidemic patterns of chronic disease resulted. This pattern has pertained from World War II to the late 1960s in regard to tobacco, animal fat, and alcohol (especially spirits) consumption, with pernicious consequences for cardiovascular health (35). Finally, the rate of production of specific substances, especially chemicals, apparently required for productivity gains has also tended to exceed society's knowledge of disease risks and ability to control environmental contamination (38,39).

Economic recession is indicated by increases in unemployment and business failure rates, declines in overall income and stock market prices, and decreased labor force participation. In general, recession has the reverse effect on the health of economic growth. In the short to medium term it brings about a cluster of some of the most severe stresses that are common in modern society: occupational failure, status loss, income loss, and finally forced downward mobility.

The key problems thought to result from such stresses are (a) psychophysiological illness affecting cardiovascular and immune systems (54,97,101); (b) classic "psychosomatic" illness, i.e., perception of transient or chronic pain or ill health in the absence of diagnosable physical illness (82,83); (c) lapse in concentration (affecting, for example, accidents) depression, aggression, and other mental disturbances (95); and (d) "alienation," i.e., a severe decline in motivation linked to loss, frustration, and antagonism (43,47).

These psychophysiological and behavioral responses obviously threaten to greatly disrupt social functioning and therefore social integration, i.e., the supportive networks of family, friendships, and community (27). However, more directly and immediately injurious to social integration is the recessional loss of jobs and the loss and financial damage to work organizations. In addition, lack of social integration in itself is now understood to be a significant risk to physical and mental health (25,58). Recession is also a principal source of work stress, involving major anxiety to workers and management over losses of job, career, and income in a situation they are unable to control because the economic decline is industry-wide, nationwide, or even international.

Over the long term the output of recession is downward mobility of the population that does not fully recover during the immediately subsequent national economic "recovery." A substantial proportion of this population is reemployed but at a significantly lower level of job status and income (7,42,52,57,106). Over the longer term they suffer relative income loss compared with their age-peers and the remainder of society who were not as injured by the recession. A major segment of this group must migrate to a new employment source. They leave behind their families and friends and their former work associates. Like themselves, many of those left behind experience the loss of community and social integration that is crucial to social support and thus to health and longevity.

The long-term health effects of recession on mortality are also indirect and stem from the well known (29,71) impact of ill health on subsequent income deterioration. The impact of serious physical and mental health problems stemming from recession involves additional economic losses due to lowered job performance, discriminatory practices, continued unemployment, and early retirement.

Finally, whether the recessional stresses fall on those at work or those ejected from the labor force, some of the coping mechanisms may be emotional, e.g., withdrawal, denial, aggression, or they may involve behavioral patterns such as alcohol or tobacco abuse. In those cases the long-term risks to health are compounded by family disruption or biochemical changes. It is traditionally found that the first peak of mortality following recession occurs approximately 2 to 3 years after the peak of unemployment or business failure rates (8,16,17,20,23). Cumulative economic and social status losses among those who do not recover and a keen sense of increased inequality, as most of society experiences economic gain during the subsequent economic recovery and expansion, are thought to explain this lagged phenomenon. An additional explanatory factor is undoubtedly the fact that the major causes of overall mortality are chronic diseases. Severe negative mental health responses to economic recession, as are indicated by suicide rates and mental hospital admissions, increase *within* the year of recession (14,16,19).

In addition to the 2 to 3-year lag between recession and the overall mortality increase, there is at least a 1-year lag between economic growth and the decline in mortality. It is hypothesized that this short lag partly reflects the difficulty of adjustment to the technological changes that make productivity increases possible.

Two factors are hypothesized to be operating here. First, consistent with classic formulations, the introduction of technology frequently threatens to make obsolete the skills and orientation of specified groups of workers and managers. This threat of obsolescence and the subsequent unemployment or downward mobility, is realized if the employees are *not* retrained for work in the new technology. This situation may occur because the employees resist the technological change or because the firm prefers to invest in the training or hiring of new, younger staff.

The second factor is in line with the demand-control model of job stress and diminished health. Adjustment to the use of new technology may both heighten work intensity and, at least temporarily, diminish the sense of control employees have over the work process. The interaction of environmental stress and relative absence of control has been found to be predictive in morbidity and mortality studies (3,30,61,62,99).

Following the approximately 1-year process of adjustment to the social changes involved in economic growth, i.e., technological change, work reorganization, work relocation through migration, and restructuring of social networks, the benefits of economic growth for health and longevity are manifest, substantial, and lasting.

EMPIRICAL RELATIONS BETWEEN NATIONAL ECONOMIC CHANGE AND HEALTH/LONGEVITY

In the post-World War United States, interest in the relation between economic change and health appears to have developed most rapidly in the mental health field. The classic studies in psychiatric epidemiology had demonstrated the basic inverse relation between social class and the prevalence of mental disorders (55,67). At the micro level, however, two opposing explanations seemed possible: (a) the stresses, vulnerabilities, and poorer resources of lower social group life increased the likelihood of mental disorder; and (b) mental disorder during early life led to decreased social/economic competence and subsequent decline in socioeconomic status.

However, the business cycle literature in economics had indicated that individual socioeconomic position was greatly influenced by national economic changes. In addition, it was well known that individuals of low socioeconomic status were at high risk for unemployment and economic losses related to recession. The enigma of causal direction in the social group/mental disorder relation could be partially unraveled if it were shown that population rates of mental disorder (i.e., symptoms) were related to the economic losses of recession. This possibility was, in fact, strongly suggested by data showing that increases in admission rates to mental hospitals in New York State were greatly influenced by employment declines during both the nineteenth (1841–1899) and twentieth (1900–1967) centuries (11).

Extension of the employment/mental disorder relation at the community level was subsequently demonstrated for Kansas City. Using aggregate measures for a city-wide area, over time, Catalano and Dooley (28) demonstrated a relation between life events and the rate of unemployment. This finding provided a link to previous research showing a connection between life events and psychiatric impairment (27,34,88,96).

Moving from psychiatric morbidity to mortality, the relation between recession and the suicide rate was demonstrated in several studies (8,14,19,53) and the extensive review by Platt (94) continuing a theoretical tradition that had originated with Durkheim (36). The relation between recession and other important sources of stress-related mortality was documented for the early twentieth century to the late 1960s. The causes of mortality included cardiovascular disease, homicide, cirrhosis, and diseases of infancy (8–10,12).

In 1976 a study sponsored by the Joint Economic Committee of Congress estimated the overall impact of economic change on mental and physical health and criminal aggression (13). This study, covering 1941 to 1974, examined the impact of unemployment, real per capita income, and inflation on pathological indices: age- and sex-specific overall mortality, cause-specific mortality (cardiovascular, cirrhosis, suicide, homicide), mental hospitalization, and imprisonment for the United States and three states. It was found that over a 6-year (distributed) lag period the unemployment rate was virtually always related to increased pathology; the trend in real per capita income usually related to decreased pathology; and no stable relation could be observed between inflation and pathology rates.

It was subsequently observed for the United States that, whereas the economic growth trend was vital to the trends of decline in age-specific mortality and recession had short- to medium-term damaging implications for mortality rates, the *first* year of rapid economic growth (i.e., following recession) was associated with higher mortality rates (17). The damaging early impact of economic growth was then understood to reflect (a) processes of urbanization and industrialization that involved large-scale changes—and therefore discontinuities—in social networks, and (b) reintegration of a portion of the population that had been unemployed during the previous recession (i.e., a year earlier) into jobs of lower socioeconomic status—a situation of forced downward mobility.

The analysis was replicated for England and Wales covering the period 1936 to 1976 in an age-specific analysis of mortality (15). For all age groups the long-term beneficial effect of economic growth and damaging effects of recession—measured by the impact of unemployment over a 10-year distributed lag period—could be observed. However, for England and Wales the hypothesized effect of rapid economic growth was not observed.

The early model, presented in the analysis of mortality in England and Wales (15), was also replicated successfully using an unemployment series that avoided problems specific to the official unemployment statistics (49), but the authors also questioned whether the basic relations could be measured for other periods. Nonetheless, in detailed studies of England, Wales, and Scotland using alternate models and time periods, for cause-specific mortality over 1955 to 1976 (18,24) and 1955 to 1979 (18,24), the basic relations for economic growth and recession continued to be observed. In addition, Bunn in Australia (26) and Forbes and Player in Scotland (45) had observed similar relations for unemployment and coronary heart disease mortality covering other periods.

Variations in the stability of the basic relations in nine countries (18,79) made clear that it would be necessary to take into account epidemiological risk factors originally associated with increased national purchasing power and industrial development. Such risk factors—alcohol, cigarette, and animal fat consumption; automobile use; chemical production—were offsetting the beneficial aspects of economic growth by contributing to mortality due to chronic diseases, accidents, and mental health problems.

The major statistical problem was that the patterns of relation between the consumption/production epidemiological risks and real income per capita were changing over time. The consumption risks, in particular, were positively related to real income growth only until the late 1960s in the United States. Therefore epidemiological risks could no longer be assumed to be a regular (or necessary) cost of economic growth and had to be measured separately (18,24).

A formulation that included basic economic indices—economic growth, economic instability (i.e., recession), economic inequality—as well as epidemiological risks initially associated with economic growth and random shocks was developed in a second study for the Joint Economic Committee of Congress in 1984 (20). This study included income, unemployment, labor force participation, and business failure rates as economic indices and showed for 1950 to 1980 the beneficial effects of long-term growth and damaging effects of recession for major causes of mortality, mental health care use, and criminal justice indices. This approach was successfully replicated with

Swedish data over 1950 to 1980 (21), for total and cardiovascular mortality in Scotland over 1952 to 1985 (22), and for heart disease in nine industrialized countries (23). The adverse mental health consequences and short-term physical symptoms of unemployment have been the subject of study on the individual level of analysis since at least the 1930s and have been amply reviewed (24,90,109). Stimulated in part by the macrostudies and by the persistence and extent of unemployment during the 1980s, a large number of individual, or micro, level studies have been undertaken, and several have measured the longer-term strength of this relation.

These studies have basically confirmed findings observed earlier at the national level in terms of types of health response and lag relations. Most recently, in the United States the study emphases have been on anxiety, depression, and general health (65,74) and on psychophysiological responses and learned helplessness (5). Canadian reports have focused on psychological distress and health services utilization (32).

It is in Britain, however, that we find the most precise analyses of causal relations linking unemployment and mortality rates. Studies by Moser et al. (86,87) have shown a long-term (i.e., at least 10 years cumulative lag) effect of unemployment on elevated mortality rates controlling for social group. They found that unemployed male subjects and their wives showed significantly elevated mortality rates in relation to the unemployment of the men. They further were able to determine that the adverse effects of unemployment, rather than initial poor health of those who become unemployed, accounted for the excess mortality of the unemployed. These analyses have been supported by studies of heightened long-standing illness among the unemployed compared to the employed (3).

ECONOMIC POLICIES AFFECTING RECESSION AND PRODUCTIVITY GROWTH

We have identified long-term economic growth (via productivity enhancement) and recession (or economic instability) as two of the key macroeconomic factors affecting socioeconomic status and thus health. It is critical, however, to understand that national *policy* pertaining to recession is a principal influence on productivity rates. Federal intervention can routinely improve or seriously damage the performance of the national economy. Nor is there any inevitability to recession that is inherent in the business "cycle." There have been no "accidental" recessions in the United States since 1960 to 1961; each recession since then resulted from deliberate acts of policy intended to control inflation (50; 92, p. 35; 107, p. 152). Since 1948, for example, the United States has had nine recessions, whereas Japan has had only two (105, p. 203).

The frequency and severity of recessions have substantial damaging effects on productivity growth (63). First, policies that minimize economic contractions and promote growth (without accelerating inflation) foster capital formation, economies of scale, and overall productivity increases (64, p. 310). Second, recession leads to substantial layoffs, high labor turnover, job insecurity, and strained labor–management relations, which considerably reduce the potential for productivity growth.

Layoffs adversely affect the training of the labor force, which leads to critical shortages of skilled laborers. Skilled blue collar workers are at high risk of being laid off during recessions, which obviously interrupts on-the-job training. The resulting shortage of blue collar workers during the subsequent economic expansion not only cuts short the potential for further expansion but provides foreign competitors an entry into American markets (78, p. 347; 105, p. 201). Additionally, the competition among employers for skilled blue-collar workers can lead to a wage-price spiral before full employment is achieved. Federal policy may then mandate the use of fiscal and monetary stringency to prevent further acceleration of inflation. This situation, in turn, produces recession. Investment is also reduced in this vicious cycle because a substantial stock of available capital remains idle in order to control inflation (105, p. 200).

High layoff rates also mean that although workers can be fired during business downturns they are encouraged and likely to leave for somewhat better job opportunities. Investment in training, which is therefore risky for employer and employee, is minimized, which obviously results in a less well trained work force. Altogether, the United States has an unusually high labor turnover rate compared with Europe (105, p. 343) and Japan (78). The relatively high labor turnover rate, which adversely affects long-term commitment to the firm, also results in short personal and corporate time horizons and foreshortening of the strategic planning required for improved productivity trends (105, p. 149).

High layoff rates clearly mean that the economic climate and the firm do not respect job security. In such an environment, there is realistic fear by workers and managers that technological change to improve productivity will eliminate jobs (78, p. 345; 105, p. 157). This situation leads to employee resistance to change through, for example, the use of restrictive work rules to increase predictability. There is evidence that resistance to change is the single most important restraint to increased productivity in the workplace and that such resistance is in turn strongly related to the firm's use of layoffs (80).

Yet another implication of recession is that it damages labor–management relations. Industrial disputes and working days lost during the disputes increase during recession. Significant relations have been found between the number of grievances and strikes, the time spent settling contracts, and decreases in productivity (78, p. 151).

ECONOMIC CHANGES AND MORTALITY DURING LATE MIDDLE AGE: SUMMARY REPORT OF A STUDY 1950–1985

We have examined, for the recent past, the relations between economic and behavioral factor changes for the United States using standard multivariate time series methodology and econometric modeling techniques (unpublished data). In this analysis, which updates U.S. findings for 1950 to 1980, we focused on annual changes in the mortality rate of the 55- to 64-year age group over the period 1950 to 1985. Concentration on this age group was for purposes of examining a population that at once shows a relatively high age-specific mortality rate and, at least for male heads of households, is essentially a working population. The latter point makes meaningful the analysis of unemployment, labor force participation, productivity, and work stress.

The study examined the impact of changes in income distribution on mortality rates. Increased economic concentration (i.e., inequality) and decreased age-specific median family income ratios were related to increased mortality rates within 1 to 2 years. National or regional studies of this type point to the importance of the *economic environment* in which individual firms must operate as a principal factor that determines the levels of work stress in American industry.

Conclusions of the Study: Economic Productivity, Work, and Health

We can now identify several of the broad economic factors that, operating through changes in socioeconomic status at the individual level, substantially alter population health and longevity patterns. They include elements of economic growth, recession, and inequality. Economic growth, through its direct effect on incomes and social mobility and its potential for investment in science, education, infrastructure, and health technology, is the fundamental source of improvement in a society's health.

Increased productivity (the source of economic growth) not only shows long-term benefits to health via increased real per capita income; even after a year of increased productivity, mortality rates begin to decline, controlling for other business cycle activity and life style risk factors dependent on purchasing power. It is likely, however, that adaptation to the first year of productivity increases—involving new technologies or organizational restructuring—involves some work stress but apparently not sufficient to adversely affect mortality rates in the late-middle-aged population. These and earlier (19,20) findings resolve questions raised about the "health risks" of prosperity (40) that continue to be cited in the research literature (37).

Economic recession—as indicated by decreased labor force participation, unemployment (over the short and long term), stock market price declines, and business failure rates—engenders patterns of elevated mortality, in part through short-term as well as permanent downward mobility. A particularly harsh aspect of the downward mobility is its imposition of relative deprivation (in addition to absolute economic and social status losses), especially during periods where much of the population experiences the benefits of economic growth.

Firms must respond to their economic environment by altering their production, investment, and marketing strategies as well as their plans for employment and unemployment, salaries/wages, career advancement, and working conditions. All of these factors depend on the relative success of the firm in managing the economic environment.

Individual-level studies of work stress, therefore, clearly need to take into account the economic environment and the financial status of the firm and its industry in order to correctly assess the significance of, for example, specific technology or work organization on health. The specific technology and work structure may be less important than *changes* in those factors, especially in relation to the financial success of the organization.

At the same time, individual-level studies of, for example, unemployment must account for comparison groups of non-unemployed persons in terms of whether they are undergoing other major work stresses related to the survival of economic organizations during recession and industrial decline.

Finally, the results of studying the implications of changing economic inequality in health show that relative deprivation may be as important as absolute socioeconomic level for mortality. Thus although economic growth is key to a nation's long-term health, the distribution of the fruits of that growth exerts a powerful moderating effect that must be considered fundamental to health policy.

REFERENCES

1. Antonovsky, A. (1967). Social class, life expectancy and overall mortality. *Milbank Memorial Fund Quarterly, 45,* 31–73.
2. Antonovsky, A. (1977). Social class and infant mortality. *Social Science and Medicine, 11,* 453–70.
3. Baker, D. B. (1985). The study of stress at work. *Annual Review of Public Health, 6,* 367–81.
4. Bassett, M. T., & Krieger, N. (1986). Social class and black-white differences in breast cancer survival. *American Journal of Public Health, 76,* 1400–3.
5. Baum, A., Raymond, F., & Reddy, D. M. (1986). Unemployment stress: loss of control, reactance and learned helplessness. *Social Science and Medicine, 22,* 509–16.
6. Billette, A., & Hill, G. B. (1978). Risque relatif de mortalite masculine et les classes sociales au Canada 1974. *L' Union Medicale du Canada, 107,* 583–90.
7. Bluestone, B., & Harrison, B. (1988). *The great U-turn.* New York: Basic Books.
8. Brenner, M. H. (1971). Economic changes and heart disease mortality. *American Journal Public Health, 61,* 606–61.
9. Brenner, M. H. (1971). *Time-series analysis of the relationship between selected economic and social indicators* (Department of Labor Manpower Administration). Washington, DC: U.S. Government Printing Office.
10. Brenner, M. H. (1973). Fetal, infant and maternal mortality during periods of economic instability. *International Journal of Health Services, 3,* 145–59.
11. Brenner, M. H. (1973). *Mental illness and the economy.* Cambridge: Harvard University Press.
12. Brenner, M. H. (1975). Trends in alcohol consumption and associated illnesses. *American Journal of Public Health, 65,* 1279.
13. Brenner, M. H. (1976). *Estimating the social costs of national economic policy: implications for mental and physical health and criminal aggression* (U.S. Congress, Joint Economic Committed). Washington, DC: U.S. Government Printing Office.
14. Brenner, M. H. (1979). Influence of the social environment on psychopathology: the historical perspective. In J. E. Barrett, R. M. Rose, and G. L. Klerman (eds.). *Stress and mental disorder* (pp. 161–79). New York: Raven Press.
15. Brenner, M. H. (1979). Mortality and the national economy: a review and the experience of England and Wales, 1936–1976. *The Lancet,* September 15, 568–73.
16. Brenner, M. H. (1980). Impact of social and industrial changes on psychopathology: a view of stress from the standpoint of macro societal trends. In L. Levi (ed.). *Society, stress and disease: working life* (Vol. 4, pp. 249–60). Oxford: Oxford University Press.
17. Brenner, M. H. (1980). Industrialization and economic growth: estimates of their effect on the health of populations. In M. H. Brenner, A. Mooney, and T. J. Nagy (eds.). *Assessing the contributions of the social sciences to health* (pp. 65–115). AAAS Symposium 26. Boulder, CO: Westview Press.
18. Brenner, M. H. (1983). Mortality and economic instability: detailed analyses for Britain and comparative analyses for selected industrialized countries. *International Journal of Health Services, 13,* 563–620.
19. Brenner, M. H. (1984). Economic change and the suicide rate: a population model including loss, separation, illness, and alcohol consumption. *Stress in health and disease* (pp. 160–85). New York: Brunner Mazel.
20. Brenner, M. H. (1984). *Estimating the effects of economic change on national mental and social well-being.* U.S. Congress, Joint Economic Committee. Washington, DC: U.S. Government Printing Office.
21. Brenner, M. H. (1987). Relation of economic change to Swedish health and social well-being, 1950–1980. *Social Science and Medicine, 25,* 183–95.
22. Brenner, M. H. (1987). Economic instability, unemployment rates, behavioral risks, and mortality rates in Scotland, 1952–83. *International Journal of Health Services, 17,* 475–84.
23. Brenner, M. H. (1987). Economic change, alcohol consumption and heart disease mortality in nine industrialized countries. *Social Science and Medicine, 25,* 119–31.
24. Brenner, M. H., & Mooney, A. (1982). Economic change and sex-specific cardiovascular mortality in Britain 1955–1976. *Social Science and Medicine, 16,* 431–42.
25. Broadhead, W. E., Kaplan, B. H., James, S. A., et al. (1983). The epidemiologic evidence for a relationship between social support and health. *American Journal of Epidemiology, 117,* 521–37.
26. Bunn, A. R. (1979). Ischaemic heart disease mortality and the business cycle in Australia. *American Journal of Public Health, 69,* 772.
27. Burman, P. (1988). *The experiences of unemployment.* Toronto: Wall and Thompson.
28. Catalano, R., & Dooley, D. (1977). Economic predictors of depressed mood and stressful life events in a metropolitan community. *Journal of Health and Social Behavior, 18,* 292–307.
29. Cooper, B., & Rice, D. (1976). The economic cost of illness revisited. *Social Security Bulletin, 39,* 21–36.
30. Cooper, C., & Payne, R. (eds.). (1988).

Causes, coping, and consequences of stress at work. New York: Wiley.

31. Dahlgren, G., & Diderichsen, F. (1986). Strategies for equity in health: report from Sweden. *International Journal of Health Services, 16,* 517–37.

32. D'Arcy, C. (1986). Unemployment and health: data and implications. *Canadian Journal of Public Health, 77*(suppl. 1), 124–31.

33. Dayal, H. H., Power, R. N., & Chiu, C. (1982). Race and socio-economic status in survival from breast cancer. *Journal of Chronic Diseases, 35,* 675–83.

34. Dohrenwend, B. S. (1973). Social status and stressful life events. *Journal of Personality and Social Psychology, 28,* 225–35.

35. Doll, S. R. (1987). Major epidemics of the 20th century: from coronary thrombosis to AIDS. *Journal of the Royal Statistical Society, 150,* 373–95.

36. Durkheim, E. (1951). *Suicide: a study in sociology* (translated by J. A. Spaulding & G. Simpson; edited, with an introduction, by G. Simpson). Glencoe, IL: Free Press (originally published in Paris: F. Alcan, 1897).

37. Dutton, D. B. (1986). Social class, health and illness. In L. H. Aiken & D. Mechanic (eds.). *Applications of social science to clinical medicine and health policy.* New Brunswick, NJ: Rutgers University Press.

38. Epstein, S. (1979). *The politics of cancer.* New York: Anchor/Doubleday.

39. Epstein, S. (1989). Losing the war against cancer: who's to blame and what to do about it. *International Journal of Health Services, 20,* 53–71.

40. Eyer, J. (1977). Does unemployment cause the death rate peak in each business cycle? A multifactor model of death rate change. *International Journal of Health Services, 7,* 625–62.

41. Faris, R., & Dunham, H. W. (1939). *Mental disorders in urban areas.* New York: Hafner.

42. Flaim, P. O., & Sehgal, E. (1985). Displaced workers of 1979–83: How well have they fared? *Monthly Labor Review,* June, 3–16.

43. Fletcher, B. (1988). The epidemiology of occupational stress. In C. Cooper & R. Payne (eds.). *Causes, coping, and consequences of stress at work* (pp. 3–50). New York: Wiley.

44. Forbes, J. F., & Pickering, R. M. (1985). Influence of maternal age, parity and social class on perinatal mortality in Scotland, 1960–82. *Journal of Biosocial Science, 17,* 339–49.

45. Forbes, W., & Player, D. (1981). Scottish unemployment and the public health. Presented at the Ninth Scientific Meeting, International Epidemiological Association, Edinburgh.

46. Fox, A. J., Goldblatt, P. O., & Jones, D. R. (1985). Social class mortality differentials: artifact, selection or life circumstances? *Journal of Epidemiology and Community Health, 39,* 1–8.

47. Frese, M. (1989). Theoretical models of control and health. In S. L. Sauter, J. J. Hurrell, & C. L. Cooper (eds.). *Job control and worker health* (pp. 107–28). New York: Wiley.

48. Gortmaker, S. L. (1979). Poverty and infant mortality in the United States. *American Sociological Review, 44,* 280–97.

49. Gravelle, M., Hutchinson, G., & Stern, J. (1981). Mortality and unemployment: a critique of Brenner's time-series analysis. *The Lancet, 2,* September 26, 675–9.

50. Greider, W. (1987). *Secrets of the temple.* New York: Simon and Schuster.

51. Haan, M., Kaplan, G. A., & Camacho, T. (1987). Poverty and health: prospective evidence from the Alameda County study. *American Journal of Epidemiology, 125,* 989–98.

52. Harrington, M., & Levinson, M. (1985). The perils of a dual economy: a growing trend in the American occupational structure. *Dissent, 32,* 417–26.

53. Henry, A. F., & Short, J. F. (1954). *Suicide and homicide.* Glencoe, IL: Free Press.

54. Henry, J. (1982). The relation of social to biological processes in disease. *Social Science and Medicine, 16,* 369–80.

55. Hollingshead, A., & Redlich, R. (1958). *Social class and mental illness.* New York: Wiley.

56. Holme, I., Helgeland, A., Hjermann, I., Leren, P., & Lund-Larsen, P. A. (1980). Four-year mortality by some socioeconomic indicators: the Oslo study. *Journal of Epidemiology and Community Health, 34,* 48–52.

57. Horvath, F. W. (1987). The pulse of economic change: displaced workers of 1981–85. *Monthly Labor Review,* June, 3–12.

58. House, J., Landis, K., & Umberson, D. (1988). Social relationships and health. *Science, 241,* 540–5.

59. Kagamimori, S. (1981). Occupational life tables for cerebrovascular disease and ischemic heart disease in Japan compared with England and Wales. *Japanese Circulation Journal, 45,* 195–201.

60. Kagamimori, S., Iibuchi, Y., & Fox, J. (1983). A comparison of socioeconomic differences in mortality between Japan and England and Wales. *World Health Statistics Quarterly, 36,* 119–28.

61. Karasek, R., & Theorell, T. (1990). *Healthy work.* New York: Basic Books.

62. Karasek, R., Baker, D., Marxer, F., Ahlbom, A., & Theorell, T. (1981). Job decision latitude, job demands, and cardiovascular disease: a prospective study of Swedish men. *American Journal of Public Health, 71,* 694–705.

63. Kendrick, J. W. (1980). Productivity trends in the United States. In S. Maital & N. M. Meltz (eds.). *Lagging productivity growth* (pp. 9–31). Cambridge: Ballinger.

64. Kendrick, J. W. (1986). *Productivity: the key to future prosperity* (Joint Economic Committee of the U.S. Congress). Washington, DC: U.S. Government Printing Office.

65. Kessler, R., House, J., & Turner, J. B. (1987). Unemployment and health in a community sample. *Journal of Health and Social Behavior, 28,* 51–59.

66. Kitagawa, E. M., & Hauser, P. M. (1973). *Differential mortality in the United States.* Cambridge: Harvard University Press.

67. Langner, T., & Michael, S. (1963). *Life stress and mental health: the midtown Manhattan study.* London: Free Press of Glencoe.

68. Leclerc, A., Lert, F., & Goldberg, M. (1984). Les inegalites sociales devant la mort en Grande-Bretagne et en France. *Social Science and Medicine, 19,* 479–87.

69. LeMarchand, L., Kolonel, L. N., & Nomura, A. M. Y. (1984). Relationship of ethnicity and other prognostic factors to breast cancer survival patterns in Hawaii. *Journal of the National Cancer Institute, 73,* 1259–65.

70. Lerner, M., Stutz, R. N. (1978). Mortality by socioeconomic status, 1959–61 and 1969–71. *Maryland State Medical Journal,* December, *27,* 35–42.

71. Levine, D., & Wilner, S. (1976). *The cost of mental illness—1974* [statistical note 125, DHEW publication (ADM) 76-158]. Bethesda: National Institute of Mental Health.

72. Levy, C., & Vallin, J. (1981). La mortalite par categorie socioprofessionnelle un essai de calcul direct. *Population, 36,* 938–45.

73. Liem, R., & Liem, J. (1978). Social class and mental illness reconsidered: the role of economic stress and social support. *Journal of Health and Social Behavior, 19,* 139–56.

74. Linn, M. W., Sandifer, R., & Stein, S. (1985). Effects of unemployment on mental and physical health. *American Journal of Public Health, 75,* 502–6.

75. Logan, W. P. D. (1982). *Cancer mortality by occupational and social class, 1851–1971.* London: H. M. S. O.

76. Marmot, M. G., & McDowall, M. E. (1986). Mortality decline and widening social inequalities. *The Lancet, 2,* August 2, 274–6.

77. Marmot, M. G., Kogevinas, M., & Elston, M. A. (1987). Social/economic status and disease. *Annual Review of Public Health, 8,* 111–35.

78. Marshall, R. (1986). *Obstacles to increasing real wages* (Joint Economic Committee of the U.S. Congress, pp. 325–59). Washington, DC: U.S. Government Printing Office.

79. McAvinchey, I. D. (1984). Economic factors and mortality: some aspects of the Scottish case 1950–1978. *Scottish Journal of Political Economy, 31,* 1.

80. McKersie, R. B., & Klein, J. A. (1985). Productivity: the industrial relations connection. In W. J. Baumol & K. McLennan (eds.). *Pro-*

ductivity growth and U.S. competitiveness (pp. 119–59). New York: Oxford University Press.

81. McMichael, A. J., & Hartshorne, J. M. (1982). Mortality risks in Australian men by occupational groups, 1968–78. *Medical Journal of Australia, 1,* 253–56.

82. Mechanic, D. (1976). *The growth of bureaucratic medicine.* New York: Wiley.

83. Mechanic, D. (1979). *Future issues in health care: social policy and the rationing of medical services.* New York: Free Press.

84. Mechanic, D. (1989). Socioeconomic status and health: the problem. In J. P. Bunker, D. S. Gomby, & B. H. Kehrer (eds.). *Pathways to health: the role of social factors* (pp. 3–25). Menlo Park, CA: The Henry J. Kaiser Family Foundation.

85. Millar, W. J. (1983). Sex differentials in mortality by income level in urban Canada. *Canadian Journal of Public Health, 74,* 329–34.

86. Moser, K. A., Fox, A. J., & Jones, D. R. (1984). Unemployment and mortality in the OPCS longitudinal study. *The Lancet, 2,* December 8, 1324.

87. Moser, K. A., Goldblatt, P. O., Fox, A. J., & Jones, D. R. (1987). Unemployment and mortality: comparison of the 1971 and 1981 longitudinal study census samples. *British Medical Journal (Clinical Research Ed.), 294,* 86–90.

88. Myers, J., Lindenthal, J., & Pepper, M. (1974). Social class, life events, and psychiatric symptoms: a longitudinal study. In B. S. Dohrenwend & B. P. Dohrenwend (eds.). *Stressful life events: their nature and effects* (pp. 191–206). New York: Wiley.

89. Nayha, S. (1977). Social group and mortality in Finland. *British Journal of Preventive and Social Medicine, 31,* 231–7.

90. O'Brien, G. E. (1986). *Psychology of work and unemployment.* New York: Wiley.

91. Pamuk, E. R. (1985). Social class inequality in mortality from 1921 to 1972 in England and Wales. *Population Studies, 39,* 17–31.

92. Pearce, N. E., Davis, P. B., Smith, A. H., & Foster, F. H. (1983). Mortality and social class in New Zealand. I. Overall male mortality. *New Zealand Medical Journal, 96,* 281–5.

93. Pearce, N. E., Davis, P. B., Smith, A. H., & Foster, F. H. (1985). Social class, ethnic group and male mortality in New Zealand 1974–78. *Journal of Epidemiology and Community Health, 39,* 9–14.

94. Platt, S. (1984). Unemployment and suicidal behaviour: a review of the literature. *Social Science and Medicine, 19,* 93–115.

95. Rabkin, J. (1982). Stress and psychiatric disorders. In L. Goldberger & S. Breznitz (eds.). *Handbook of stress: theoretical and clinical aspects* (pp. 566–84). New York: Free Press.

96. Rabkin, J., & Struening, E. (1976). Life events, stress, and illness. *Science, 194,* 1013–20.

97. Rozanski, A., Bairey, C. N., Krantz, D. S., et al. (1988). Mental stress and the induction of silent myocardial ischemia in patients with coronary artery disease. *The New England Journal of Medicine, 318*, 1005–12.

98. Salonen, J. T. (1982). Socioeconomic status and risk of cancer, cerebral stroke, and death due to coronary heart disease and any disease: a longitudinal study in eastern Finland. *Journal of Epidemiology and Community Health, 36*, 294–7.

99. Sauter, S. L., Hurrell, J. J., & Cooper, C. L. (eds.). (1989). *Job control and worker health.* New York: Wiley.

100. Seltzer, C. C., & Jablon, S. (1977). Army rank and subsequent mortality by cause: 23-year follow-up. *American Journal of Epidemiology, 105*, 559–66.

101. Solomon, G. (1987). Psychoneuroimmunology: interactions between central nervous system and immune system. *Journal of Neuroscience Research, 18*, 1–9.

102. Srole, L., Langnes, T. S., Michael, S. T., Opler, M. K., & Jennie, T. A. C. (1962). *Mental Health in the Metopolis* (Vol. 1). New York: Blakiston Division, McGraw-Hill.

103. Stockwell, E. G., & Wicks, J. W. (1980). Patterns and variations in the relationship between infant mortality and socioeconomic status. *Social Biology, 31*, 28–39.

104. Stockwell, E. G., Swanson, D. A., & Wicks, J. W. (1988). Economic status differences in infant mortality by cause of death. *Public Health Reports, 103*, 135–42.

105. Thurow, L. (1985). *The zero-sum solution.* New York: Simon & Schuster.

106. Thurow, L. (1987). A surge in inequality. *Scientific American, 256*, 30–7.

107. Tobin, J. (1986). *Fiscal and monetary policy under the Employment Act* (pp. 150–172). Washington, DC: Joint Economic Committee of the U.S. Congress, U.S. Government Printing Office.

108. Valkonen, T. (1982). Psychosocial stress and sociodemographic differentials in mortality from ischaemic heart disease in Finland. *Acta Medica Scandinavica, 660*, 152–64.

109. Warr, P. (1987). *Work, unemployment, and mental health.* Oxford: Clarendon Press.

110. Wilkinson, R. (ed.). (1986). *Class and health.* London: Tavistock.

111. Wise, P. H., Kotelchuck, M., Wilson, M. L., & Mills, M. (1985). Racial and socioeconomic disparities in childhood mortality in Boston. *New England Journal of Medicine, 313*, 360–6.

112. Yeracdris, C. A., & Kim, J. H. (1978). Socioeconomic differentials in selected causes of death. *American Journal of Public health, 68*, 342–351.

17
Health Promotion at the Worksite

Jonathan Fielding

Employers have increasingly recognized the close associations between employee health and productivity. Faced with increased aging of the population with higher rates of chronic conditions, difficulty in controlling health benefit costs, increased frequency of employee morale problems, and growing epidemiological data relating definable health risks to future health problems, many employers have turned to worksite health promotion programs with the hope that they will have a positive impact on all of these (9,13).

While reported reasons for initiating worksite health promotion programs vary, most observers agree that rapid escalation in employer-borne health benefits costs have been a principal motivator. The grand total for these costs was estimated to exceed $125 billion dollars in 1987 in the United States (35; see also Chapter 15). Legislation at the federal and state levels has gradually increased employer responsibility for employee health-related costs in a country that in 1990 will spend about 12% of its gross national product (GNP) on health care (21). In sharp contrast to all other industrialized countries, many American employers, including the vast majority of large employers, pay for health care costs based primarily on their own experience through experience-rated insurance and self-insurance. A significant portion of total benefit payments made by employers on behalf of employees is health-related (9), as is evident in Table 17–1.

A significant fraction of the costs of illness—direct costs such as health care under health benefits and workers' compensation and indirect costs such as absenteeism, disability, increased turnover, and diminished quality and quantity of work—are related to preventable or postponable diseases and injuries whose toll may be substantially reduced through screening and early treatment (10; see also Chapter 15). Table 17–2 lists some of the most common of these health conditions and the estimated years of potential life lost from each before age 65. Worksite health promotion programs are established in the hope of reducing the toll of preventable illness and improving productivity.

DEFINITIONAL PROBLEMS

For purposes of this discussion, health promotion is defined broadly, subsuming both activities designed to assess and reduce future health risks and maximize individual health. The definition applies to some services delivered by usual providers of health

Table 17–1. Health-Related Employee Benefits: Expense per Week, 1987

Type of benefit	Employer's expense per 40-hour work week ($)
Old-age, survivors, disability, and health insurance (FICA taxes) and Railroad Retirement Tax	32.32
Insurance premium (e.g., life, hospital, surgical, medical, dental, retiree, other)	41.60
Workers' compensation	5.68
Paid sick leave	7.12
Short-term disability	2.60
Salary continuation or long-term disability	0.88
Total health-related benefits	90.20
Total employee benefits	205.04
Average weekly salary	528.42
Health-related benefits as a percentage of total benefits	44%
Health-related benefits as a percentage of average weekly salary	17.1%

Source: Data from Employee Benefits 1988 (U.S. Chamber of Commerce) (34).

care services, such as physicians, hospitals, and occupational medicine clinics, and services provided through organizations and individuals specifically providing non-medical assessment and counseling to maintain or improve health status through behavioral approaches (e.g., exercise, nutrition counseling, stress management classes). It can be argued that an important distinction exists between disease prevention, health promotion, and health protection. The first may be considered to include clinical services, such as periodic health examinations, mammography, and immunizations. Health promotion encompasses all other health risk assessment and reduction activities aside from those related to worksite exposures, be they safety, chemicals, or ergonomic, which together would comprise health protection. However, these distinc-

Table 17–2. Estimated Years of Potential Life Lost Before Age 65 (YPLL-65), United States, 1987 and 1988

Cause of death	YPLL-65 for persons dying in 1987	YPLL-65 for persons dying in 1988
All causes (total)	12,074,193	12,281,741
Unintentional injuries	2,305,508	2,319,400
Malignant neoplasms	1,816,927	1,809,289
Diseases of the heart	1,519,962	1,466,629
Suicide/homicide	1,326,968	1,361,473
Congenital anomalies	641,827	671,709
Human immunodeficiency virus infection	363,494	472,800
Prematurity	428,087	432,342
Cerebrovascular disease	248,026	245,722
Chronic liver disease and cirrhosis	235,135	236,944
Pneumonia/influenza	172,009	172,712
Diabetes mellitus	122,837	130,666
Chronic obstructive pulmonary disease	131,880	128,126

Source: Centers for Disease Control, 1987, 1988 (6).

tions are easily blurred in the context of a worksite. A comprehensive health promotion program will often include hypertension screening and assessing potential stressful aspects of the work environment. An occupational physician counseling employees to wear their safety equipment and to reduce fat intake, and providing tetanus boosters, based on those distinctions, is engaging in health promotion, disease prevention, and health protection during the same visit. In practice, worksite occupational medicine programs that deal primarily with worksite safety and other environmental issues are usually organizationally or programmatically distinct from general health promotion and disease prevention activities. The two latter categories of activities thus form the functional definition for health promotion programming.

Another issue of boundaries is what constitutes a health promotion "program." Does a single distribution of a leaflet on how to do breast self-examination constitute a program? What about annual participation in the Great American Smokeout? As a starting point for further discussion, worksite health promotion programs are considered to exist when the following criteria are met: (1) the activities are designed to improve or maintain health of employees, dependents, and retirees; (2) participation is voluntary; (3) programs involve activities in addition to the provisions of educational materials; (4) programs address one or more factors reasonably demonstrated to alter personal health risk; and (5) programs are offered on a periodic or continuing basis.

PROGRAM PREVALENCE AND GENERAL CHARACTERISTICS

Statewide Surveys

A number of random sample surveys of health-promotion programs in worksites within a single state, conducted during the early 1980s, revealed that most large and medium-size employers (i.e., more than 100 employees) had one or more health-promotion activities. The frequency of various types of health-promotion activities as well as the percentage of employers planning new programs in a California survey are summarized in Table 17–3. The average number of activities increased directly with employer size, from 1.0 activities in worksites with 100 to 249 employees to 3.9 in the 5,000+ employee worksites. Most frequently cited reasons for not having a program in the California study included "too costly" (100%), "no need/employees healthy" (94.7%), "too difficult to implement" (29.8%), and "high employee turnover" (21.3%). From patterns of when specific activities had been implemented, a clear pattern of accelerating program initial adoption and expansion has emerged (Table 17–4).

National Survey

The only nationwide survey of worksite health-promotion programs was undertaken in 1985 by the Health Promotion Division of U.S. Corporate Health Management (now merged into Johnson & Johnson Health Management, Inc.). The study, sponsored by the Office of Disease Prevention and Health Promotion in the Office of the Assistant Secretary for Health and the Office of the Assistant Secretary for Planning and Evaluation in the Department of Health and Human Services (DHHS), was conducted with the assistance of Research Triangle Institute. The primary objective of the National Survey of Worksite Health Promotion Activities was to determine the nature and extent of health-promotion activities in worksites with 50 or more employees (16). Worksites

Table 17–3. Health-Promotion Activities of California Employers, 1981

Health-promotion activity	Currently offering program Percent of programs (*n* = 938)	Percent of employers[a] (*n* = 332)	Planning new programs (% of programs) (*n* = 217)
Hypertension screening	4.6	13.0	11.1
Smoking cessation	3.7	10.5	9.7
Weight control	3.4	9.6	7.8
Mental health counseling	8.3	23.5	3.7
Nutrition training	2.3	6.6	6.0
CPR, choke saver	23.9	67.5	11.1
Exercise/fitness	5.2	14.8	12.0
Drug/alcohol abuse	8.4	23.8	8.3
Stress management	5.9	16.6	14.3
Accident prevention	29.2	82.5	4.6
Cancer risk reduction	2.9	8.1	4.1
Other	2.1	6.0	7.4

Source: Fielding and Breslow (15).
[a]With at least one activity.

were defined as geographically contiguous settings. The December 1984 Dun & Bradstreet list of businesses was used to develop the survey samples. For worksites with 100 or more employees, 3,000 sites were selected with equal probability stratified by geographic region, worksite size, and industry type. The corresponding sample size for worksites with 50 to 99 employees was 600, drawn in a similar manner except that size of worksite was not used as a stratifying variable.

Interviewing lists of 20 sites for smaller worksites (50 to 99 employees) and 100 sites for larger worksites (100 or more employees) were created in a manner that respondents would constitute a valid probability sample. A ratio adjustment, which varied across several poststratification classes, was applied to the sampling weight to reduce the effect of nonresponse on survey estimates.

Survey instrument questions covered the following: (a) the presence of nine common types of health-promotion activities during the prior 12 months; (b) information on each type of activity present; (c) characteristics of the overall health promotion

Table 17–4. Chronology of Health-Promotion Activity Initiation Among California Employers

Time interval	No. of activities initiated[a]	Activities added per year (av. No.)
Prior to 1961	68[b]	—
1962–1971	113	11.3
1972–1974	45	15.0
1975–1977	188	62.7
1978–1981	446	111.5
Total	860	

Source: Fielding and Breslow (15).
[a]Based on 860 activities for which duration was provided.
[b]Of 68 activities, 52 were accident prevention.

effort such as budget, sources of assistance, and use of outside providers; and (d) demographic characteristics of the worksite.

Survey Results

Overall, data were collected on 1,038 worksites with 100 or more employees and 320 worksites with 50 to 99 employees. The final completion rate was 83.1%, including worksites that could not be found or where no respondent was identified, and 87.3% for worksites contacted. Interviewer contact results are summarized in Table 17–5.

Prevalence of the nine target activities are summarized in Figure 17–1. Overall 65.8% of worksites had one or more of these activities, with smoking control the most common, followed closely by health risk assessment, back care, and stress management.

The prevalence of activities increased with worksite size, whereas rank order of activities demonstrated considerable consistency. Notable exceptions include (a) the sharp increase in health risk assessment activities with size, two-thirds of all worksites with 750+ employees having such an activity and placing this activity in first rank; (b) stress management achieving a higher rank order with increasing worksite size such that three of five worksites with more than 750+ employees reported such activities; and (c) only one activity, off-the-job accident prevention, achieving significantly less than 50% prevalence in the group of largest worksites.

Almost 30% of all worksites offered physical examinations, periodic health assessments, various screening tests alone or in combination, or health risk appraisals. Of worksites with any of these activities, about one-fourth provided health risk appraisal, and 77.4% offered some type of health examination (14). The relative frequency of screening tests is summarized in Figure 17–2.

Almost three-fourths (73%) of worksites reported no written goals or objectives for their health-promotion activities. According to respondents, the most frequently provided reason for offering health-promotion activities was "to improve employee health" (28%), followed by "because management wanted it" (17.6%). Less fre-

Table 17–5. Interviewer Contact Results

Parameter	Large worksites (>100 employees)		Small worksites (<100 employees)		Total worksites	
	No.	%	No.	%	No.	%
Original sample	1,300	100	400	100	1,700	100
Active worksites at time of data collection[a]	1,235[a]	100	400	100	1,635	100
Total interviews completed	1,038	100	320	80	1,358	83.1
Unable to complete interview[b]	190	15.4	67	16.9	257	16.2
Other[c]	7	0.6	13	3.3	20	1.2

Source: Fielding and Piserchia (16).
[a]Sixty-five large worksites went out of business after selection but before name/address files were received.
[b]Out of business, unable to contact, refusal.
[c]Incorrect worksite size from Dun & Bradstreet list.

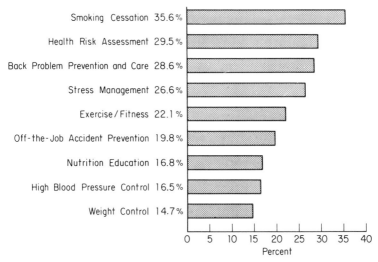

Figure 17–1. Prevalence (percent) by type of activity. From ODPHP (28).

quently advanced reasons included "to increase productivity/output," "to improve employee morale," "because the employees wanted it," "to reduce insurance costs/medical utilization," "to reduce disability claims and lost time," and "to reduce accidents" (12).

Each respondent was asked a set of forced choice questions about the perceived benefits of implementing any activities they reported. The categories included: (a) improved employee morale; (b) improved employee health; (c) increased productivity; (d) reduced health care costs; and (e) no benefits (Table 17–6). Although the results should be interpreted with caution as only one-fourth of the respondents reported having any formal evaluation activities, the perceptions of benefit should be reflective of implicit or explicit employer objectives. For only two of the activities—off-the-job accident prevention and back care activities—were reduced health care costs the most frequently perceived benefit. Increased productivity was the most commonly perceived benefit only for stress management activities. Improved employee health was the most

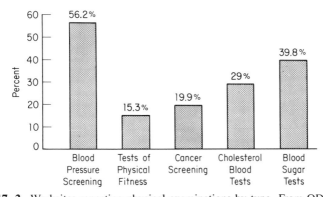

Figure 17–2. Worksites reporting physical examinations by type. From ODPHP (28).

Table 17–6. Perceived Benefits by Health-Promotion Activity

	Health risk asssessment	Smoking cessation	High blood pressure control and treatment	Exercise and fitness	Weight control	Nutrition education	Stress management	Back problem prevention and care	Off-the-job accident prevention
Improved morale	14.2	9.0	17.7	39.6	33.0	20.8	29.9	3.6	3.9
Improved health	47.1	41.1	57.5	54.2	53.4	59.9	20.3	26.4	19.6
Increased productivity	24.2	16.1	31.5	25.5	29.4	25.2	46.5	24.3	23.4
Reduced health cost care	14.1	7.9	13.7	4.5	6.5	5.8	4.2	40.8	25.0
No benefits	9.3	10.3	0.8	9.2	12.1	7.2	7.9	3.2	4.7
Other	30.6	42.7	32.3	24.1	21.3	29.6	36.1	39.8	48.4

Source: Fielding (12).

Data are given as the percent of worksites that offered *that* activity.

Note: Worksites could select up to three perceived benefits. Benefits cannot be compared across activity categories.

commonly cited benefit for all other activities, usually followed by improved employee morale or improved productivity (12).

The impetus for establishing health-promotion activities came at almost one-half of the worksites from top management, whereas employee impetus was primary in about 15% of worksites, head of personnel/employee relations in 12.5%, and top management at a higher corporate level in 11.4%. In worksites that were part of a larger company, the impetus for starting the health-promotion program came from someplace other than the worksite queried in 41.3% of cases (12).

The site for employer-sponsored health-promotion activities exhibited substantial variation. Individual counseling as well as group classes or workshops were most often provided at the worksite, whereas screenings/examinations were more equally divided, with slightly more than one-half of worksites reporting these activities to occur exclusively or primarily off-site (12).

For each type of reported activity the employer was the primary funding source in 70 to 90% of cases. Cost sharing for individual counseling occurred in 15.9% of worksites, 13.1% for group classes or workshops, and in only 8.9% of cases for screening or examinations. Participants paid exclusively for various activities at no more than 3.3% of worksites. Company funding was most likely to come from the personnel or benefits budget (55.2%), with considerably less frequency from the medical department budget (17.5%) or through insurance benefits (16.1%). About 40% of company funding was from other corporate budget accounts. Funding came from voluntary health organizations in 8.7% of worksites, presumably where there were limited programs (12,16).

Health-promotion activities were coordinated entirely in house (41.8%) or through combined in-house and outside resources (36.5%) (16). Use of outside assistance to present programs was the rule, as shown in Table 17–7. Most sources of assistance became more frequent with increasing worksite size, although insurance company assistance was reported in 40 to 50% of worksites regardless of size. Local hospitals, private providers or consultants, and voluntary organizations frequently had an important role in existing activities.

Problems of establishing health-promotion activities were cited overall by approximately 25% of respondents. Most commonly cited were high costs, lack of employee interest, and time limitations. Four of five worksites (81.3%) indicated moderate or

Table 17–7. Worksites Using External Sources of Program Assistance, By Worksite Size and Source of Assistance

Source of program assistance	Percent, by worksite size			
	< 100	100–249	250–749	750+
Voluntary	48.0	55.3	64.0	76.6
Government	17.0	24.2	23.6	26.4
Private providers or consultants	43.0	54.7	52.6	59.5
Local hospitals	35.4	46.9	42.0	61.2
Unions	6.6	5.8	10.0	15.7
Insurance companies	41.0	48.2	45.4	47.4

Source: Fielding (12).

extreme concern about health care cost management, with 43% reporting that they had implemented a health care cost management strategy during the previous 3-year period. The likelihood of implementation of such a strategy was directly correlated with worksite size (12).

The first National Survey of Worksite Health Promotion Activities revealed that two-thirds of worksites with 50 or more employees had one or more health-promotion activities. Decision makers at most worksites seemed to believe that some level of investment to improve employee health is appropriate, even if the dollar savings associated with that investment cannot be easily estimated and without the perceived need for a formal evaluation. However, the variation in the level of activity associated with a particular health-promotion opportunity is tremendous. The presence of an activity does not mean that it is well coordinated, publicized, attended, or effective. Additional surveys, possibly including site visits, would serve to better define such variables as participation rates, corporate commitment, budgetary resources devoted to the activities, and coordination of various offerings. This initial survey provides an important baseline for assessing trends over time, for gauging the effectiveness of public and private sector health-promotion initiatives, and for assessing progress compared to explicit national health objectives developed by the DHHS.

PROGRAM EVALUATION

The results of the first National Survey of Worksite Health Promotion Activities highlights the small percentage of worksites that report incorporating formal evaluations into their programming (16). Employers may not wish to incur the extra expense, or they may have enough faith that the program is meeting their objectives to not require validation. Lack of evaluation of these efforts seems anomalous in business, where success often depends on tracking the results of every investment. Most businesses willing to consider a large investment in health promotion programming are interested in the results of other evaluations, and often use this information in deciding whether to move ahead or even what components the program should have.

Effective worksite health promotion evaluation must be responsive to the stated objectives. Objectives of these programs vary considerably, from increasing awareness of a health problem to reducing absenteeism, from decreasing perceived stress to reducing the rate of first heart attacks. Frequently the criteria for program success require measurement of worksite program effectiveness with respect to eight categories of variables, as modified from DeMuth et al. (7):

1. Participation rates.
2. Employee satisfaction with programs.
3. Management satisfaction with programs.
4. Health status changes measured via changes in knowledge, attitudes, behaviors, risk levels for specific diseases, and expected longevity.
5. Economic benefits, such as effects on health benefit costs, short- and long-term disability, worker's compensation.
6. Program costs (dollar costs and administrative effort required).
7. Productivity measures: rarely direct measurement of output or quality; often

morale, job satisfaction, satisfaction with employer, satisfaction with benefit packages, turnover rates, recruiting ease.
8. Employer image in community or compared with competition.

The literature on health-promotion program evaluation has grown at an accelerating rate. Many initial evaluations of programs were anecdotal, and few were published in well known peer reviewed journals. Increasingly, researchers have discovered that worksites can be appropriate laboratories to test health-promotion intervention strategies. To date, most reports of worksite health-promotion programs have been of single component programs such as smoking cessation, weight management, or high blood pressure control. The interventions models tested in the worksite are often adapted from programs previously tested in clinical settings.

The study design in published evaluations of worksite interventions has undergone considerable evolution. Initial studies rarely employed a control group; a second wave of studies utilized nonrandomized control groups; and more recent studies have increasingly employed random assignment to groups. Comprehensive review of this literature is beyond the scope of this chapter, but a sense of the research base for single component interventions is presented below through the example of hypertension control programs. Data suggesting reasonable expectations for an effective intervention are also provided for that example.

Appropriate questions to be answered for any intervention include the following:

1. Is it clear that the health risks targeted by health-promotion programs cause significant increases in morbidity and mortality?
2. Are these health risks found with significant frequency in working populations?
3. Can these increased risks be mitigated or eliminated by changes in habits or specified treatments?
4. Have health-promotion activities (including clinical disease prevention) in any setting been shown to change the target behavior or to alter biochemical or physiological measures of risk, and have these changes endured?
5. Have studies linked specific health-promotion strategies with superior results?
6. Have studies quantified intervention costs and benefits?
7. Have studies demonstrated program effectiveness in employer-sponsored programs?

Hypertension

Programs to assess and control blood pressure are used as an example of how the literature on evaluation has developed and to illustrate some of the challenges in mounting effective evaluations and in generalizing the results of studies. Elevated blood pressure is a firmly established risk factor, although the appropriate level above which drug treatment should be instituted remains controversial (36,38). Compared to normotensive individuals, hypertensives develop approximately three times as much coronary heart disease, six times as much congestive heart failure, and seven times as many strokes (37,38). Lowering high blood pressure reduces the excess risk of hypertension-related morbidity and mortality in a dose-response fashion (38).

Hypertension is prevalent in workforce populations, with blood pressures in excess of 140/90 mm Hg found in 15 to 25% of the worksite population (27). Employer-sponsored hypertension detection and management programs have reported considerable success in identifying and controlling high blood pressure in employees. During the initial program year at the home office of the Massachusetts Mutual Life Insurance Company, the percentage of hypertensives under control increased from 36% to 82% (26).

A Michigan study of four alternative methods of hypertension management at Ford Motor Company plants reported that, at the three sites where the intervention incorporated follow-up activities, 56 to 62% of employees identified as hypertensive had follow-up blood pressure readings below 140/90 mm Hg and 86 to 90% had readings below 160/95 mm Hg. Corresponding control rates were only 21 to 47% in employees screened without follow-up (17).

Effective worksite blood pressure control models include the establishment of special off-site blood pressure control programs. For example, among 218 Chicago area hypertensive employees attending a special high blood pressure control clinic near their workplace, diastolic blood pressure fell from an average level of 102.6 mm Hg at initial screening and 98.8 mm Hg on repeat screening to 83.1 mm Hg at the end of the first year of treatment (33).

In the debate over how much health care should be delivered through the worksite, it is relevant that well designed worksite hypertension control programs appear to yield better control rates than usual primary care arrangements (17,24). For example, in a study of Toronto area workers assigned randomly to worksite or community (regular) care, specially trained nurses at the worksite were associated with 48.5% control over the first 6 months of treatment compared to 27.5% in the usual care group.

Evidence regarding cost-effectiveness and relative costs versus benefits of hypertension screening programs associated with the worksite is limited. However, the Toronto study results suggest that worksite treatment can be more cost-effective. Although the average cost of care did not differ significantly between the two groups (worksite $243 and community $211—both in Canadian dollars), the incremental cost-effectiveness of the worksite-treated groups ($5.63/mm Hg reduction) was well below the base cost-effectiveness ratio for the regular care groups ($32.51/mm Hg reduction) (24).

The other reported economic variable from worksite hypertension studies is absenteeism. Reported results are conflicting. A study of 8,467 union members undergoing hypertension screening and control either at the worksite or through their physician found that disability days in treated hypertensives decreased 25.3 and 30.9 days, respectively, over the next 2 years, compared to an increase of 9.2% in the overall employee population (1). In contrast, an increase of 5.2 days per year (80%) in absenteeism was reported in newly diagnosed hypertensive male employees at Dominion Foundries and Steel (Canada) (20). This level of increase was not affected by institution of antihypertensive drug treatment or degree of control achieved. Authors speculate that informing employees that they had a health problem induced sick role behavior.

In the multicenter Hypertension Detection and Follow-up Program, newly identifying a hypertensive individual was not, on average, associated with any changes in absenteeism. However, the subgroup of newly identified hypertensives referred to their usual source of care did have an increase in absenteeism. Previously treated hypertensives referred to special hypertensive clinics experienced reduced absenteeism (29). Given the conflicting results of three well-controlled studies, drawing conclusions about the impact of hypertension screening and control programs is premature. There are suggestions, however, that the way in which information regarding the condition is presented and the interaction between a hypertensive patient and his or her physician may condition the degree to which an individual regards his or her condition and the propensity to use this condition as a reason for absence from work.

Although the health benefits of treatment are clear for most categories of hypertensives, the overall relationship between costs and monetary benefits of a comprehensive worksite hypertension detection and control program from the perspective of the employer is less clear. Modeling of either side of the cost:benefit equation requires using assumptions based on limited information for a number of the terms (11). For example, the percentage of previously undiagnosed hypertensives is declining, despite the aging of the population, as is the yield from broad-based screening programs at the worksite. At the same time, the installation of more comprehensive worksite health-promotion programs into which hypertensive screening is integrated effectively decreases the cost of each detection. Integrated follow-up programs for a variety of high risk characteristics also reduces the unit cost of follow-up to ensure adequate control.

The longevity of effects has been well addressed in a follow-up study four years after discontinuation of a 3-year controlled study of hypertension detection and control. At the end of the 3 year study, study site employees who had received routine follow-up monitoring of blood pressure had significantly better levels of control than at their initial screening, as well as better control than employees without follow-up monitoring. Four years after discontinuation of the follow-up services, the blood pressure levels in the experimental sites were no better than at the control sites, and both sets had no better control than would have been predicted in the absence of the original intervention program. These results suggest that effectiveness for some programs require indefinite continuation. In these situations, significant initial investment may be wasted if the program is discontinued (8).

MULTICOMPONENT PROGRAMS

While most of the evaluation literature has addressed single component programs, results of surveys suggest that multicomponent programs are frequent and likely to become the most common type. Few rigorous evaluations of comprehensive worksite health promotion programs have been reported. Barriers to conducting such evaluations can be significant, and include:

1. High cost of evaluation given the number of dependent variables that should be collected and analyzed.
2. More difficulty standardizing the intervention than for single component health promotion programs.
3. Difficulty predicting effect size and therefore sample size.
4. Need for considerable data manipulation to deal with interactive effects of different intervention components.
5. Difficulty obtaining comparable control groups.

Although these challenges also must be confronted in single component studies, they are magnified in comprehensive interventions.

Comprehensive programs generally include a planning phase, often involving an interested employee group, orientation to the program via print media, large group presentations or videotapes, a health assessment including a computerized health profile, a standard set of physiological and often biochemical measures, feedback to the employee of the results, a series of behavioral change programs directed at common deleterious health habits, and various promotional activities and incentives to maximize participation within a worksite. However, comprehensive programs differ considerably in many critical respects, such as level of effort, sophistication in selling the program to employees, quality control in delivery, and expertise of personnel. Program objectives may also differ.

Programs that have been frequently described in the literature include those of the Control Data Corporation (25), AT&T Communications Division (32), Blue Cross and Blue Shield of Indiana (19), Blue Cross and Blue Shield of Michigan (3), and Johnson & Johnson (5,40).

To date, the Johnson & Johnson program has been the subject of the most reports and is the only one on which there has been peer-reviewed articles covering the impact of the program on both health risks and health-related costs. When designing the program, it was decided to make the target of intervention the entire worksite rather than those employees who chose to participate in a specific set of activities. Because of this approach, an entire worksite had to be either a study or control group.

After considerable planning, LIVE FOR LIFE® programs were initiated at selected sites in 1979. The program has gradually been phased in at Johnson & Johnson companies in the United States and nine other countries, and it currently covers approximately 31,200 employees. The first evaluation of this program involved a quasi-experimental design involving seven Johnson & Johnson plants in New Jersey and Pennsylvania (41). Study and control group characteristics are summarized in Table 17–8. In general, the three study and four control companies' employees have similar demographic and health habit characteristics with some exceptions, such as smoking (26.9% in study plants versus 35.0% in controls). The average age of the workforce was about 35 years, with no significant differences in the average age of men and women.

The LIVE FOR LIFE® program has been described in detail elsewhere (40). The program is coordinated by an account executive for each participating Johnson & Johnson company. The process begins with a presentation to that company's management board and a request that the company commit financial resources, management time, and responsiveness to requests by employees for improvements in the health environment at the worksite. Responsibility for the program is vested in a member of the management board, who in turn chooses a LIVE FOR LIFE® administrator, often from within the personnel function but sometimes from finance or other parts of the company. Volunteers from the company participate in task forces organized around key health areas.

All employees are encouraged to take a nurse-administered Health Profile, which includes behavioral, attitudinal, and biometric measures (blood pressure, blood lipids, body fat, height and weight, bicycle ergometry). The Health Profile, which takes approximately 1 hour to complete, is offered on company time.

Table 17–8. Selected Baseline Characteristics of Health Screen Volunteers by Treatment and Sex

Parameter	Women		Men	
	Control	Treatment	Control	Treatment
No. of volunteers	751	1272	518	971
Volunteer rate (%)	73.5	79.3	77.3	77.7
Mean age (years)	34.8	33.7	36.1	34.3*
Age distribution (%)				
18–24	24.3	22.4	8.1	11.1
25–34	35.1	41.0	43.6	48.2
35–44	14.7	16.8*	28.8	25.9
45–54	19.0	12.6	14.1	10.5
55+	6.9	7.2	5.4	4.3
Total	100.0	100.0	100.0	100.0
Ethnicity (%) minority	9.8	16.4*	10.0	15.1*
College graduates (%)	11.6	20.7*	58.4	61.8
Smoking distribution (%)				
Never smoker	40.5	49.7	40.7	50.1
Former smoker	17.4	19.6	32.3	26.8
Current smoker	42.1	30.7*	27.0	23.1*
Total	100.0	100.0	100.0	100.0
Mean cigarettes per day (current smokers)	18.3	18.5	23.3	21.9
Mean total ethanol per week (oz)	2.4	23.8	4.6	4.0
Mean systolic blood pressure (mm Hg)	116.3	114.4	126.7	124.8*
Mean diastolic blood pressure (mm Hg)	75.1	73.3*	81.5	80.8
Hypertensive (% with SBP of 140 or DBP of 90)†	8.4	6.3	22.1	16.5*
Mean % above ideal weight[a]	15.1	11.7*	16.9	15.9
Mean total activity (kcal/kg/day)[b]	34.4	34.8	36.9	36.9
Mean general well-being[c]	76.8	77.2	82.0	81.5
Mean Framingham type A behavior scale[d]	6.1	6.0	5.3	5.3
Mean No. of self-reported sick days	6.1	5.6	2.7	3.8*
Mean job satisfaction with growth opportunities	59.5	61.0	63.8	62.9
Mean satisfaction with supervision	66.9	65.7	64.3	63.1
Mean satisfaction with working conditions	71.3	71.6	70.9	62.9

Source: Wilbur et al. (41).
[a]Ideal weight is 5 lb more than the values in the Metropolitan Life Insurance tables.
[b]Estimated from a previously validated, 7-day physical activity recall interview (Blair et al. [2]).
[c]Scale based on a series of 18 questions developed from the National Center for Health Statistics (18).
[d]A scale based on a series of ten questions developed for the Framingham Study (Haynes et al. [20]).
*Difference between the treatment and control with sex group is statistically significant at $p = 0.01$.
†SBP = systolic blood pressure; DBP = diastolic blood pressure.

Employees who have taken the Health Profile participate in the Lifestyle Seminar, which is an effective way to introduce them to all aspects of the LIVE FOR LIFE® program over a 3-hour period. The Health Profile is returned, and recommendations are provided for participation in a variety of programs. Life style improvement activities include behaviorally oriented programs dealing with nutrition, exercise, weight control, smoking cessation, stress management, high blood pressure control, and others. These programs are supplemented with a panoply of special health programs on such subjects as breast self-examination, AIDS, dealing with menopause, caring for elders, or dealing with a child who has a behavior problem. Wherever possible, demonstrations and participation by employees are incorporated.

An extensive program of incentives is provided to reward participation and encourage enhanced involvement in various aspects of the program. It is one stratagem to make the entire worksite environment more healthy. An abbreviated list of others is included in Table 17–9.

The outline of the LIVE FOR LIFE® program in place during the time of the initial epidemiological and economic evaluations has evolved based on program experience. For example, today the results of the Health Profile are immediately available. A comprehensive alcohol and other drug awareness module has been added. Contests have been employed to catalyze behavioral change, and behavioral change programs are delivered not only in group session but using self-paced manuals and via telephone.

Epidemiological Evaluation Results

For the epidemiological evaluation, Lifestyle Questionnaire and Health Profile data were collected from employee volunteers in both study and control companies at baseline (preintervention), 1 year, and 2 years. Sample sizes were 1,272 for employees completing two Health Profiles in 1979 and 1981 in study companies and 751 employees in control companies. A random nonvolunteer sample of 53% of nonrespondents were sampled and asked to take a nonrespondent questionnaire administered by the interviewer. Comparisons between these groups indicated similar health habits with the exception that nonrespondents were more likely to have smoked, significantly more female nonrespondents reported current smoking, respondents were less likely to exer-

Table 17–9. Incentives to Make Entire Worksite More Healthy

Fitness
    Shower and locker facilities on-site
    Exercise facilities either on-site or rented from local organization
Weight control/nutrition
    Scales in restrooms
    Availability of convenient nutrition information where food is sold
    Availability of nutritious foods in the company cafeteria and vending machines
Stress management
    Employee assistance program to provide professional treatment and referral services to troubled employees
    Availability of management training programs designed to improve boss–subordinate relations
    Flextime
    Carpooling
    Self-administered blood pressure equipment
Smoking cessation
    Smoking policy
    Availability of LIVE FOR LIFE® Program Thank-You-For-Not-Smoking signs
Publicity and promotions
    Incentive prizes and awards for participation in LIVE FOR LIFE® activities
    LIVE FOR LIFE® Program newsletter
    LIVE FOR LIFE® Program bulletin board and information display area
    Comprehensive recruitment brochure
    Health fairs
    Poster displays for upcoming programs

Source: Wilbur et al. (41).

cise regularly, and male respondents were less likely to have been told they had high blood pressure (Table 17–10). Overall it was judged that volunteers taking the Health Profile in both sets of companies constituted an accurate reflection of the health status and health habits of the entire work force (30).

Important differences between study and control groups include LIVE FOR LIFE® employees having a significantly higher smoking cessation rate (23% versus 17%), based on self-report with biochemical validation (31). LIVE FOR LIFE® employees lost significantly more weight or gained less weight than control employees. Overweight employees in study sites lost an average of 1.1 lb, and overweight controls gained an average of 0.5 lb. The program impact on weight per employee includes all employees, regardless of whether they participated in any aspect of LIVE FOR LIFE® that might have affected their weight.

Similar groups were used to assess exercise changes over the same 2-year period (2). Physical activity and fitness were assessed using a variety of measures. Direct assessment of fitness was performed using a submaximal bicycle ergometry and extrapolating to maximum oxygen uptake. The nature and level of physical activity were also assessed using three questionnaires. Participants were queried regarding their level of activity compared to their peers and if they regularly performed activities corresponding to a minimum of 1,000 kcal/week (for a 70-kg individual); they also were asked to complete a 7-day physical activity recall.

During the 2-year study period, almost 20% of women and 30% of men in LIVE FOR LIFE® companies initiated regular vigorous exercise, compared to 7% and 19% for men and women, respectively, in control companies (2) (Figure 17–3). In study com-

Table 17–10. Respondents and Nonrespondents Answering "Yes" to Health Screen Items Included in the Nonrespondent Questionnaire

Variable	Men answering "yes" (%)		Women answering "yes" (%)	
	Respondents	Nonresp.	Respondents	Nonresp.
Ever smoked cigarettes?	56.3*	66.7	54.0	63.6
	(662/1,175)	(86/129)	(593/1,098)	(89/140)
Currently smoke cigarettes?	28.0	34.1	35.0**	46.4
	(327/1,168)	(44/129)	(447/1,095)	(65/140)
Engage in regular exercise	29.0**	46.5	15.2**	31.4
activities?	(342/1,180)	(60/129)	(168/1,109)	(44/140)
Ever had a myocardial	1.2	2.3	0.4	2.1
infarction?	(15/1,223)	(3/129)	(5/1,146)	(3/140)
Ever told had high blood	16.3**	27.1	12.7	17.1
pressure?	(199/1,222)	(35/129)	(146/1,150)	(24/140)
Ever treated for high blood	8.0	11.9	7.5	9.4
pressure?	(86/1,079)	(15/126)	(74/982)	(13/138)
Currently treated for high	5.0	8.6	4.2	5.9
blood pressure?	(57/1,129)	(11/128)	(44/1,050)	(8/136)
Ever, or now, diabetic?	1.0	2.3	0.7	1.4
	(12/1,221)	(3/129)	(8/1,149)	(2/138)

Source: Settergren et al. (30).
Numbers in parentheses are the number of subjects answering "yes"/total.
*Difference between respondents and nonrespondents is statistically significant at $p < 0.05$. **Difference between respondents and nonrespondents is statistically significant at $p < 0.01$.

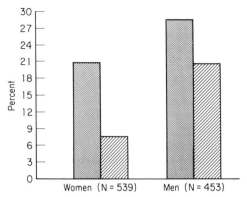

Figure 17–3. Percent of participants who started vigorous exercise by year 2. These individuals did not participate in vigorous exercise at baseline. Solid bars = health-promotion program employees; hatched bars = health-screen-only employees. From Blair (2).

panies, maximum oxygen consumption per employee, regardless of participation in LIVE FOR LIFE® sponsored exercise activities, increased an average of 8.4% during year 1 and 10.5% during year 2, versus 1.5% and 4.7%, respectively, for the controls.

Maximum oxygen uptake was not affected by demographic factors, and attrition bias was excluded as a source of intergroup differences. Large increments in maximum oxygen uptake were significantly correlated with reduction in body weight, percent body fat, and systolic blood pressure but not diastolic blood pressure or blood lipid concentrations (2) (Table 17–11).

Economic Evaluation Results

Potential program impacts on economic variables such as health care utilization and related costs may be expected to be slowly exerted, mediated through a reduction in quantifiable risks for many serious diseases. However, a direct impact of improved

Table 17–11. Changes in CHD Risk Factors From Baseline to Year 2 in VO_2max Change Categories: Health-Promotion Program Companies Only

| Change in CHD Risk Factors, Baseline to Year 2 | Changes in VO_2max[a](%) | | | |
	< 5 (n = 337)	5–15 (n = 111)	> 15 (n = 270)	Significance (p value)
Body weight (lb)	3.30	−0.12	−0.29	< 0.01
Body fat (%)	−1.50	−2.46	−2.85	< 0.01
Systolic BP (mm Hg)	−3.96	−3.55	−5.80	< 0.05
Diastolic BP (mm Hg)	−0.42	−1.61	−1.82	NS
Cholesterol level (mg/dl)	−10.51	−17.54	−14.22	NS
HDL cholesterol level[b] (ml/dl)	−1.73	−3.57	−2.55	NS
CHD risk[c]	0.003	−2.070	0.035	NS

Source: Blair et al. (2).
[a]VO_2max = maximum oxygen uptake. Values are least-squares mean differences, adjusted for age, sex, and all other variables in the table. Overall change using multivariate analysis of covariance, Wilk's, $F = 4.26$, $p < 0.001$.
[b]HDL = high-density lipoprotein.
[c]Risk of CHD in 8 years (from Framingham multiple logistic equation).

morale and general well-being could also be reflected by a reduction over a shorter period in health care utilization and costs. To test whether the program could have an impact on these variables over a several-year period, health care claims paid by Johnson & Johnson on behalf of their employees were analyzed for three groups of companies: (a) those with no program as of December 1983; (b) those with the program for 18 to 30 months as of that data; and (c) those with more than 30 months of program experience as of that data (4). Employees in these three groups, which numbered between 3,000 and 5,000, were included in the analyses only if they had been continuously employed by participating Johnson & Johnson companies during the entire study period. Analysis of covariance was employed to adjust for intergroup differences in age, gender, job classification, location, and baseline health care utilization levels.

Inpatient and outpatient costs were analyzed separately. Although there were no significant differences in the per-employee costs for covered outpatient services among the groups, there was a striking difference with respect to inpatient services (4) (Table 17–12). The average employee in companies with LIVE FOR LIFE® groups experienced significantly slower increases in inpatient costs than the control group counterparts. Mean annual cost increases (constant dollars) were $43 and $42 respectively, for the two groups with the program compared with $76 for the control group. Live for Life groups also experienced slower increases in per capita admissions and hospital days in acute care facilities.

Table 17–12. Medical Claims, 1979–1983[a]

Year	Unadjusted means, by group			Adjusted means, by group		
	1	2	3	1	2	3
Inpatient costs per employee ($)						
1979	89	78	87	—	—	—
1980	102	131	111	110	144*	100
1981	158	164	150	167	171	149
1982	177	195	224	190	207	229
1983	233	212	424	265**	258**	403
Admissions per 1,000 employees						
1979	67	81	87	—	—	—
1980	84	94	78	91	97	77
1981	87	94	83	95	99	83
1982	102	107	116	109	109	120
1983	127	106	154	143	118*	156
Hospital days per 1,000 employees						
1979	405	408	406	—	—	—
1980	428	553	440	461	593	393
1981	724	745	527	814	854	407
1982	613	619	569	607	551	674
1983	831	750	1,090	877	765	1,125

Source: Bly et al. (4).

[a] Adjusted means for 1980 to 1983 include adjustments to raw means based on age, sex, job class, Now Jersey status, and baseline (1979) differences. Standard errors of estimate related to the adjusted means ranged from $7.16 in 1980 to $15.75 in 1983 for inpatient costs. For days of hospitalization, the standard errors ranged from 28.0 days/1,000 to 54.6/1,000 in 1983. For admissions, the standard errors ranged from 3.2/1000 in 1980 to 5.6/1,000 in 1983.
*p = 0.01 to 0.05.
**p = 0.001 to 0.005. Comparisons are made to group 3.

Absenteeism and Employee Attitudes Evaluation Results

In addition to direct health care costs, the indirect health care costs which are reflected in employee morale, productivity, or job satisfaction have been evaluated using LIVE FOR LIFE® data. Examination of absenteeism data over a 3-year period revealed that hourly workers who participated in the LIVE FOR LIFE® programs had significantly lower absence rates ($p<.01$) than their peers, although this difference was not found for salaried workers (23).

An extensive, 2-year quasi-experimental evaluation of employee attitudes found significant favorable changes at LIVE FOR LIFE® companies compared to companies without this program. Attitudes toward the company that were favorably changed were commitment to the organization, perception of job competence, feelings about supervision, working conditions, pay and fringe benefits, and job security (22).

FUTURE EVALUATION PRIORITIES

There is considerable need for additional evaluation efforts. High priorities for these efforts include the following.

1. Assessment of program impact on different subpopulations of employees, e.g., blue collar versus white collar, urban versus rural, different cultural groups, high risk versus low risk for a particular health problem, union versus nonunion, native English speakers versus those who speak English as a second language, single versus married.

2. Assessment of the process for implementing worksite health-promotion programs in different settings. What aspects of the planning and implementation process appear to correlate with program effectiveness? What are the characteristics of the worksite that influence the effectiveness of a planning and implementation process?

3. Rigorous cost-benefit and cost-effectiveness analysis from several perspectives: the individual, the employer sponsoring the program, and society in general. A literature review prior to the publication of the LIVE FOR LIFE® economic results revealed that in only two of ten health-promotion program areas—hypertension control and individual smoking cessation programs—could information on economic impact be considered suggestive (39).

4. Assessment of relative effectiveness of the same intervention over time. For example, if the same weight management or smoking cessation program is repeatedly offered over a 3-year period, what is the impact on enrollment?

5. What are the major factors affecting participation, both initially and over time?

6. What is the impact of establishing specific health relevant policies, e.g., a smoking policy or requiring the use of seat belts in company-owned vehicles?

7. What programmatic activities are most attractive to different types of employees? Are there methods to target particular program configurations or modes of delivery to the subsegment of the employee population most amenable to that approach?

8. How can programs be easily extended to dependents and retirees? What models lead to efficient delivery and best program impact with each of these groups?

Investigation of the interrelation of health and productivity at work is a final high priority. Although acceptance of this relationship is universal, there have been few efforts to quantify the relations beyond the most obvious first order effects. A worker who is not on the job owing to ill health may be assumed to cost the company an amount equivalent to his salary, benefits, and related overhead expenses during that period. Much more difficult is to impute a cost due to health-related reduced productivity while on the job. A depressed worker, a smoker who takes frequent cigarette breaks, a coworker breathing in second-hand smoke, an overweight worker concerned about how to avoid overeating at lunch have in common a potential impact on productivity, but the tools available to measure this loss have yet to be developed. Some of the impacts are not on output but on the quality of the product or service provided. Whereas the cost of lack of quality can be assessed at a gross level, the attribution of what portion of this cost may derive from lack of health is entirely speculative.

The Johnson & Johnson experience and that of a few other worksite health-promotion programs have documented an improvement in employee relations based on such measures as satisfaction with the job and with the employer, a sense of job security, and a feeling that the company cares about employees as individuals. However, there is no accepted method available to translate those improvements into dollars. Nonetheless, those making decisions about implementing worksite health promotion programs seem willing to use their own calculus to decide that those changes, coupled with demonstrable improvements in risk factors, are sufficient to justify investment in health-promotion programs. The challenge is to provide them the database to decide which programs have the greatest likelihood of achieving their stated health and economic objectives while providing program developers with the tools to refine interventions to maximize both efficiency and effectiveness.

REFERENCES

1. Alderman, M. H., & Davis, T. K. (1976). Hypertensive control at the work site. *Journal of Occupational Medicine, 18,* 793–6.
2. Blair, S. N., Piserchia, P. V., Wilbur, C. S., & Crowder, J. H. (1986). Public health intervention model for work-site health promotion. *Journal of the American Medical Association, 228,* 921–26.
3. Blue Cross and Blue Shield of Michigan. (1983). *Go to health: final report.* Detroit: Michigan Health Care Education and Research Foundation.
4. Bly, J. L., Jones, R. C., & Richardson, J. E. (1986). Impact of worksite health promotion on health care costs and utilization. *Journal of the American Medical Association, 26,* 3235–40.
5. Breslow, L., Fielding, J., Herrmann, A. A., & Wilbur, C. S. (1990). Worksite health promotion: Its evolution and the Johnson & Johnson experience. *Preventive Medicine, 19,* 13–21.
6. Centers for Disease Control. (1990). Years of potential life lost before ages 65 and 85—United States, 1987 and 1988. *Morbidity and Mortality Weekly Report, 39,* 20–22.
7. DeMuth, N. M., Fielding, J. E., Stunkard, A. J., & Hollander, R. B. (1986). Evaluation of industrial health promotion programs: return-on-investment and survival of the fittest. In M. F. Cataldo & T. J. Coates (eds.). *Health and*
industry—a behavioral medicine perspective. New York: Wiley.
8. Erfurt, J. C., & Foote, A. (1990). Maintenance of blood pressure treatment and control after discontinuation of work site follow-up. *Journal of Occupational Medicine, 32,* 513–20.
9. Fielding, J. E. (1984). *Corporate health management.* Reading, MA: Addison-Wesley.
10. Fielding, J. E. (1984). Health promotion and disease prevention at the worksite. *Annual Review of Public Health, 5,* 237–65.
11. Fielding, J. E. (1986). Evaluations, results and problems for worksite health promotion programs. In M. F. Cataldo & T. J. Coates (eds.). *Health & industry—a behavioral medicine perspective* (pp. 373–96). New York: Wiley.
12. Fielding, J. E. (1988). Results of the first national survey of worksite health promotion activities. Unpublished data.
13. Fielding, J. E. (1989). Corporate health cost management. *Occupational Medicine: State of the Art Reviews, 4,* 121–44.
14. Fielding, J. E. (1989). Frequency of health risk assessment activities at U.S. worksites. *American Journal of Preventive Medicine, 5,* 73–81.
15. Fielding, J. E., & Breslow, L. (1983). Health promotion programs sponsored by California employers. *American Journal of Public Health, 73,* 538–42.

16. Fielding, J. E., & Piserchia, P. V. (1989). Frequency of worksite health promotion activities. *American Journal of Public Health, 79,* 16–20.

17. Foote, A., Erfurt, J. C. (1983). Hypertension control at the worksite. *The New England Journal of Medicine, 308,* 809–13.

18. Frazio, A. F. (1977). *A concurrent validation study of the NCHS General Well-Being Schedule.* DHEW Publication No. HRA 78-1347. Data Evaluation and Methods Research, Series 2, No. 73 (pp. 1–52). Washington, DC: U.S. Government Printing Office.

19. Gibbs, J. O., Mulvaney, D., Henes, C., & Reed, R. W. (1985). Work-site health promotion. *Journal of Occupational Medicine, 27,* 826–30.

20. Haynes, R. B., Sackett, D. L., Taylor, D. W., Gibson, E. S., & Johnson, A. L. (1978). Increased absenteeism from work after detection and labeling of hypertensive patients. *The New England Journal of Medicine, 299,* 741–44.

21. Health Care Financing Administration, Division of National Cost Estimates. (1990).

22. Holzbach, R. L., Piserchia, P. V., McFadden, D. W., Hartwell, T. D., Herrmann, A., & Fielding, J. E. (1990). Effect of the Johnson & Johnson LIVE FOR LIFE® Program on employee attitudes. *Journal of Occupational Medicine, 32* 973–78.

23. Jones, R. C., Bly, J. L., & Richardson, J. E. (1990). A study of a work site health promotion program and absenteeism. *Journal of Occupational Medicine, 32,* 95–99.

24. Logan, A., Milne, B., Achber, C., Campbell, W., & Haynes, R. B. (1981). Cost effectiveness of work site hypertension treatment program. *Hypertension, 3,* 211–19.

25. Naditch, M. P. (1984). The Staywell program. In J. D. Matarazzo, S. M. Weiss, J. A. Herd, & N. E. Miller (eds.). *Behavioral health: a handbook of health promotion and disease prevention* (pp. 1071–8). New York: Wiley.

26. National Heart, Lung, and Blood Institute. (1980). National high blood pressure education program, At Mass Mutual: off-site care and good monitoring reduce medical costs, *Re: High blood pressure control in the worksetting.* Bethesda: National Heart, Lung and Blood Institute.

27. National Heart, Lung, and Blood Institute. (1981). *Cardiovascular primer for the workplace.* Health Education Branch, Office of Prevention, Education and Control NIH publication 81-2210. Bethesda: National Heart, Lung, and Blood Institute.

28. Office of Disease Prevention and Health Promotion. (1987). *National survey of worksite health promotion activities: a summary.* Department of Health and Human Services, ODPHP Monograph Series.

29. Polk, F. B., Harland, L. C., Pozner-Cooper, S., Stromer, M., Ignatus, J., Mull, H., & Blaszowski, T. P. (1969). Disability days associates with detection and treatment in a hypertension control program. *American Journal of Epidemiology, 119,* 44–53.

30. Settergren, S. K., Wilbur, C. S., Hartwell, T. D., & Rassweiler, J. (1983). Comparison of respondents and non-respondents to a worksite health screen. *Journal of Occupational Medicine, 25,* 475–80.

31. Shipley, R. H., Orleans, C. T., Wilbur, C. S., Piserchia, P. V., & McFadden, D. W. (1988). Effect of the Johnson & Johnson program on employee smoking. *Preventive Medicine, 17,* 25–34.

32. Spilman, M. A., Goetz, A., Schultz, J., Bellingham, R., & Johnson, D. (1986). Effects of a corporate health promotion program. *Journal of Occupational Medicine, 28,* 285–9.

33. Stamler, R., Gosch, F. C., Stamler, J., Lindberg, H., & Hilker, R. (1979). A hypertension control program based on the workplace. *Journal of Occupational Medicine, 20,* 618–25.

34. U.S. Chamber of Commerce. (1988). *Employee Benefits, 1988 Edition.* Washington, DC: U.S. Chamber of Commerce.

35. U.S. General Accounting Office. (1990). Health Insurance. Cost Increases Lead to Coverage Limitations and Cost Shifting. GAO/HRD-90-68. Washington, DC: U.S. General Accounting Office.

36. Veterans Administration Cooperative Study Group on Antihypertensive Agents. (1967). Effects on morbidity in hypertension, results in patients with diastolic blood pressures averaging 15 through 129 mm Hg. *Journal of the American Medical Association, 202,* 1028–34.

37. Veterans Administration Cooperative Study Group on Antihypertensive Agents. (1970). II. Results in patients with diastolic blood pressures averaging 90 through 114 mm Hg. *Journal of the American Medical Association, 213,* 1143–52.

38. Veterans Administration Cooperative Study Group on Antihypertensive Agents. (1972). Effects in treatment on morbidity in hypertension. IV. Influence of age, diastolic pressure, and prior cardiovascular disease: further analysis of side effects. *Circulation, 45,* 991–1004.

39. Warner, K. E., Wickizer, T. M., Wolfe, R. A., Schildroth, J. E., & Samuelson, M. H. (1988). Economic implications of workplace health promotion programs: review of the literature. *Journal of Occupational Medicine, 30*(2), 106–12.

40. Wilbur, C. S. (1983). The Johnson & Johnson Program 1983. *Preventive Medicine, 12,* 672–81.

41. Wilbur, C. S., Hartwell, T. D., & Piserchia, P. V. (1986). The Johnson Live for Life program: its organization and evaluation plan. In M. F. Cataldo & T. J. Coates (eds.). *Health and industry—a behavioral medicine perspective* (pp. 538–50). New York: Wiley.

VI

CONCLUSIONS AND ISSUES FOR FUTURE WORK

This section has two purposes: to draw general conclusions based on the material presented in this book and to identify research that is still needed on work, health, and productivity. There are two underlying premises of the book: (a) that the productivity or success of a work enterprise and the health of workers are interdependent; and (b) that this relation persists, though the issues change, in the shift from industrial to postindustrial work.

Because the work environment and workforce are currently undergoing extensive change, it is timely to explore how the health of workers interacts with the work environment.

18
Conclusions

Gareth M. Green and Frank Baker

Originally, industrialization brought about a decline in the quality of the work environment. The nature, methods, and rate of work became dependent on the pace of machines rather than the natural rhythm of human effort. The industrial process tended to produce an environment that was filled with hazards, including exposure to toxic substances and increased risk of accidental injuries. Mechanization and power multiplied the capacity of productive work and its attendant waste products.

The recent shift in the workplace away from basic industries such as steel, chemicals, and textiles has changed the nature of productivity. The products, the means of production, and the basic organization of work have changed. Information-age technology based on the microcomputer has changed the manufacturing process and the organizational controls in ways that are only beginning to be understood.

In postindustrial societies, with their emphasis on information and service industries, attention has been shifting from the physical, chemical, and biological hazards of the work environment to problems with the psychosocial environment. The meaning of productivity is changing; the means of achieving productivity is changing; and new measures by which the product is evaluated (e.g., durability, effects on the environment, and health effects) are emerging.

CHANGE IN MEASURES OF PRODUCTIVITY

A number of issues related to the measurement of productivity require further explication. Ideas about the purpose of work are broadening from the production of goods and services to the fulfillment of a range of personal and social goals. Jobs and economic development have become the means to promote individual and social goals, rather than to serve only the goals of the employer. The workplace is seen as a setting of personal fulfillment as well as a means of earning a living. The notion that "people work to live" is being tempered by the reverse dictum that "people live to work." The job increasingly provides not only pay but access to essential services and supports.

Productivity is conventionally defined as the quantity of output in goods and services per unit of input in capital and labor (P = O/I). However, because organized work has become the locus of economic resources, various social objectives have been "tacked on" as "fringe benefits," e.g., education, health insurance, and medical care. These benefits obviously cost money (often more than the cost of raw materials), and such costs appear in the denominator of the productivity equation. However, the value of these benefits as outputs of work does not appear in the numerator and productivity appears to decline. Unless these benefits of work are incorporated in the numerator as their costs appear in the denominator, the value of these costs is lost and productivity appears to decline. This principle extends to other "value added" "external" factors, such as health during old age from disease prevention programs, improved environmental quality through pollution control, and decreased risk of injury through hazard controls (4). These values as work objectives have evolved with economic development, differ considerably among societies at different stages of industrialization, and become important considerations in cross-cultural comparisons of productivity. A society that is raising its expectations in terms of quality of life for the worker as well as quality of product demands a different set of measures in the productivity equation from a society that is overcoming bare survival and exploits its workers for 10 to 20 years, only to discard them as waste by-products of the production process at the end of their useful lives.

A central theme of this book is that the variable of health must be incorporated in the productivity equation as an output in order to accurately measure workplace productivity. Because productivity is currently measured by an incomplete set of variables, it appears to be declining, or at least not increasing competitively. If environmental measures, as well as health measures, were incorporated into the equation, it might turn out that productivity has actually increased. Perhaps there is a false feeling about productivity because the "wrong" early industrial age measures for productivity are being used during an era when different measures are required. For example, we might speculate that the fall in productivity after 1968, rather than being related to changes in economic policy or the poor quality of work or labor demands, was instead due to marked increases in regulation to improve environmental quality and reduce the health risks of toxicants. These costs are incurred to meet societal values, but the benefits need to be incorporated as outputs in the productivity measures. If they are not, how then do we measure their value as goals of the workplace?

CHANGE IN GOALS AND PRIORITIES

A substantial portion of the population has expressed a willingness to alter behavior and to pay money to address the value of environmental quality. Like health, that value needs to be incorporated into the numerator of the productivity equation. It may be worth exploring how values such as personal health and questions of environmental pollution affect the calculations of costs and benefits to society at work. These common human values may have a greater or lesser priority in a society depending on how well off the people are, or how close they are to starvation, or how far the societies have evolved in their economic climb. However, even in poor countries, the population verbalizes these values and enacts statutes to enforce environmental quality. For example, India has begun a massive initiative to clean up the Ganges despite the urgency of other short-term needs.

These major themes relate to health and have emerged during the last quarter-century at the same time productivity has been slowed in those countries that have been concerned with those issues. If, in the fashion of Brenner (see Chapter 16), we draw time-lag graphs to correlate drops in productivity with, for example, increases in regulatory legislation, their association might tell us something about changing societal goals of health and environmental quality and perhaps something about the hypotheses relating these goals to productivity.

The more advanced industrialized and postindustrialized societies set different goals; they incorporate factors such as health and safety into their policies that affect the outcomes of societal productivity. By applying the old measures of productivity, societies that are just becoming industrialized appear to be more productive because they have not set these new goals.

The thrust of this discussion involves the *units of analysis* issue and whether it is the society, a particular organization, or some sector of the society or occupational group that is taken as the unit of measurement. The question is *whose productivity is being measured, what factors are to be included in productivity, and should that measurement be aggregated* to include factors of health or environmental quality. If this measure is to be disaggregated, what are the distortions? A key part of the problem of comparing productivity across cultures or social units lies with the decisions of what is to be included in the productivity equation and what excluded.

CHANGES AND EFFECTS ON WORKERS

The feedback effect on the worker population of changing productivity measures also has to be considered, particularly as it plays a part in the long-term equation of productivity. If the health of workers is destroyed, they are not in a position to be productive later. In the same sense, if a society does not educate its workers to the technology levels that are necessary to compete, the society is not going to be productive. For example, if the Japanese should educate more engineers and the United States more lawyers, there will be different effects on the two societies. Each is preparing people to take certain roles in its society, and the impact of these decisions affects the human resources available to contribute to the overall balance of productive output of the society.

A related point concerns issues of aging of the population. Will the United States be more productive as a result of the 1984 decision to lift the retirement age? Will it make a difference to keep people on the job who in the postindustrial age are able to be productive because of well maintained mental abilities? These issues require consideration.

In the information age, white collar productivity and health have increasing significance. By the turn of the century, more than 85% of the U.S. labor force will be comprised of white collar workers compared to 30% in 1950 and 53% in 1985 (3). This change in the nature of work is accompanied by changes in the technology of work. Work with computers and other high technology equipment has been found to be contributory to office worker stress. In particular, the video display terminal (VDT), has been identified as a source of psychological stress, fatigue, and eye strain (5,11,14).

This issue of increased stress is complicated by the fact that the introduction of new technologies leads to changes in the degree of control workers have over their lives. Research has shown that high demand/low control conditions in the workplace are particularly prone to engendering poor health outcomes (8,9).

COSTS OF STRESS

Stress seems to be on the increase, and accompanying stress are a number of health-related problems. Stress is a costly business expense, affecting both employee health and company profits. It is associated with work-related accidents due to psychological and psychosomatic problems that contribute markedly to long-term employee disability. Stress clearly seems to be related to cardiovascular disease (2), and there is increasing evidence of stress negatively affecting the body's immune system (10); moreover, it is related to mental health problems and drug and alcohol abuse (13). Stress also has implications for litigation regarding corporate responsibility for stressing workers and affecting their long-term health status (1).

STRESS AND PERSON/ENVIRONMENT INTERACTIONS

Stress in the work organization results from the transactions between persons and their environments. The environment presents dynamic conditions (potential stressors) that can be perceived as opportunities, constraints, or demands. There are significant individual differences in what and how environmental factors affect persons related to their internal dispositions and resources, including their needs, values, and coping skills as well as their external resources such as social support (6,7).

Apparently, stress is additive in its effects across time and across situations (12). Therefore one must consider not only stress on the job but also its interaction with stress in other domains of the individual's life. Demographic changes in the labor force described in Chapter 1 make it necessary to reexamine the linkages between home and work. Traditionally, work and family (and leisure) were considered separate worlds. Men occupied the work world, and women were responsible for the family. There was little impetus to study the relation between work and the rest of life's domains. This separation was supported by a split in academic research disciplines and the life spheres they "owned." Values are also changing within both men and women. For example, self-expression is considered important by what has been called the "new breed" workers who want more in their lives than just work. (15).

VALUES AND WORK ENVIRONMENT DECISIONS

Cross-cultural comparisons of the effects of patterns of work organization on health can be particularly informative. Such comparisons allow examination of differences in worker orientations and values. Changes in health technology result in other differences as well, such as allowing for screening of risk. (Screening raises its own ethical issues for hiring practices.) Improvement in the ability to assess susceptibility raises other concerns about fitting workers to the appropriate work environment to minimize potential risks to health in susceptible workers and the development of work-related problems. A related issue is whether employees have reasonable and accurate perceptions of risks to health they face on the job. The concept of "acceptable risk" is a cultural and personal value judgment that raises questions regarding the right of employers and government to gamble with workers' health without their consent. The key issue here is informed consent. At present, workers and those concerned with employee health are not making these decisions. The values underlying such decisions are likely to show substantial cross-cultural variation.

Another set of questions about values and work environment decisions relates to industries' efforts to improve the health status of workers. Health promotion activities in the workplace emphasize a strategy of educating workers to their responsibility to be aware of risk factors and, if necessary, to change their life styles to lower their own risks, e.g., changing diet, stopping smoking, and reducing and managing stress. This strategy is inconsistent with the passive acceptance role of workers implied in the "acceptable risk" approach of both government (Occupational Safety and Health Administration) and business. There is also a major need to evaluate the health promotion programs that are proliferating in industry, most of which have never been adequately evaluated as to cost-effectiveness.

MULTIPLE CONSTITUENCIES

Finally, this volume points out the dangers in paternalistically assigning too much responsibility for health to the corporate entity. Many constituencies are affected by the relation of work, health, and productivity, including the workers and their organizations, managers, governmental officials, health care professionals, and researchers. Developing solutions to the problems of worker health and productivity requires the cooperation of all these interest groups.

GENERAL CONCLUSIONS

1. *Both the physical/chemical environment and the psychosocial environment are critical to the health of workers.* Arguments have been presented that (a) the work environment constitutes a set of real and potential hazards that affect health; (b) there is an important interaction between this physical/chemical/biological environment and the psychosocial environment in the impact this interaction has on individual and worker group health; and (c) *research and possible interventions require focusing by considering interactions of the physical environment and the psychosocial environment.* Examples are offered in accident prevention, the use of protective clothing, and health behaviors in the psychosocial environment that protect against the hazards of the physical environment.

2. *There is a need to work together across disciplinary boundaries to bring together social/behavioral scientists and environmental health scientists.* There is such a degree of separation in the fields of concentration and their research and theory that people who work with the more physical aspects of the environment are not aware of behavioral science and the behavioral irregularities that can take place; likewise, behavioral scientists have not adequately considered the physical hazards in the environment. Recognition of the need to involve professionals from these different fields is symbolized in the editorship and the contributors to this book.

3. *People are a central component of productivity. There is a need for the focus to be on the "people component,"* with a primary concern for human health, concern about the impact of the whole environment on the individual, concern about people as they interact with technology, and concern about people as they interact with the environments they have created to make the product. Attention to the changing issues of future productivity calls for the central focus to be on the human dimension and on human health.

4. *The problems of productivity can be dealt with at many analytical and conceptual levels; more needs to be done to understand the translation of conclusions from one analytical level to another.* Analysis at the economic or macrosociological approach attempts to understand the relation of economic policy, growth-recession cycles, employment-unemployment, socioeconomic status, and health and productivity. Work at the organizational, group, and individual levels tends to use different variables, although sometimes there is a useful attempt to use the same or at least counterpart variables. Issues of demand and control, which are variables at the lower social system levels, and the use of psychological or social psychological mechanisms to explain the effects of economic policy must be represented in the equations one uses to avoid a discontinuity in the analytical levels. There are a number of interesting, though difficult, questions to be raised concerning the use of psychological or social psychological theories to explain something that is being observed at a macrosociological level.

Whether those broad societal analyses are too focused on post hoc explanations, some regularities are observed. There may be concomitant changes occurring, e.g., changes in health research and application, that produce changes in individuals and health. These changes may not be a result directly of economic policy but, rather, concomitant variables that are not considered in the equation. These models must be used carefully in extrapolations among levels and in being predictive rather than offering post hoc explanations. There is a need for the development of a standard science base that can be used to test hypotheses from these social system level analyses as they apply to the individual, group, or organizational level. More and better communication is required across the disciplines that are involved and the opportunities for testing such cross-level hypotheses have to be developed.

5. *Health is important because of personnel costs; personnel represent a major cost, a major input factor to productivity.* It is not clear how the costs of maintaining or improving health affect productivity in the short and long term. When studying these issues, one needs to look not only at immediate costs but also at longer-term costs. The assumption is that if healthy behaviors are increased workers will cost less in terms of the health care they require. If workers eat right, exercise, and deal with stress, they are less likely to get sick, and it is thus less costly to provide whatever curative or medical care is required. Those assumptions have not been adequately tested for long-term effects. It may be that in terms of the economics involved short-term costs do go down; however, long-term costs may go up because people live longer and die of more "expensive" diseases.

However, old age is not inevitably expensive. Often, expensive old age is the product of poor health during middle age. There may be a gain by maintaining and promoting health during the working years to increase autonomy and the ability to carry on independently and less expensively in older age. Although the elderly living in nursing homes may be expensive if in poor health, there are many elderly persons who live healthily and at home close to the time of death. The growing number of healthy octogenarians and nonagenarians is impressive. Individuals over age 80 form the fastest growing segment of the population and do not by any means all reside in nursing homes (3).

6. *A final general conclusion is the need for research.* In Chapter 19 we make specific recommendations regarding needed research as part of a general discussion

about issues for future work. Few researchers cross disciplinary boundaries, and research rarely takes a programmatic approach to consider the broad range of variables involved when studying the health of workers as affected by their work environment. Even when the latter is studied comprehensively, not enough attention is paid to the other aspects of a worker's life, with the carryover of problems from the home and family.

REFERENCES

1. Adams, G. T. (1987). Preventive law trends and compensation payments for stress-disabled workers. In J. C. Quick, R. S. Bhagat, J. E. Dalton, & J. D. Quick (eds.). *Work stress: health care systems in the workplace* (pp. 235–45). New York: Praeger.

2. Balick, L. R., & Herd, J. A. (1986). Assessment of physiological indices related to cardiovascular disease as influenced by job stress. *Journal of Organizational Behavior Management, 8,* 103–15.

3. Bezold, C., Carlson, F. J., & Peck, J. C. (1986). *The future of work and health.* Dover, MA: Auburn House.

4. Brief, R. S. (1989). Benefits vs cost—a tool for industrial hygiene management. *American Industrial Hygiene Journal, 50,* 289–92.

5. Dainoff, M. J., Hupp, A., & Crane, P. (1981). Visual fatigue and occupational stress in VDT operators. *Human Factors, 23,* 421–38.

6. Gore, S. (1986). Perspectives on social support and research on stress moderating processes. *Journal of Organizational Behavior Management, 8,* 85–101.

7. Hurrell, J. J. (1987). An overview of organizational stress and health. In L. R. Murphy & T. F. Schoenborn (eds.). *Stress management in work settings* (pp. 31–45). Washington, DC: U.S. Government Printing Office.

8. Karasek, R. (1979). Job demands, job decision latitude, and mental health: implications for job redesign. *Administrative Science Quarterly, 24,* 285–398.

9. Karasek, R., Baker, D., Marxer, F., Ahlbom, A., & Theorell, T. (1981). Job decision latitude, job demands, and cardiovascular disease: a prospective study of Swedish men. *American Journal of Public Health, 71,* 694–705.

10. Kiecolt-Glaser, J. K., & Glaser, R. (1987). Behavioral influences on immune function: evidence for the interplay between stress and health. In T. Field, P. M. McCabe, & N. Scheiderman (eds.). *Stress and coping across development.* Hillsdale, NJ: Lawrence Erlbaum Associates.

11. Matula, R. A. (1981). Effects of visual display units on the eyes: a bibliography (1972–1980). *Human Factors, 23,* 581–6.

12. Taylor, S. E. (1986). *Health psychology.* New York: Random House.

13. Warshaw, L. J. (1986). Occupational stress. In J. LaDou (ed.). *Introduction to occupational health and safety* (pp. 135–54). Chicago: National Safety Council.

14. Wineman, J. (1982). Office design and evaluation: an overview. *Environment and Behavior, 14,* 271–98.

15. Yankelovich, D., Zetterberg, H., Strümpel, B., et al. (1984). *The world at work.* New York: Octagon Books.

19
Issues for Future Work

Gareth M. Green and Frank Baker

A principal conclusion of this book is that the health of workers is important to issues of industrial productivity, particularly at the organizational level. There is also some evidence that unemployment at a macrosocietal level influences health. How these micro- and macrolevel studies relate to each other in regard to understanding the interdependence of productivity and health requires additional research and clarification. Such studies are not easy because of theoretical, measurement, and analytical inadequacies, but there is much to be gained by coordinating efforts across disciplines and levels of analysis.

One of the major concerns that must be underscored is the paucity of theory and research that encompasses the range of variables of concern in the interaction of worker health and industrial productivity. A barrier to that research is the necessarily broad span of involvement across the borders of public health, medicine, economics, sociology, psychology, and management.

There is a need to develop funding for the required interdisciplinary research and to develop field laboratory opportunities where relevant variables can be studied. Some existing experiments with new arrangements of work, such as participatory management, offer opportunities for piggybacking new research on existing studies. There is a need for further study of *how management policy interacts with health*. Far-reaching decisions are made at the societal level, but managers also make significant decisions that affect health. Some of those experiments are on-going, as in quality circles that would improve the quality of work life. There is a need to look at the health outcomes of these initiatives and the effects on promoting productivity.

TECHNOLOGICAL CHANGES

Some recommendations for future work are directed to issues of the organization and management of the workplace. Given the evidence for stress due to change in the work environment, changes at work might be introduced in a more deliberate fashion. Some technological changes in the workplace occur so rapidly that the rate of change itself becomes a problem.

The introduction of computerization as a major technological innovation of the new information age requires that more consideration be given to the reeducation of workers. With regard to the social organization of work, care must be given to the possible alienation of workers. Some have suggested that the "electronic cottage," in which people work at home using their computers to connect with the work organization, may be considered the new "sweat shops," given their removal from the protection of visibility and the benefits of union assistance. As noted in Chapter 1, there is the possibility that computers in the office may be used by management who do not value or trust their employees to deskill white collar work and make workers more easily replaceable.

WORK SCHEDULES AND CIRCADIAN RHYTHMS

There is still much work to be done to understand the effect of work schedules on productivity. Research is needed on innovative work schedules including compact work weeks and "flex-time" schedules. Some of the research on these topics so far reflects only attitudes and subjective estimates. Research using well controlled designs and "harder" performance measures is called for.

There is also a pressing need for more research on how circadian rhythms affect workers as round-the-clock operations to increase productivity and to meet the requirements of emergency services lead to more alterations or inversions of normal activity cycles in workers. Many human processes have been shown to follow a 24-hour (i.e., "circadian") rhythm in relation to the diurnal activity cycle (12). They range from basic physiological processes such as enzyme production, respiration, and heart rate to psychological and behavioral functions such as memory, vigilance, and reaction time (7). It appears that disruption of these processes in key workers can result in major industrial disasters. A group of researchers on circadian rhythmicity has suggested that it was not by chance that the accidents at Chernobyl, Three Mile Island, and Bhopal occurred between midnight and 6:00 A.M. Focusing on accidents among a wide variety of workers, including truck drivers, commercial pilots, and manufacturing plant operators, Moore-Ede and colleagues have studied the effects of rotating shiftwork schedules on the circadian cycles of sleep and wakefulness (14). Their research indicated that such accidents are related to a loss of employee alertness during these early morning hours.

In addition to contributing to accidents, work schedules that require an individual to reverse normal sleep and waking patterns are difficult to adjust to and may have major negative health effects (4). Field studies suggest that there are more sleep and digestive disorders among workers on rotating shifts, and some workers cannot tolerate such schedules. Animal studies show decreases in length of life due to light-dark phase shifts (6), but research remains to be done to determine the long-term effects of such phase shifts in humans (4).

Some laboratory research has indicated that bright light may have a direct effect on the human circadian oscillator, and that disorders resulting from shiftwork, jet lag, and other work that disrupts sleep-wake patterns may be treated through therapeutic exposure to light (2,3). The practical implications of such research are obvious. Certainly, more laboratory research on such treatments is needed, but available data suggest that it might be useful to undertake field experiments that attempt to reset the human circadian pacemaker that controls daily variations in physiological, cognitive, and behavorial functions through the use of exposure to bright light.

HEALTH PROMOTION PROGRAM EVALUATION

One type of research which is essential for the future is rigorous evaluation of health promotion efforts carried out in the workplace to reduce risks of disease for workers. While a considerable amount of health promotion activity has been undertaken in various industries and businesses, there has been relatively little evaluation of the effectiveness of these efforts in reaching their stated goals. To improve the state of the art of health promotion program evaluation the following needs must be addressed:

1. Implementation of studies which follow workers over time.
2. Inclusion of comparable worker control groups as part of experimental research designs.
3. Establishment of the effectiveness of different interventions, such as nutritional programs, which have not been adequately studied previously.
4. Conducting evaluations of comprehensive programs which allow the sorting out of the contributions of various program elements acting together and separately.
5. Development of more cost-effectiveness and cost-benefit studies.

AGING AND HEALTH

There has been considerable research on the relation between childhood disease and adult illness. There is also a need to study the effects of adult health on elderly illness, especially the relation of health during the working life. Do people who have been healthy throughout their lives live longer? If so, is it due to genetics or environment? These questions require the study of healthy aging and its relation to the workplace, e.g. if people who maintain employment after retirement, as volunteers or part-time workers, are healthier.

WORK ENVIRONMENT RESEARCH

As noted in Chapter 1, the primary attention of much of the research on adaptation of the individual in the work situation has been on work morale and job satisfaction. However, the adaptation of the employee in terms of overall well-being and health is also of primary concern, as these variables interact with the individual's work morale/satisfaction in influencing the level of performance (the individual level of productivity). A conclusion of this review of contemporary research and theory must be that there is a need to focus further research on the interdependence of the work environment, worker health, individual performance, and aggregate organizational productivity.

The work environment system may be usefully conceptualized in four domains of variables:

1. Physical environment, including the biological, chemical, and architectural features.
2. Organizational structure and management policies, including the size, shape, centralization, differentiation, formalization, and span of control.
3. Aggregate of the members' personal characteristics, including their physical

characteristics and their psychological characteristics, e.g., values, norms, abilities, and personality traits.

4. Work group social climate, including the way in which individuals in a setting relate to each other, the goal orientation toward which that setting is oriented, and its amount of structure and openness to change (13).

There has been extensive exploration of the social psychology of the workplace in field studies in industry and the controlled settings of laboratory experiments. However, for the most part, this work has neglected the relation between employee health and productivity. It is time to focus scientific research on the health and productivity impacts of particular work environments. The right kind of research could translate into recommendations for redesign of the work environment and revisions in management and regulatory agency policies. There is a clear need for research findings and policy recommendations based on well controlled work environment research to be disseminated widely to improve worker health and productivity.

Such research should explore the interactions of each of the major variable domains mentioned above. Previous research has tended to focus on bivariate relations rather than examining the multivariate interactions. For example, there is a considerable amount of research on the effects of particular chemical and biological hazards on the health of workers (although it is surprising how little is known about the effects of many work environmental toxins on humans); there is much less knowledge of the differences in individual susceptibility of particular workers. Also, there is little research on the interactions of psychosocial variables with physical environmental variables. For example, the effects of psychosocial variables on individual health and well-being through such phenomena as "mass psychogenic illness" in "sick building syndrome" situations have been discovered only after the failure to find any physical causes for feelings of illness in large groups of employees working in those buildings (1).

The complicated interrelations among the work group climate, the organization of work, and the effects on physical health and productivity may be illustrated in studies of workers who operate under high demand schedules with little opportunity for social support from fellow workers or a feeling of being able to exercise any control over their work situation (8,9). For example, bus drivers have to meet the demands of a tight schedule over which they usually have little control (10). Cardiovascular disease has been found to be unusually high in these workers, but evidence is developing that giving them an opportunity to believe that they exercise some control over some aspects of their work lives can ameliorate these negative health effects without substantially losing productivity (5).

Work can provide a goal or meaning to life and can help to structure life for individuals. Work not only provides material means but provides social support. In situations where the fit between the workers and their work environment is bad—if they are unable to control work conditions, if they are not able to cope effectively and lack social support—conditions are ripe to produce pathogenic reactions that can lead to disease (11).

Although there is much that we do not know about work, health, productivity, and their relations, there is more known than has been applied. There is much to be clarified in transference of what is known to those who can use it most effectively.

Industry and labor should be more involved with academia when considering this broad study of health and productivity. International groups would be useful for considering the lessons learned in different countries and cultures.

QUESTIONS FOR RESEARCH

Research is needed at many levels: epidemiological studies to identify the environmental correlates of health problems at an aggregate level; retrospective cross-sectional studies to examine relations between work environment and individual characteristics and morbidity or mortality at an individual level; intensive, interdisciplinary, longitudinal studies of high risk occupational groups; and laboratory and field experimental studies of environmental, work group, and behavioral patterns that affect health and productivity. With regard to the latter type of study, among the interesting kinds of work environment research that might be undertaken are field and laboratory studies of the following:

1. Effects of stressful work environments on changes in cardiovascular, neuroendocrine, and immunological functioning of workers.
2. Impact of stress from the nonwork environment as it carries over into the workplace, affecting the cardiovascular, neuroendocrine, and immunological functioning of workers.
3. Effects of stigmatizing job-related health problems (e.g., occupational dermatitis) on work productivity.
4. Role of psychosocial factors in personal and professional assessments of occupational risks.
5. Factors affecting the effectiveness of risk communication concerning job-related hazards.
6. Individual, social, and environmental factors in changing health-related behaviors to reduce risk, prevent illness, and promote health in the work situation.
7. Effects of child day care at the worker's place of employment on the stress and health of the parent as well as the health of the child.
8. Evaluation of workplace health-promotion programs through controlled experimental designs.
9. Controlled studies of various social and physical work environments on employee well-being and productivity.
10. Studies of person/environment fit in relation to health and productivity outcomes.

METHODOLOGICAL PROBLEMS

There are methodological problems to be dealt with when moving forward on the study of health, work, and productivity.

1. How health can serve as a proxy measure of productivity.
2. How to adequately model the interactions of the work environment (chemical, physical, biological, psychosocial) and worker characteristics as they affect health and productivity outcomes.

3. How to effectively translate hypotheses from one level of analysis to another.
4. How to adequately evaluate changes in the workplace and in health education efforts to change workers in their long-term effects on health.
5. What natural experiments, case–control studies, and so on, are available for studying workplace environmental effects on worker health and productivity.

There is a need to accomplish the following:

1. Achieve greater integration of field epidemiological, experimental, and laboratory studies to consider unresolved issues and research agendas.
2. Set up natural field experiments to study how the interaction of people and the environment produce health effects.
3. Conduct studies that follow cohorts of people through time, such as picking up worker populations and following them through retirement into old age, or doing case–control studies of people who do have healthy aging and those who do not to determine to what extent employment or activity is related.

Focus on the interactions of different hazards in different work environment systems would be useful but would require consideration of a number of variables. Clearly, consideration of the impact of changing technology and the work environments created by these changes on workers' health requires multiple disciplines and numerous methodologies.

ETHICAL QUESTIONS FOR STUDY

Aside from the biological questions and the technical issues addressed in these chapters, a host of ethical issues of great current concern are generated by these considerations. In view of the numerous behavioral and environmental risk factors for health and thereby for productivity, consider these questions.

1. What are the cultural expectations and obligations of the employer to minimize the environmental factors and of the employee to minimize the host factors (e.g., alcohol, smoking, physical sickness) in reducing these risk factors for dysfunction and disease in the effort to minimize risk due to factors of susceptibility and environment?
2. What are the obligations of the employee and the employer to reveal workplace hazards (e.g., through right to know procedures) or to find out aspects of worker susceptibility (e.g., through screening) versus rights of privacy and confidentiality and the necessity for productivity and health maintenance?
3. When does improved accuracy of biological over environmental monitoring justify the invasion of personal privacy in the best interests of worker health and corporate productivity?
4. What are the obligations of the individual versus the employer in regulating associated personal exposures (e.g., to drugs, alcohol, and smoking) that can alter susceptibility and therefore responsivity to workplace exposures and can alter the results of screening and health surveillance?
5. What are the relative responsibilities of the employer and employee for the resultant health effects and the control of risk? (Indeed, the U.S. Supreme Court

has enunciated the principle of attributable risk in attempting to distribute these responsibilities equitably among the employers and employees.)

The current answers to these ethical dilemmas are still far from satisfactory. Worker selection, behavior modification, and environmental regulation and control are the three levers for promoting the appropriate relation between optimal health and productivity. If health of the workforce should become recognized as a corporate goal equivalent to its material productivity, it is likely that these ethical dilemmas would be alleviated through a more cooperative rather than adversarial engagement of the participants in achieving common goals.

REFERENCES

1. Colligan, M., Pennebaker, J., & Murphy, L. (eds.). (1982). *Mass psychogenic illness: a social psychological analysis.* Hillsdale, NJ: Lawrence Erlbaum Associates.
2. Czeisler, C. A., Allan, J. S., Strogatz, S. H.,et al. (1986). Bright light resets the human circadian pacemaker independent of the timing of the sleep-wake cycle. *Science, 233,*667–71.
3. Czeisler, C. A., Kronauer, R. E., Allan, J. S. Duffy, J. F., Jewett, M. E., Brown, E. N., & Ronda, J. M. (1990). Bright light induction of strong (Type O) resetting of the human circadian pacemaker. *Science, 244,* 1328–33.
4. Czeisler, C. A., Moore-Ede, M. C., & Colean, R. M. (1982). Rotating shift work schedules that disrupt sleep are improved by applying circadian principles. *Science, 217,* 460–63.
5. Gardell, B. (1987). Efficiency and health hazards in mechanized work. In J. C. Quick, R. S. Bhagat, J. E. Dalton, & J. D. Quick (eds.). *Work stress: health care systems in the workplace* (pp. 50–71). New York: Praeger.
6. Halberg, F., Nelson, W. L., & Cadotte, L. (1977). *International Conference Proceedings of the International Society of Chronobiology, 12,* 133.
7. Hurrell, J. J., & Colligan, M. J. (1986). Machine pacing and shiftwork: evidence for job stress. *Journal of Organizational Behavior Management, 8,* 159–275.

8. Karasek, R. (1979) Job demands, job decision latitude, and mental health: implications for job redesign. *Administrative Science Quarterly, 24,* 285–398.
9. Karasek, R., Baker, D., Marxer, F. Ahlbom, A., & Theorell, T. (1981). Job decision latitude, job demands, and cardiovascular disease: a prospective study of Swedish men. *American Journal of Public Health, 71,* 694–705.
10. Kolata, G. (1986) Reducing risk: a change of heart? *Science, 231,* 669–70.
11. Levi, L., Frankenhaeusar, M., & Gardell, B. (1982). Work stress related to social structures and processes. In G. Elliott & C. Eisdorfer (eds.). *Stress and human health* (pp. 119–46). New York: Springer.
12. Luce, G. G. (1970). *Biological rhythms in psychiatry and medicine,* Washington DC: Public Health Service Publication 2088, U.S. Government Printing Office.
13. Moos, R. H. (1986). Work as a human context. In M. S. Pallak & R. O. Perloff (eds.). *Psychology and work: productivity, change and employment* (pp. 9–52). Washington, DC: American Psychological Association.
14. Staff.(May 29, 1986). Loss of alertness and technical failure: Dr. Moore-Ede seeks physiological determinants of human error. *Harvard Medical Area Focus,* pp. 2–3.

Author Index

293

Subject Index